D1523443

MULTISYSTEM ORGAN FAILURE

PATHOPHYSIOLOGY AND CLINICAL IMPLICATIONS

MULTISYSTEM ORGAN FAILURE

PATHOPHYSIOLOGY AND CLINICAL IMPLICATIONS

VIRGINIA BYRN HUDDLESTON, RN, MSN, CCRN

Adjunct Faculty, Vanderbilt University,
Nashville, Tennessee;
Critical Care Consultant,
Barbara Clark Mims Associates,
Lewisville, Texas

With **84** illustrations

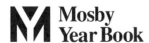
Mosby
Year Book

St. Louis Baltimore Boston Chicago London Philadelphia Sydney Toronto

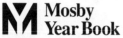

Mosby
Year Book
Dedicated to Publishing Excellence

Publisher: Alison Miller
Editor: Terry Van Schaik
Developmental Editor: Janet Livingston
Project Manager: Karen Edwards
Production Editor: Jim Russell
Production Assistants: Kathy Teal, Ginny Douglas
Book and Cover Design: Gail Morey Hudson

Printed in the United States of America

Mosby–Year Book, Inc.
11830 Westline Industrial Drive, St. Louis, Missouri 63146

Library of Congress Cataloging in Publication Data
Multisystem organ failure   :   Pathophysiology and clinical implications
  /   [edited by] Virginia Byrn Huddleston.—1st ed.
      p.   cm.
   Includes bibliographical references and index.
   ISBN 0-8016-6754-2
   1. Multiple organ failure—Pathophysiology.   2. Multiple organ
failure—Nursing.   I. Huddleston, Virginia Byrn.
   [DNLM: 1.   Critical Care—nurses' instruction.   2.   Multiple Organ
Failure—complications—nurses' instruction.   3. Multiple Organ
Failure—physiopathology—nurses' instruction.   QZ 140 M96158]
   RB150.M84M88   1992
   616'.028—dc20
   DNLM/DLC
   for Library of Congress   92-8668
                                                              CIP

92 93 94 95 96 GW/MY 9 8 7 6 5 4 3 2 1

Contributors

TALLY N. BELL, RN, MN, CCRN

Manager, Clinical Education,
HCA Wesley Medical Center;
Adjunct Clinical Coordinator,
Wichita State University, Wichita, Kansas

SANDRA J. CZERWINSKI, RN, MSN, CCRN

Education Coordinator, Pediatric Critical Care,
Tampa General Hospital, Tampa, Florida

VENITA DASCH, RN, BSN

Critical Care Consultant,
Barbara Clark Mims Associates,
Lewisville, Texas;
Staff Nurse, Surgical Intensive Care Unit,
Parkland Memorial Hospital, Dallas, Texas

DORIS M. GATES, RN, MS, CCRN

Critical Care Educator, Sharp Memorial Hospital,
San Diego, California

VIRGINIA BYRN HUDDLESTON, RN, MSN, CCRN

Adjunct Faculty, Vanderbilt University,
Nashville, Tennessee;
Critical Care Consultant,
Barbara Clark Mims Associates,
Lewisville, Texas

JOY DAVIS KIMBRELL, RN, MSN, CCRN

Critical Care Clinical Nurse Specialist,
HCA Donelson Hospital;
Adjunct Faculty,
Vanderbilt University,
Nashville, Tennessee

LARRY E. LANCASTER, RN, MSN, EdD

Associate Professor,
Vanderbilt University School of Nursing,
Nashville, Tennessee

JO-ELL M. LOHRMAN, RN, BSN, CCRN

Assistant Head Nurse,
Surgical and Trauma Intensive Care Unit,
Parkland Memorial Hospital, Dallas, Texas

JANICE McMILLAN, RN, MSN, CCRN

Clinical Nurse Specialist, The Heart Group;
Adjunct Faculty, Vanderbilt University,
Nashville, Tennessee

BARBARA CLARK MIMS, RN, MSN, CCRN

Coordinator,
Critical Care and Trauma Nurse Internship,
Parkland Memorial Hospital, Dallas, Texas;
Director, Barbara Clark Mims Associates,
Lewisville, Texas;
Adjunct Faculty, University of Texas at Arlington,
Arlington, Texas

PATRICIA A. MOLONEY-HARMON, RN, MS, CCRN

Clinical Nurse Specialist,
Women and Children's Services,
Sinai Hospital of Baltimore,
Baltimore, Maryland

MARGARET T. MORRIS, RN, MSN, CCRN, CEN, EMT

Flight Nurse,
Vanderbilt Lifeflight Helicopter Program;
Staff Nurse, SICU,
Vanderbilt University Medical Center,
Nashville, Tennessee

PAMELA LASH O'NEILL, RN, CCRN

Staff Nurse,
Neurosurgical Intensive Care Unit,
Harborview Medical Center,
Seattle, Washington
Formerly Assistant Head Nurse,
Surgical Intensive Care Unit,
Parkland Memorial Hospital, Dallas, Texas

ELAINE V. ROBINS, RN, MS

Staff Education Instructor, Burn/Trauma Unit,
Emergency Services, Ambulatory Practices,
Brigham and Women's Hospital,
Boston, Massachusetts

Consultants

JILL ADAMS, RN, MS

Education Specialist, Emergency Room,
Tampa General Hospital, Tampa, Florida

ROBERT BARKER, MD

Medical Director, Medical Intensive Care Unit,
Kettering Medical Center, Kettering, Ohio

GORDON R. BERNARD, MD

Associate Professor of Medicine,
Vanderbilt University Medical School;
Director, Medical Intensive Care Unit,
Vanderbilt University Medical Center,
Nashville, Tennessee

MARTHA McDANIEL BUCKNER, RN, MSN, CNSN

Project Director, Center for Nursing Research,
Vanderbilt University School of Nursing;
Formerly Clinical Nurse Specialist,
Nutrition Support Team,
Vanderbilt University Medical Center,
Nashville, Tennessee

ANGELA COLLINS, RN, MSN, CCRN

Doctoral Candidate,
University of Alabama at Birmingham,
Birmingham, Alabama

ANNE DALEIDEN, RN, BSN

Assistant Trauma Coordinator,
Sharp Memorial Hospital, San Diego, California

DAVID R. DANTZKER, MD

Chairman, Department of Medicine,
Professor of Medicine,
Albert Einstein College of Medicine,
Long Island Jewish Medical Center,
New Hyde, New York

COLE GILLER, MD

Assistant Professor of Neurosurgery,
University of Texas Southwestern Medical Center at Dallas;
Attending Neurosurgeon,
Parkland Memorial Hospital, Dallas, Texas

NANCY GILLIUM, RN, MS

Education Coordinator,
Tampa General Hospital, Tampa, Florida

BETTY K. GREEN, RD, CNSD

Clinical Dietitian, Nutrition Support Team,
HCA Donelson Hospital, Nashville, Tennessee

BRIAN JASKI, MD

Associate Director,
San Diego Cardiac Center, San Diego California

CHERYL LaLONDE, BS

Senior Research Associate,
Longwood Area Trauma Center,
Boston, Massachusetts

W. EVAN SECOR, PhD

Research Fellow, Harvard School of Public Health,
Department of Rheumatology and Immunology,
Brigham and Women's Hospital,
Boston, Massachusetts

WILLIAM C. SHOEMAKER, MD

Chief, Department of Emergency Medicine,
King-Drew Medical Center,
UCLA School of Medicine,
Los Angeles, California

PATRICIA SRNEC, RN, MS, CCRN, CNA

Nurse Manager, Pediatric Intensive Care Unit,
University of Maryland Medical System,
Baltimore, Maryland

GREGORY G. STANFORD, MD

Assistant Professor of Surgery,
University of Texas Southwestern Medical,
Center at Dallas, Dallas, Texas

PENNY VAUGHAN, RN, MSN

Associate Director, Critical Care Program,
University of Tennessee, Nashville, Tennessee

JOHN A. WEIGELT, MD, FACS

Professor of Surgery,
Chief, Section of Surgical Critical Care and
Trauma Surgery, University of Texas,
Southwestern Medical Center at Dallas;
Medical Director, Department of Trauma,
Parkland Memorial Hospital, Dallas, Texas

This book is dedicated to my parents

Mr. and Mrs. Robert Alvis Huddleston, Jr.

for their constant and generous support of all my endeavors,
for the example they set, and for their love.

V.B.H.

Foreword

"To act is easy, to think is hard"
JOHANN WOLFGANG VON GOETHE

In 1992 critical care nurses not only must be able to act, they also must be able to think. Competent actions are a primary component of nursing practice. Yet, actions must be based on critical thinking—the ability to apply information from a broad knowledge base to complex patient care situations to effect a positive patient outcome. Careful reading of this comprehensive text on multisystem organ failure is one way that critical care nurses can broaden their knowledge base and acquire a better understanding of the syndrome that has been called "the final common pathway to death."

I would suggest that the nurse who reads this book do so carefully. The subject is not a simple one, and the material present is advanced. Topics are not covered superficially, but with completeness and sophisticated integration.

Multisystem Organ Failure: Physiology and Clinical Implications thoroughly addresses the subject of multisystem organ failure. In doing so, the book also addresses many aspects of general critical care. Information presented in the text is applicable to a variety of patients, including those with shock, trauma, coagulopathies, respiratory failure, cardiac failure, liver failure, gastrointes-

tinal dysfunction, and sepsis. In the decade ahead, this book will serve as a valuable resource to advanced practitioners, educators, and other health team members involved in the care of critically ill patients, especially those with multisystem organ failure.

Twenty years ago, when critical care nursing was in its infancy, complex pathophysiologic concepts, as described in this text, would not have been found in nursing literature; rather, such information would have appeared only in medical writings. To have the subject of multisystem organ failure described in such a thorough, well-documented work written solely by nurses is a major step forward in nursing literature and an advancement for the nursing profession. I applaud the advanced practitioners who have combined their personal clinical experiences with well-documented medical and nursing research to produce this comprehensive text.

Vee Rice, RN, PhD

Critical Care Coordinator
Critical Care Program
The University of Tennessee
Nashville, Tennessee

Preface

With the advancement of sophisticated modes of treatment, more patients are surviving the initial phase of a critical illness or injury only to have the stage set for the development of multisystem organ failure (MSOF). This complex phenomenon, once thought to be a clinical presentation stemming solely from cardiovascular instability and poor oxygen delivery, is now recognized as a systemic disturbance mediated by a sustained inflammatory response. No longer viewed as a series of isolated failures, MSOF represents a complex interaction between organ systems in both their functioning and pathophysiologic states. Each organ may be a target of the syndrome or a significant factor in the development and progression of MSOF.

The purpose of this text is to provide the experienced critical care nurse and other health care team members with the pathophysiologic background and understanding of MSOF necessary to develop an effective plan of care and anticipate events associated with this syndrome. The text not only presents *what* you see but also *why* you see it. The information presented assumes that the reader possesses a working knowledge of basic critical care assessment parameters, hemodynamic monitoring, and routine standards of care for the critically ill population; therefore basic nursing care is not included. The focus is on integration of clinical assessment into a pathophysiologic knowledge base so that decision making is based on a foundation of science and research rather than tradition.

Section I provides an overview of the syndrome, along with a complete chapter on the inflammatory/immune response (IIR) and its impact on the critically ill. The inflammatory mediators playing a principal role in sepsis and MSOF are presented in Chapter 3. Because coagulation and the endothelium are closely related to the IIR, the role of disseminated intravascular coagulation (DIC) in the potentiation of MSOF has been given individual attention in Chapter 4.

Section II presents the major pathophysiologic derangements occurring in sepsis* and MSOF. As major etiologic factors in MSOF, sepsis and shock are common threads running through the text. Many of the pathophysiologic changes present in sepsis parallel the development and progression of MSOF. Detail is given to the source of these changes as well as the clinical presentation accompanying each change. Section III then presents each organ as a piece of the entire MSOF puzzle. Damage sustained, clinical evidence of failure, and the ensuing impact that each organ's failure produces are discussed. Although individual organ support continues to be a major element of the therapeutic regimen, it is no longer the primary focus of care.

Section IV provides an overview of MSOF and associated therapeutic interventions. Special concerns for the pediatric patient are also addressed in a separate chapter. As the leading cause of late mortality in the critical care unit, MSOF presents a tremendous challenge to the health care team caring for the critically ill patient. A collaborative approach to management serves as the foundation for discussing assessment and intervention in this text. As case management moves to the forefront of health care delivery and the one set of goals/one plan of care approach (Critical Path) becomes more common, patient goal attainment will depend on the ability to collaborate and work together rather than in isolation.† In a unique study, Knaus et al‡ reported a decrease in expected mortality

---

*Due to inconsistent use in the literature of the terms *septicemia, septic shock,* and the *septic syndrome,* the term *sepsis* will be used in this text to refer to all three syndromes as a group. The terms *shock* and *syndrome* will be used and defined in specific discussions when applicable.

†Zander K. Nursing case management: Strategic management of cost and quality outcomes. J Nurs Admin 1988;18(5):23-30.

‡Knaus WA et al. An evaluation of outcome from intensive care in major medical centers. Ann Intern Med 1986;104:410-418.

rates in those intensive care units that demonstrated a high degree of nurse/physician collaboration.

Because nurses are at the bedside 24 hours a day, they play a key role in early intervention and successful management of the patient with MSOF, including coordination of the numerous disciplines involved. Nursing care of the patient with MSOF requires a great degree of knowledge, independent judgment, and skill. Accurate monitoring, astute assessment, and genuine compassion all combine to enhance the care and comfort of the critically ill patient.

Section IV also provides an overview of current investigational therapies. The study of MSOF is an explosive area of research both in pathogenic mechanisms and in therapeutic modalities. New data become available almost daily concerning the numerous mediators that have been implicated in the pathogenesis of this complex phenomenon. Present investigational therapies are aimed at inhibiting the IIR and minimizing tissue damage after inflammation.

Because MSOF can strike any patient in any type of critical care area, knowledge of MSOF and its associated clinical conditions is imperative for the critical care nurse. It is beyond the scope and purpose of this text to comprehensively cover all areas of critical care. However, remember that every aspect of the patient's condition and treatment, from tube feedings to mechanical ventilation, has the potential to affect the MSOF process. By understanding the etiologic factors and pathophysiologic mechanisms operating in MSOF, the nurse can more effectively assess the patient, implement an individualized plan of care, and evaluate the patient's response to the therapeutic regimen.

How to use this text

This text is one of a rare number of books in the nursing literature that focuses on a single clinical syndrome and its pathophysiologic background. Although written at an advanced level and primarily intended for an experienced audience, the format of this text does allow for use by the less experienced reader.

Level of reader

For the experienced reader with a strong background in basic anatomy, physiology, and pathophysiology, Sections I and II provide an in-depth pathophysiologic discussion on prevailing systemic alterations that actually set the stage for damage in the individual organs. For the reader without a strong background in pathophysiologic mechanisms or without enough time to cover the entire text, most of the organ chapters (Section III) provide an overview of normal physiology and then proceed to discuss pathophysiology, significant assessment parameters, and management strategies for each major organ system. The organ chapters are the clinical "meat" of the text.

For the reader new to the critical care arena, reading the introduction (Chapter 1) and conclusion (Chapter 16), which emphasize the sequence of events, will offer a baseline understanding of MSOF and its management. Reading the text "in reverse" (Section IV to Section I) may actually enhance understanding of the more difficult material. Begin with the concluding overview in Section IV, then delve a little deeper into normal anatomy and physiology and pathophysiology in the various organ chapters in Section III, applying that information to clinical assessment and management. When a grasp of the material is acquired, move to the in-depth pathophysiologic derangements in Section II. Keep in mind that these pathophysiologic changes actually incite the organ damage discussed in Section III.

Points of notice

Because Chapter 3 extensively examines the physiologic role and the pathophysiologic impact of the principal inflammatory mediators thought to be involved in the organ dysfunction observed in MSOF, each chapter author focuses only on the mediators' roles within his or her topic. The reader is referred to Chapter 3 for additional background information, such as each mediator's source, activation, and biologic activity. Appendix A also provides a quick reference to the major mediators.

Many charts and flow diagrams have been included in the text to give the reader an overall view of the cascade of events occurring in the various systems. In material of this depth, it is easy to get lost in the details and lose sight of the overall process as it affects the patient. The charts and diagrams assist the reader in integrating complex physiologic concepts into the reader's clinical practice and decision making, often showing the sequence of events that leads to a particular clinical presentation. An extensive reference list at the end of each chapter provides bibliographic support for that chapter's presentation, but the reference lists were also developed to furnish source material for those who choose to research a particular area in more depth.

Acknowledgments

My deepest appreciation goes to the contributing authors of this text. Their attention to detail, knowledge of the subject matter, and interest in providing state-of-the-art information have produced a text that is both physiologically based and clinically relevant. I would like to extend my gratitude to the expert reviewers for sharing their expertise, valuable time, and helpful suggestions to ensure the accuracy of this text. A special thank you goes to Sheila Easley, RN, for her detailed artistic depiction of bacterial translocation in Chapter 9. To the editors and staff at Mosby–Year Book, specifically Terry Van Schaik, Editor; Janet Livingston, Developmental Editor; and Jim Russell, Production Editor, I offer my sincere appreciation for their many helpful suggestions, unending patience, and skill in the preparation and review of this text.

On a more personal note, I warmly thank Joan King, RN, PhD; Vee Rice, RN, PhD; and Penny Vaughan, RN, MSN for showing interest in me and my endeavors and providing recommendations for this text and its contributing authors. They serve as consummate role models for critical care nursing education. I am indebted to Mrs. Richard D. Williams for her provision of constant support, endless encouragement, and, not least importantly, a place to live during the preparation of this text. Her knowledge of the English language, gift of teaching, and commitment to the Word are a constant source of inspiration to me. I cannot imagine these last two years without her. To W. Evan Secor, PhD, I extend my love and sincere appreciation for his invaluable assistance in the review of chapters, discussion of immune mechanisms, laborious proofing of this text, and above all, providing a source

of strength, humor, and stability in the midst of it all.

I would be remiss if I did not acknowledge the Critical Care and Trauma Nurse Internship Program and the nursing staff of the SICU at Parkland Memorial Hospital in Dallas, Texas, particularly those present during my tenure there from 1983 to 1986. Their incredible expertise, commitment to high-quality care, and search to understand why we do what we do were and still are a continual motivation to me and the inspiration for this text. To them and to all other critical care nurses interested in an increased understanding of both physiology and pathophysiology and its application at the bedside, this text is for you.

On a final note, I would like to pay tribute to June Buckingham, RN (1943–1992). I believe most of us can look back and identify at least one person that played a central role in our decision to choose nursing as a career. For me that person was June. She was not only a consummate professional but a dear friend as well, and her death represents a significant loss to her family, friends, and the nursing community. June was a "good nurse." Although that phrase sounds so plain, it is one of the highest compliments we as nurses give to each other. It intimates an understanding of health and disease, meticulous technique but not obsessiveness, assertiveness but not rudeness, and ultimate concern for the patient's welfare. May we all be such good role models to future generations.

In the relatively young study of MSOF, we seek to describe the syndrome as a unique clinical entity. I hope this text will provide you with a new appreciation for the complexity of the syndrome, challenge you to an increased awareness of the role of the inflammatory/immune response in critical illness, and enhance your understanding of the assessment and interventions required to care for the patient with MSOF.

Virginia Byrn Huddleston

Contents

SECTION THREE

Organ Involvement and Clinical Presentation

14 Pancreatitis, 251

Janice McMillan

Special Considerations and Management

15 The Pediatric Patient, 265

Patricia A. Moloney-Harmon
Sandra J. Czerwinski

SECTION ONE

Primary Events and Mediator Release

Multisystem organ failure ultimately results from the body's response to physiologic insult such as trauma, shock, sepsis, and ischemia. Various biologic systems activate as the body attempts to protect itself and repair the damage. The inflammatory/immune response, along with neuroendocrine activation and endothelial damage, triggers the release of numerous mediators specifically targeted to maintain host defense, hemodynamic stability, and physiologic homeostasis. Localized to the site of injury, these mediators elicit changes in the microcirculation and white blood cell activity necessary for wound healing, tissue repair, and organ protection. However, overwhelming activation and loss of regulatory control of these same systems shift activity from the local site to the systemic circulation and distant tissue.

1 Multisystem Organ Failure: Background and Etiology

Virginia Byrn Huddleston

Once used only to label the patient at end-stage experiencing failure of all major organ systems, multisystem organ failure (MSOF) has come into its own as a distinct clinical syndrome.[1-13] Although the literature refers to multisystem organ failure (MSOF) by various names—multiple organ failure,[1,4,14] remote organ failure,[15] sequential organ failure,[16] or hypermetabolism organ failure complex[17]—the definition remains the same. MSOF is a nonspecific expression of critical illness involving progressive failure of two or more organ systems, which is driven by the presence of numerous circulating mediators and clinical conditions (see box on the right). MSOF often follows successful resuscitation after severe trauma, major surgery, intraabdominal sepsis, and other forms of critical illness, and the organs involved are often remote from the site of injury or inflammation.[18-21]

HISTORY AND BACKGROUND

In the 1950s and 1960s, single organ failure was the leading cause of death following major traumatic and surgical insults. Renal failure and, more predominantly, respiratory failure had mortality rates greater than 70%.[3] With the advent of sophisticated modes of resuscitation and invasive monitoring, more patients are surviving previously lethal insults. With this increase in survival, new patterns of morbidity and mortality have emerged in the intensive care unit (ICU). Although respiratory failure, namely the adult respiratory distress syndrome (ARDS), still occurs early in the process, the cause of death today is not usually failure of gas exchange, as seen in the 1960s and early 1970s, but rather sepsis-related complications and multisystem organ failure.[3] As our therapies and understanding of disease processes such as sepsis and shock improve, the appearance of "new" compli-

---

TRIGGERS OF THE INFLAMMATORY/IMMUNE RESPONSE

Mechanical tissue damage

Burns
Crush injuries
Surgical procedures

Abscesses

Intraabdominal
Intracranial
Other

Ischemic/necrotic tissue

Myocardial infarction
Pancreatitis
DIC

Microbial invasion

Immunosuppressed states
Surgery/trauma
Community exposure
Nosocomial exposure

Endotoxin release

Gram-negative sepsis
Translocation of bacteria from gut

Global perfusion deficits

Shock states
Cardiopulmonary arrest

Regional perfusion deficits

Vascular injury
Vascular repair procedures
Thromboembolic events

cations and syndromes has kept pace.[22] As Pinsky[22] states: "Patients rarely die of their disease but of complications related to it." MSOF may be considered the final common pathway to death in the 20th-century ICU and is the leading cause of late mortality.[18,19]

Several early reports described an association between impaired function of multiple organs and gram-negative sepsis or shock,[23-25] but reports in the mid-1970s by Tilney, Bailey, and Morgan,[26] Baue,[16] Eiseman, Bealt, and Norton,[14] and Polk and Shields[15] actually described a distinct clinical syndrome characterized by *sequential* organ failure. This *sequential* organ failure, or MSOF, in contrast to the simultaneous failure of numerous

organs commonly seen after severe shock, was related not only to the insult itself but also to associated therapeutic interventions.[16]

CLASSIFICATION AND STAGING

Meakins[12] has described a classification system based on a single, double, and persistent hit scenario (Fig. 1-1). Lekander and Cerra[10] also describe distinct categories of MSOF (Fig. 1-2). Their Type I (early mortality) coincides with Meakins's single hit, and their Type II (late mortality) parallels the double and persistent hit presentations. In the single hit scenario, the insult itself along with resuscitative measures contributes directly to the development of rapid respiratory failure, followed by

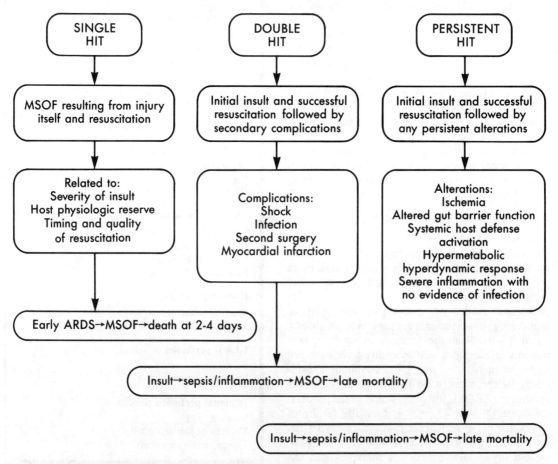

Fig. 1-1 MSOF classification according to Meakins. (Modified from Meakins JL. Etiology of multiple organ failure. J Trauma 1990;30:S165-S168.)

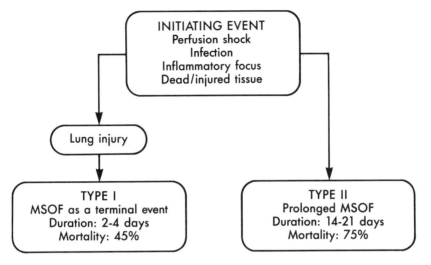

Fig. 1-2 MSOF classification according to Lekander and Cerra. (From Lekander BJ, Cerra FB. The syndrome of multiple organ failure. Crit Care Nurs Clin North Am 1990;2:331-342.)

renal and cardiovascular failure. Infection may or may not be present, and death ensues within 2 to 4 days of admission. Direct pulmonary trauma (hemothorax or pneumothorax, pulmonary contusion, and aspiration), severe head injury, and delayed or inadequate resuscitation measures greatly contribute to the single hit or early, rapid MSOF picture.[10,12]

In the double hit and persistent hit scenarios, secondary complications and persistent inflammation and ischemia contribute to loss of gut barrier function,[12,27-29] activation of host defense systems,[1,3,5,30,31] hypermetabolism,[2,10,17,32] and overwhelming inflammation.[33-36] MSOF is the ultimate sequela.[1,12] Pulmonary failure usually occurs first, followed by liver or gastrointestinal (GI) dysfunction, renal failure, and cardiovascular instability. The central nervous system and hematologic system may also be involved. Late mortality (defined as 14 to 21 days after insult) is the final outcome. DeCamp and Demling[3] have staged the MSOF continuum (Table 1-1).

The incidence of MSOF is difficult to document because different institutions and research protocols use varying criteria to define the syndrome. Overall mortality rates of 60% to 90% have been reported, and MSOF is the major cause of death

following septic, traumatic, and burn insults.* More recent research reports a high correlation between the number of organs involved and mortality. Mortality approaches 100% when three or more organs have failed.[6,11,19,39]

FINAL COMMON PATHWAY

On autopsy, the involved organs in the MSOF patient display similar patterns of tissue damage and are often remote from the initial injury site or septic source[35]; therefore theories concerning the pathophysiologic mechanism involved in MSOF focus on common pathways and interactions between the organ systems, rather than on isolated processes. If the organs are suffering similar injury, could their damage be related and could it be caused by systemic alterations rather than isolated derangements in each organ? The search for a "final common pathway" to the development of MSOF has been the primary goal of recent research. The availability of more advanced biochemical instrumentation and techniques in recent years has provided the foundation for more extensive research into the processes associated with the MSOF complex. Once thought to be related solely to cardio-

*References 14, 25, 26, 33, 37, 38.

Table 1-1 Clinical Progression of Multisystem Organ Failure

Stage	Onset after injury	Clinical observations
Sepsis	2 to 7 days	Fever and leukocytosis
		Decreased systemic vascular resistance
		Increased cardiac output and oxygen consumption
Early MSOF	7 to 14 days	Acute respiratory failure
		Impaired oxygen extraction
		Hypermetabolism with or without jaundice
		Ileus and thrombocytopenia
		Leukocytosis or leukopenia
		Possible mental status changes
Established MSOF	2 weeks to months	Progressive adult respiratory distress syndrome
		Hemodynamic instability
		Hypermetabolism and lactic acidosis
		Jaundice and azotemia with or without oliguria
		Possible stress and gastrointestinal tract bleeding
		Disseminated intravascular coagulation
Preterminal MSOF	Weeks to months	Hypodynamic cardiovascular state refractory to inotropic or alpha-adrenergic support
		Minimal oxygen extraction
		Worsening lactic acidosis

From DeCamp MM, Demling RH. Posttraumatic multisystem organ failure. JAMA 1988;260:532. Copyright 1988, American Medical Association.

vascular instability and poor oxygen delivery, MSOF is now recognized as a systemic syndrome mediated by numerous plasma enzyme cascades, cellular elements, and biochemical mediators commonly released and activated in inflammation and/or infection* (see Chapter 3 and Appendix A).

INFLAMMATION VERSUS INFECTION

As numerous investigators have described the syndrome over the last two decades, an interesting finding is becoming increasingly evident: positive blood cultures and clinical infection are not needed to initiate the MSOF process. Although septic shock remains the most common single etiologic factor in the development of MSOF, 40% to 50% of MSOF patients do not have positive blood cultures or a septic focus.[3,4,18] Other major conditions, including perfusion deficits and persistent inflammatory foci, are also associated with the development of MSOF (see box on triggers of the inflammatory/immune response on p. 3). Abscesses, ischemic tissue, necrotic tissue, and endotoxin continually trigger the inflammatory/immune response

*References 5, 19, 34, 36, 40, 41.

(IIR), causing further liberation of inflammatory mediators.[31,42,43]

The common pathway in all these clinical conditions is triggering of the IIR and release of mediators, even in classically "noninfectious" states such as hypovolemic shock or cardiac arrest. As tissue perfusion decreases, cellular oxygen metabolism is altered, and by-products of anaerobic metabolism and numerous mediators are released, including lactic acid, proteases, oxygen-derived free radicals, catabolic hormones (epinephrine, glucagon, glucocorticoids), opioids, arachidonic acid metabolites, and cytokines.[44-46]

Nonbacteremic sepsis and the septic syndrome are two terms commonly applied to the patients who demonstrate a classic septic presentation, yet no source of infection can be found.[3,13,47] Even on autopsy, inflammation is present, often without infection or septic focus.[4,35] Because of these findings, inflammation and inflammatory mediators are becoming a focal point of clinical research and attention. Any process that triggers the body's inflammatory response, whether it be microbial, ischemic, or mechanical, has the potential to incite the MSOF process.

These patients, with or without positive cultures, are in a hyperdynamic, hypermetabolic state. Elevated cardiac output, decreased systemic vascular resistance (SVR), leukocytosis, tachycardia, and fever are prominent. Major alterations in tissue perfusion, metabolism, and oxygen use occur. The major danger of the MSOF syndrome appears to be its self-propagating nature. Once the inflammatory process reaches a certain level of activation, minimal stimulus is necessary to keep it going.[3] This makes prevention and early identification crucial. Special attention must be given to identification of early markers of infection, inflammation, and ischemia. Whether systemic inflammation causes the ischemia or the ischemia causes the inflammation, the outcome is often the same—organ system dysfunction and failure.

Many investigators believe the presence and activity of numerous mediators provide the common pathway to the development of MSOF, with or without septicemia and shock.* But from where do these mediators come and why are they released? Following bodily insult, whether it be multisystem trauma, microbial invasion, or myocardial infarction, specific primary events occur that trigger the release of mediators into the circulation from various sources as the body seeks to protect itself and recover from the insult. The primary events are:

1. Neuroendocrine activation
2. Activation of IIR
3. Endothelial damage

PRIMARY EVENTS
Neuroendocrine activation

One of the earliest responses to injury is neuroendocrine activation. The nervous system and endocrine system are intimately linked in their control of tissue function. The nervous system generates biochemical agents that act as hormones, and the endocrine system produces substances that mediate activity within the central nervous system. Therefore the two systems are often referred to as one functional unit and given the name neuroendocrine (neurohumoral or neurohormonal).[48]

Following an insult, activation of the neuroendocrine system stimulates the release of numerous substances into the circulation, including ACTH from the anterior pituitary, glucocorticoids from the adrenal cortex, epinephrine from the adrenal medulla, and norepinephrine from sympathetic nerves.[49] Pituitary and CNS endorphin, growth hormone, and prolactin levels are also increased following exposure to stressful stimuli (Table 1-2).[50] The secretion of "stress hormones" prepares the body for fight or flight from the insult. The hormones also allow the body to compensate for complications occurring secondary to the insult, such as fluid losses, hypotension, and microbial invasion. Other changes, including increased blood flow, increased capillary permeability, and increased blood glucose, provide an environment necessary for adequate repair and healing. In the face of hemorrhage and massive third-spacing, other mediators responsible for maintaining circulating volume will also be released, such as aldosterone and renin.

The "mass discharge" of the sympathetic nervous system occurs almost instantaneously, with the autonomic centers of the brain stimulating almost all the sympathetic nerves at once.[51] The sympathetic nervous system can effect change in target organs with extreme rapidity and intensity. Heart rate can double in 3 to 5 seconds, blood pressure can double in 10 to 15 seconds, and cardiac output can increase fourfold. Sweating and involuntary bladder emptying can also occur within seconds.[51]

Inflammatory/immune response

Activation of the IIR represents a major physiologic event in the body. Following an insult, multiple immune mechanisms are activated to protect the host from invading microorganisms, to limit the extent of injury, and to promote rapid healing of involved tissues. A series of complex interactions occurs with numerous activating and inhibiting feedback loops and redundant pathways. These interactions occur through humoral, cellular, and biochemical mediators (Appendix A). Although the process is initiated to protect the host, lack of appropriate regulation can lead to a malignant (uncontrolled) intravascular inflammation that ultimately harms the host.[13,22,34,36] Inflammatory mediators produced by white blood cells, such as tumor necrosis factor (TNF), interleukin-1 (IL-1), oxygen-derived free radicals, and proteases, are very damaging to tissues and vessels and are implicated or associated with many signs and symp-

---

*References 3, 5, 13, 19, 33-36.

Table 1-2 Neuroendocrine Hormone Activity in the Stress State[1,50,51]

Hormone	Secretory source	Activity
ACTH	Anterior pituitary	Stimulated release of cortisol from adrenal cortex
		Increased lipolysis
		Increased amino acid and glucose uptake in muscle
		Increased beta-cell release of insulin
Cortisol	Adrenal cortex	Increased gluconeogenesis
		Decreased extrahepatic cellular protein
		Increased hepatic protein synthesis
		Mobilized fatty acids
		Stabilized lysosomal membrane
		Decreased capillary permeability
		Depressed WBC activity and mediator release
		Lymphocyte suppression
Catecholamines (epinephrine and norepinephrine)	Adrenal medulla and sympathetic nerve endings	Increased sweat production
		Increased heart rate and contractility
		Increased blood pressure
		Increased respiratory rate
		Bronchodilatation
		Decreased peristalsis
		Increased gluconeogenesis and glycogenolysis
		Increased basal metabolic rate
		Increased lipolysis
Growth hormone	Anterior pituitary	Increased protein synthesis
		Increased fatty acid mobilization
		Decreased glucose utilization rate (conservation of carbohydrates)
Endorphins	Hypothalamus, anterior pituitary, pancreas, and GI tract	Regulated ACTH secretion
		Suppressed cortisol levels
		Induced analgesia
		Euphoria

MEDIATORS OF THE INFLAMMATORY/IMMUNE RESPONSE[1,40,53]

Clotting factors	Oxygen-derived free radicals
Colony-stimulating factors	Plasminogen
Complement	Plasminogen activators
Hageman factor	Platelet activating factor
Heparin	Prostaglandins*
Histamine	Proteases
Interferon	Thromboxane*
Interleukins	Tissue factor
Leukotrienes*	Tumor necrosis factor

*Arachidonic acid metabolites.

toms seen in MSOF[52-54] (see box on p. 8). A vicious, self-activating cycle can occur, and previously protective mechanisms actually contribute to maldistribution of volume, imbalance of oxygen supply and demand, and alterations in metabolism.[32,45,55-57] If these pathophysiologic changes cannot be reversed or slowed, organ dysfunction and failure ensue. For further information on this exquisite and complicated mechanism, see Chapters 2 and 3.

The wound's role in the systemic response has become a focus of recent question and investigation.[1,58] The wound produces extensive inflammation by activating large numbers of neutrophils and macrophages, which in turn produce inflammatory mediators such as TNF, oxygen-derived free radicals, and proteases.[42] These mediators can be systemically absorbed and target distant organs. The wound also makes oxygen and metabolic demands on an already stressed system.[1]

An extensive overlap exists between the IIR and coagulation. Several circulating components play a role in both processes: kallikrein/kinin cascade, complement, Hageman factor, and platelets. Activation of the IIR often leads to concomitant activation of coagulation or alterations in the hemostatic balance (Fig. 1-3). Because of this overlap, DIC and other coagulopathies are common in the septic patient or the patient experiencing a major inflammatory insult, such as soft-tissue damage, burn injury, or pancreatitis.

Endothelial damage

Coagulation abnormalities are also prevalent in the critically ill patient population because of the extensive endothelial damage that is often present. The endothelium is a major contributor to the activation and potentiation of the IIR, coagulopathies, and MSOF because of its extensive surface area (throughout the body), susceptibility to injury, and metabolic functions. Once thought to be an inert barrier between the flowing blood and the substructure of the blood vessels and tissue, the endothelium is now recognized as an active metabolic organ[59] (see Chapter 3). One of the major functions of the endothelium is *anticoagulation*.[60] When damaged, the endothelium loses many of its anticoagulant properties and may even generate and release procoagulant substances, such as tissue thromboplastin (tissue factor).[61,62]

The endothelium is very susceptible to damage by a variety of factors (see box on p. 12), especially white blood cell/endothelial cell interactions.[63,64] TNF and other inflammatory mediators also directly damage the endothelium.[43,65,66] Not only does endothelial damage potentiate coagulation abnormalities, but it can affect capillary permeability as well. Direct damage or mediator activity can significantly increase capillary permeability, thus promoting edema formation and changes in oncotic pressure gradients.[43,67,68] Whether the patient is a victim of a fresh myocardial infarction, multisystem trauma, or pneumonia, potentially toxic substances are circulating that could alter endothelial integrity and incite coagulation abnormalities or increased vascular permeability. In summary, the healthy endothelium not only aids in keeping the blood fluid but also in retaining the circulating volume within the vascular space. Both activation of the IIR and endothelial damage contribute to the coagulopathies seen in sepsis and MSOF.[43,69]

Summary

The body suffering an insult is exposed not only to direct damage by the insult but also to the actions of many activated mediators. More than 100 mediators have been implicated in the development of sepsis and MSOF.[70] The mediators released in response to the three primary events of neuroendocrine activation, IIR activation, and endothelial damage initially serve a physiologic function in host defense and repair, but the loss of regulation and the overwhelming of the clearance mechanisms lead to a pathologic buildup of many mediators. As the levels increase, previously localized responses become systemic derangements. For example, vasodilatation and erythema occurring at the local site of injury secondary to kinin and complement activity may extend to systemic vasodilatation if the mediator levels increase above a threshold value. Severe decreases in SVR and BP then ensue. Substances and systems initially primed and activated to protect and defend the host actually cause severe tissue damage, shock, and death in the form of MSOF.[22,34,36,42]

The numerous mediators provoke changes in three major areas of body function. The three pathophysiologic derangements are: (1) maldistribution of circulating volume, (2) oxygen supply and demand imbalance, and (3) metabolic alterations (Fig. 1-4). See Chapters 5, 6, and 7, respectively.

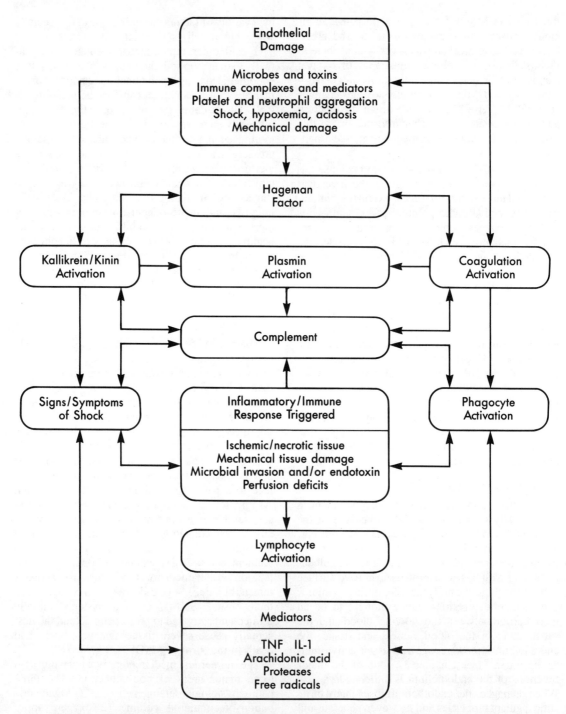

Fig. 1-3   Interrelationship between coagulation and inflammation and shock. (From Huddleston VB. Multisystem organ failure: A pathophysiologic approach, Boston, 1991;17. Abbreviations: *TNF*, Tumor necrosis factor; *IL-1*, interleukin-1.)

SEQUELAE
Determining factors

The sequelae of these three pathophysiologic changes are organ system dysfunction and failure. But why does the patient in Bed 1 develop fulminant MSOF and the patient in Bed 2 overcome the obstacles and recover? Although the exact trigger determining the fatal progression of MSOF remains elusive, the development of organ failure following insult and pathophysiologic derangements is affected by the severity of insult, host-related factors, and therapeutic interventions. These factors, in turn, influence the degree of reperfusion injury and IIR activation present. Obviously, the more severe the insult, the more likely the patient will develop complications. Host-related factors including age, chronic disease states, and immunosuppression may increase the risk of MSOF. Iatrogenic factors such as invasive lines and catheters, immunosuppressant therapy, surgical procedures, and antibiotic therapy may predispose the patient to the development of sepsis and thus MSOF. The skin and mucosal surfaces provide the first line of defense against microbial invasion. If they are breached by invasive devices and procedures, invasive colonization can occur. Invasive devices such as intravenous lines, endotracheal tubes, and urinary catheters may serve as reservoirs for the colonization and spread of organisms. See Chapter 2 for further discussion on contributing factors and immunosuppression in the ICU.

Overwhelmed clearance mechanisms and malignant IIR. In the patient with altered defense mechanisms or increased severity of insult, normal regulatory and clearance mechanisms are more likely to be overwhelmed. The body cannot clear the elevated levels of potentially toxic mediators, and the mediators begin to inflict damage on vessels and tissue. Because of the autoactivating nature of the stimulated IIR, the IIR becomes malignant and perpetuates itself in a vicious cycle requiring minimal additional stimulus. In other words, once the system becomes activated, it may keep itself running despite the removal of initial stimuli such as abscesses, microbes, or necrotic tissue[3,13] (Fig. 1-3).

Reperfusion injury. Reperfusion injury has also been shown to play a role in remote organ damage and MSOF.[71] It is especially prevalent following low-flow or ischemic events, such as shock states, arrest situations, myocardial infarctions, and aortic cross-clamping.[58,72,73] When tissues become ischemic, certain transformations occur to select enzymes and substances in the tissue. When the area is reperfused, these transformed enzymes and substances react with the freshly delivered oxygen to form oxygen-derived free radicals. These radicals, along with the lactic acid, potassium, and other substances released from reperfused tissues, are very toxic to tissues and the endothelium and may perpetuate damage that has already occurred secondary to ischemia. Increased capillary permeability, tissue edema, and microcirculatory compression may occur and cause further damage to already compromised limbs or organs. See Chapter 5 for an in-depth discussion on reperfusion injury.

Organ involvement

Although the heart, lung, liver, and kidney are most often addressed in discussions of MSOF, every organ has the potential to suffer damage. Even peripheral neuropathies are now associated with critical illness and MSOF.[74] Every organ is at risk because every organ receives a blood supply containing many of the inflammatory mediators. Not all organs have equal susceptibility to injury, nor does each organ's failure affect patient survival with the same magnitude. Factors affecting organ system involvement include: (1) sensitivity of the organ's vascular bed to mediators and hypoperfusion, (2) regional degree of inflammation and proximity to the primary site of trauma or infection, and (3) responsiveness to the therapeutic regimen: what may help one organ may harm another.[1,7,13]

Keep in mind that the damage suffered by an individual organ may be the contributing factor to the development of MSOF, or it may be the direct result of the ongoing inflammatory process. In other words, the organ may be the source of the problem or a victim of the process. For example, ARDS may potentiate the development of MSOF, or ARDS may develop secondary to mediators and toxins circulating in the blood during the MSOF syndrome and/or a sustained inflammatory response.[75] This concept, victim of the process versus source of the problem, is one of the many factors contributing to the complexity of the syndrome.

Abbreviations: *TNF*, tumor necrosis factor; *IL-1*, interleukin-1.

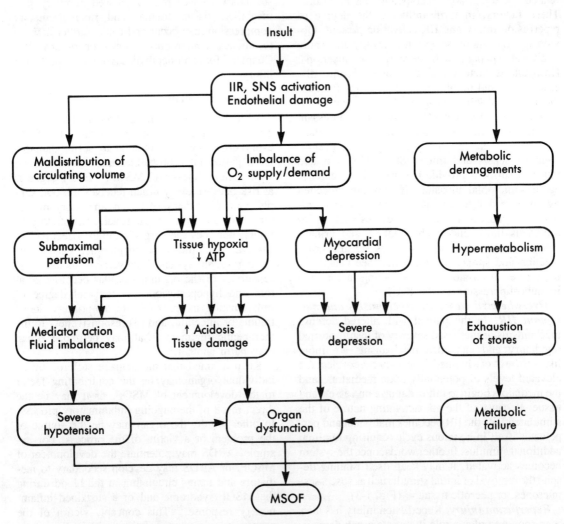

Fig. 1-4 Pathophysiologic cascade mechanism of multisystem organ failure. (From Huddleston VB. Multisystem organ failure: A pathophysiologic approach, Boston, 1991;24. Abbreviations: *IIR*, Inflammatory/immune response; *SNS*, sympathetic nervous system; *ATP*, adenosine triphosphate.)

ASSESSMENT AND MANAGEMENT

Assessment and treatment of this complex syndrome focus primarily on minimizing infectious/inflammatory stimuli, maintaining adequate preload and circulating volume, enhancing oxygen delivery and consumption, minimizing oxygen demand, and meeting metabolic requirements.[76,77] The following chapters provide pathophysiologic background, assessment parameters, and management strategies for both systemic changes and organ-specific complications and failure. The high mortality rates associated with MSOF reflect the inadequacy of even the highly technologic monitoring and interventions available to the critical care team at present. Until newer therapies (such as monoclonal antibodies to TNF[78] and endotoxin[79]) are fully developed that can control the inflammatory process without increasing the risk of infection, efforts must be focused on *prevention* and *early* identification of inflammation and infection. Understanding the disease process enhances clinical decision making as one integrates assessment findings, trends in patient response to therapy, and knowledge of underlying pathophysiologic derangements into developing an individualized plan of care that focuses on prompt recognition and treatment of secondary complications.

CONCLUSION

This complex phenomenon, once thought to be a clinical presentation stemming solely from cardiovascular instability, is now recognized as a systemic disturbance mediated by a sustained inflammatory response, hypermetabolism, hypoperfusion, and ultimately dysfunctional cellular activity and oxygen extraction/utilization defects.* No longer viewed as a series of isolated failures, MSOF represents a complex interaction of organ systems in both their physiologic and pathophysiologic states and may be the ultimate result of host defense homeostatic failure (Fig. 1-4).[1,4,8,9,13]

---

*References 1, 13, 32, 45, 55-57.

REFERENCES

1. Baue AE. Multiple organ failure: Patient care and prevention. St. Louis: Mosby–Year Book; 1990.
2. Cerra FB. Hypermetabolism, organ failure, and metabolic support. Surgery 1987;101:1-14.
3. DeCamp MM, Demling RH. Posttraumatic multisystem organ failure. JAMA 1988;260:530-534.
4. Deitch EA, ed. Multiple organ failure. New York: Thieme Medical Publishers; 1990.
5. Dorinsky PM, Gadek JE. Multiple organ failure. Clin Chest Med 1990;11:581-591.
6. Fry DE. Multiple system organ failure. Surg Clin North Am 1988;68:107-122.
7. Goodwin CW. Multiple organ failure: Clinical overview of the syndrome. J Trauma 1990;30:S163-S165.
8. Hotter AN. The pathophysiology of multi-system organ failure in the trauma patient. Clin Issues Crit Care Nurs 1990;1:465-478.
9. Huddleston VB. Multisystem organ failure. In: Mims BC, ed. Case studies in critical care nursing. Baltimore: Williams & Wilkins; 1990:494-499.
10. Lekander BJ, Cerra FB. The syndrome of multiple organ failure. Crit Care Nurs Clin North Am 1990;2:331-342.
11. Marshall JC, Meakins JL. Multiorgan failure. In: Wilmore DW, ed. American College of Surgeons: Care of the surgical patient. Volume 1. Critical care. New York: Scientific American; 1989.
12. Meakins JL. Etiology of multiple organ failure. J Trauma 1990;30:S165-S168.
13. Pinsky MR, Matuschak GM. Multiple systems organ failure: Failure of host defense homeostasis. Crit Care Clin 1989;5:199-220.
14. Eiseman B, Beart R, Norton L. Multiple organ failure. Surg Gynecol Obstet 1977;144:323-326.
15. Polk HC, Shields CL. Remote organ failure: A valid sign of occult intra-abdominal infection. Surgery 1977;81:310-313.
16. Baue AE. Multiple, progressive, or sequential systems failure: A syndrome of the 1970s. Arch Surg 1975;110:779-781.
17. Cerra FB. The hypermetabolism organ failure complex. World J Surg 1987;11:173-181.
18. Carrico CJ et al. Multiple-organ-failure syndrome [Panel discussion-Surgical Infection Society]. Arch Surg 1986; 121:196-208.
19. Crump JM, Duncan DA, Wears R. Analysis of multiple organ system failure in trauma and nontrauma patients. Am Surg 1988;12:702-708.
20. Darling GE et al. Multiorgan failure in critically ill patients. Can J Surg 1988;31:172-176.
21. Dorinsky PM, Gadek JE. Mechanisms of multiple nonpulmonary organ failure in ARDS. Chest 1989;96:885-892.
22. Pinsky MR. Multiple systems organ failure: Malignant intravascular inflammation. Crit Care Clin 1989;5:195-198.
23. Burke JF, Pontopiddan H, Welch CE. High output respiratory failure: An important cause of death ascribed to peritonitis or ileus. Ann Surg 1963;158:581-595.
24. Clowes GHA et al. Observations on the pathogenesis of the pneumonitis associated with severe infections in other parts of the body. Ann Surg 1968;167:630-650.
25. Skillman JJ et al. Respiratory failure, hypotension, sepsis, and jaundice. Am J Surg 1969;117:523-530.
26. Tilney NL, Bailey GL, Morgan AP. Sequential system failure after rupture of abdominal aortic aneurysms: An unsolved problem in postoperative care. Ann Surg 1973;178:117-122.
27. Deitch EA. The role of intestinal barrier failure and bacterial translocation in the development of systemic infection and multiple organ failure. Arch Surg 1990;125:403-404.

28. Deitch EA. Bacterial translocation of the gut flora. J Trauma 1990;30(Suppl 12):S184-S189.

29. Bounous G. The intestinal factor in multiple organ failure and shock. Surgery 1990;107:118-119.

30. Hyers TM, Gee M, Andreadis NA. Cellular interactions in the multiple organ injury syndrome. Am Rev Respir Dis 1987;135:952-953.

31. Border JR. Hypothesis: Sepsis, multiple systems organ failure, and the macrophage [editorial]. Arch Surg 1988;123:285-286.

32. Barton R, Cerra FB. The hypermetabolism, multiple organ failure syndrome. Chest 1989;96:1153-1160.

33. Goris RJ et al. Multiple organ failure: Generalized autodestructive inflammation. Arch Surg 1985;120:1109-1115.

34. Goris RJ. Multiple organ failure: Whole body inflammation? Schweiz Med Wochenschr 1989; 119:347-353.

35. Nuytinck HKS et al. Whole-body inflammation in trauma patients. Arch Surg 1988;123:1519-1524.

36. Anderson BO, Harken AH. Multiple organ failure: Inflammatory priming and activation sequences promote autologous tissue injury. J Trauma 1990;30:S44-S49.

37. Fry DE et al. Multiple system organ failure. The role of uncontrolled infection. Arch Surg 1980;115:136-140.

38. Sweet SJ et al. Synergistic effect of acute renal failure and respiratory failure in the surgical intensive care unit. Am J Surg 1981;141:492-496.

39. Rauss A et al. Prognosis for recovery from multiple organ system failure: The accuracy of objective estimates of chances for survival. The French Multicentric Group of ICU Research. Med Decis Making 1990;10:155-162.

40. Jacobs RF, Tabor DR. Immune cellular interactions during sepsis and septic injury. Crit Care Clin 1989;5:9-26.

41. Petrak RA, Balk RA, Bone RC. Prostaglandins, cyclooxygenase inhibitors, and thromboxane synthetase inhibitors in the pathogenesis of multiple systems organ failure. Crit Care Clin 1989;5:302-314.

42. Demling RH. Wound inflammatory mediators and multisystem organ failure. Prog Clin Biol Res 1987;236A:525-537.

43. Meyrick B, Johnson JE, Brigham KL. Endotoxin-induced pulmonary endothelial injury. Prog Clin Biol Res: Second Vienna Shock Forum 1989;308:91-100.

44. Shoemaker WC, Appel PL, Kram HB. Tissue oxygen debt as a determinant of postoperative organ failure. Prog Clin Biol Res: Second Vienna Shock Forum 1989;308:133-136.

45. Gutierrez G, Lund N, Bryan-Brown CW. Cellular oxygen utilization during multiple organ failure. Crit Care Clin 1989;5:271-288.

46. Schumacker PT, Samsel RW. Oxygen delivery and uptake by peripheral tissues: Physiology and pathophysiology. Crit Care Clin 1989;5:255-270.

47. Balk RA, Bone RC. The septic syndrome: Definitions and clinical implications. Crit Care Clin 1989;5:1-8.

48. Wilson JD, Foster DW. Introduction: Hormones and hormone action. In: Wilson JD, Foster DW, eds. Williams textbook of endocrinology. 7th ed. Philadelphia: WB Saunders; 1985:1-8.

49. Axelrod J, Reisine TD. Stress hormones: Their interaction and regulation. Science 1984;224:452-459.

50. Rose RM. Psychoendocrinology. In: Wilson JD, Foster DW, eds. Williams textbook of endocrinology. 7th ed. Philadelphia: WB Saunders; 1985:662-666.

51. Guyton AC. Textbook of medical physiology. 8th ed. Philadelphia: WB Saunders; 1991.

52. Mallick AA et al. Multiple organ damage caused by tumor necrosis factor and prevented by prior neutrophil depletion. Chest 1989;95:1114-1120.

53. Tracey KJ, Lowry SF. The role of cytokine mediators in septic shock. Adv Surg 1990;23:21-56.

54. Dinarello CA. Biology of interleukin 1. FASEB J 1988;2:108-115.

55. Dantzker D. Oxygen delivery and utilization in sepsis. Crit Care Clin 1989;5:81-98.

56. Bersten A, Sibbald WJ. Acute lung injury in septic shock. Crit Care Clin 1989;5:49-80.

57. Cunnion RE, Parrillo JE. Myocardial dysfunction in sepsis. Crit Care Clin 1989;5:99-118.

58. Baxter CR. Future prospectives in trauma and burn care. J Trauma 1990;30(Suppl 12):S208-S209.

59. Ryan US, ed. Pulmonary endothelium in health and disease. New York: Marcel Dekker; 1987.

60. Gimbrone MA, ed. Vascular endothelium in hemostasis and thrombosis. New York: Churchill Livingstone; 1986.

61. Müller-Berghaus G. Pathophysiologic and biochemical events in disseminated intravascular coagulation: Dysregulation of procoagulant and anticoagulant pathways. Semin Thromb and Hemost 1989;15:58-87.

62. Müller-Berghaus G. Septicemia and the vessel wall. In: Verstraete M, Vermylen J, Lijnen R, Arnout J, eds. Thrombosis and haemostasis. Leuven, Belgium: Leuven University Press; 1987:619-671.

63. Weiss SJ. Tissue destruction by neutrophils. N Engl J Med 1989;320:365-376.

64. Brigham KL. Role of free radicals in lung injury. Chest 1986;89:859-863.

65. Tracey KJ et al. Shock and tissue injury induced by recombinant human cachectin. Science 1986;234:470-474.

66. Beutler B. Cachectin in tissue injury, shock, and related states. Crit Care Clin 1989;5:353-368.

67. Freudenberg N. Reaction of the vascular intima to endotoxin shock. Prog Clin Bio Res: Second Vienna Shock Forum 1989;308:77-89.

68. Del Vecchio PJ, Malik AB. Thrombin-induced neutrophil adhesion. Prog Clin Bio Res: Second Vienna Shock Forum 1989;308:101-112.

69. Gidlof A, Lewis DH. Do endotoxinemia and sepsis impair the regulatory functions of capillary endothelial cells. Prog Clin Bio Res: Second Vienna Shock Forum 1989;308:157-162.

70. Neugebauer E et al. Mediators in septic shock: Strategies of securing them and assessment of their causal significance. Chirurg 1987;58:470-481.

71. Nelson K, Herndon B, Reisz G. Pulmonary effects of ischemic limb reperfusion: Evidence for a role of oxygen-derived radicals. Crit Care Med 1991;19:360-363.

72. Kloner RA, Przyklenk K, Patel B. Altered myocardial states: The stunned and hibernating myocardium. Am J Med 1989;86(suppl 1A):14-22.

73. Black L, Coombs VJ, Townsend SN. Reperfusion and reperfusion injury in acute myocardial infarction. Heart Lung 1990;19:274-286.

74. Witt NJ et al. Peripheral nerve function in sepsis and multiple organ failure. Chest 1991;99:176-184.

75. Hudson LD. Multiple systems organ failure (MSOF): Lessons learned from the adult respiratory distress syndrome (ARDS). Crit Care Clin 1989;5:697-705.

76. Sheagren JN. Mechanism-oriented therapy for multiple systems organ failure. Crit Care Clin 1989;5:393-409.

77. Macho JR, Luce JM. Rational approach to the management of multiple systems organ failure. Crit Care Clin 1989;5:379-392.

78. Tracey KJ et al. Anticachectin/TNF monoclonal antibodies prevent shock during lethal bacteraemia. Nature 1987;330:662-665.

79. Ziegler EJ et al. Treatment of gram-negative bacteremia and septic shock with HA-1A human monoclonal antibody against endotoxin. N Engl J Med 1991;324:429-436.

2 The Inflammatory/Immune Response: Implications for the Critically Ill

Virginia Byrn Huddleston

The inflammatory/immune response (IIR) represents one of the body's most exquisite and complicated homeostatic mechanisms. IIR activity spans all levels of physiologic interaction from the molecular to the systemic via numerous humoral, cellular, and biochemical pathways. When the body receives an insult, whether it be mechanical (surgery or crush injury), ischemic (shock or myocardial infarction), chemical (ingestion of toxic substances or drug abuse), or microbial (bacterial, viral, fungal, or parasitic), multiple systems are activated to protect the host from invading pathogens, limit the extent of injury, and promote rapid healing of involved tissues.[1] A series of complex interactions occurs with numerous activating and inhibiting feedback loops and redundant pathways.

Identifying the signs and symptoms of IIR activity date back to 3000 BC, when the Mesopotamian culture recognized fever in association with disease. In 200 BC, the Chinese and Egyptians recognized the existence of acquired immunity by practicing a process known as variolation, which introduced smallpox organisms into scratch lesions on the skin. Celsus identified the four cardinal signs of inflammation (tumor, rubor, dolor, and calor) in the first century.[2] The 1950s heralded the era of modern immunology with the recognition of histocompatibility antigen, delineation of antibody structure, and increased understanding of immunopathologic conditions.[2] On the forefront of immunologic research today are mechanisms of cellular activation and regulation, the role of genetic coding in specific immune recognition, and the nature of cellular messengers and surface receptors.

But what does this mean for the critical care patient today? For the team caring for that patient? Why is knowledge of the IIR not only helpful but necessary in caring for the critically ill patient? The IIR has been shown to play a role not only in multisystem organ failure (MSOF) but in many other areas of critical care as well. A major emphasis of research into the pathogenesis and treatment of many pathologic conditions involves the functioning of the IIR. Cancer, AIDS, organ transplantation, traumatic injury, and reperfusion injury are major examples. Even a myocardial infarction is now seen as an inflammatory event as well as an ischemic event. In addition to the pathology of many disease states, most patients in critical care areas have many risk factors for immunosuppression or dysfunction: trauma, stress, or malnutrition (Table 2-1). Because coagulation and the endothelium are intimately related to the IIR, individual attention has also been given to their activity and role in the potentiation of MSOF.

Knowledge of the IIR is vital not only in un-

Table 2-1 Risk Factors for Immune Dysfunction

Host-related	Treatment-related
Age	Invasive lines, catheters, or devices
Malnutrition	Malnutrition
Chronic diseases	Antibiotic therapy
Debilitated states	Immunosuppressant therapy
Stress	Stress
Trauma/burns	Trauma/surgery/anesthesia
Hemorrhage	Blood transfusions
Perfusion deficit	Perfusion deficit
Sepsis	Sepsis
Inflammatory foci	Inflammatory foci

derstanding the pathophysiology of disease states, but also in understanding drug therapy and assessment findings.[3] How does one safely administer interleukin-2 (IL-2) in a cancer patient if he or she does not know what IL-2 is, what it does, or what the common side effects are?[4] What is the difference between administering purified tumor necrosis factor (TNF) or the anti-TNF monoclonal antibodies? What do we monitor to assess the effectiveness of these therapeutic regimens? Confusing these two pharmacologic agents and their effects could gravely injure the patient or expedite the patient's demise.

It is beyond the scope and purpose of this text to give a comprehensive presentation of the entire IIR and associated immunopathologies in disease states. The following discussion presents a brief overview and background of major components, levels of host defense, and the orchestration of the IIR, then proceeds to a discussion on clinical conditions associated with immune dysfunction and common assessment parameters. Chapter 3 presents a comprehensive discussion of the major cells and mediators of the MSOF syndrome and their impact on the entire process. Finally, remember that the organ dysfunction or failure seen in MSOF is not a series of isolated failures, but rather a systemic process demonstrating interdependence of organs in both their physiologic and pathophysiologic states.[5,6] It is becoming increasingly evident that inflammation and malfunction of immunoregulation play a key role in the development and potentiation of MSOF. Sepsis and/or inflammatory changes are present in most patients dying of MSOF.[7,8] Although numerous hypotheses exist concerning the final common pathway of organ system dysfunction and failure, the IIR certainly plays a role (see box on p. 3). The extent of that role is yet to be defined.[5,9-12.]

INFLAMMATORY/IMMUNE RESPONSE
Components

Plasma enzyme cascades. The four interlocking plasma enzymatic cascades produce a rapid, highly amplified response to numerous stimuli such as ischemia, tissue debris, and endotoxin. Also known as humoral mediators because of their presence in the plasma, the enzymatic cascades quickly become activated because the product of one reaction is the enzymatic catalyst for the next reaction.[13] The four primary cascades play a major role in injury and the nonspecific immune response and include the complement, coagulation, fibrinolysis, and kallikrein/kinin cascades (Table 2-2).

Cellular components. The cellular components of the IIR include all the white blood cells (WBCs),

Table 2-2 Activity of Plasma Enzyme Cascades[5,13,14]

Cascade	Activity	Role in injury
Complement	Induction of inflammation Opsonization Activation of phagocytic cells Direct target cell lysis	Excessive inflammation Excessive cellular activation with mediator release
Coagulation	Hemostasis	Excessive intravascular coagulation leading to vascular obstruction, endothelial damage, and tissue ischemia
Fibrinolysis	Degradation of fibrin clot	Hemorrhage leading to decreased oxygen delivery and tissue ischemia
Kallikrein/kinin (bradykinin)	Enhanced IIR activity Enhanced fibrinolytic cascade Possible role in renal blood flow and blood pressure regulation	Massive vasodilatation Increased microvascular permeability Bronchoconstriction Excessive inflammation Excessive cellular activation

Abbreviation: *IIR*, Inflammatory/immune response.

Table 2-3   Cellular Mediators of the Inflammatory/Immune Response[1,5]

Cell	Mediators
Neutrophil	Arachidonic acid metabolites
	Interleukins
	Oxygen-derived free radicals
	Platelet activating factor
	Proteases (collagenase, elastase)
	Tissue thromboplastin (tissue factor)
Macrophages	Arachidonic acid metabolites
	Coagulation factors
	Colony stimulating factors
	Complement proteins
	Interferon
	Interleukins
	Oxygen-derived free radicals
	Plasminogen activators
	Platelet activating factor
	Proteases
	Tumor necrosis factor
Lymphocytes	Antibodies
	Colony stimulating factors
	Gamma-interferon
	Interleukins
	Tumor necrosis factor
Mast cells	Arachidonic acid metabolites
	Heparin
	Histamine
	Interleukins
	Platelet activating factor
	Proteases
Platelets	Arachidonic acid metabolites
	Chemotactants
	Histamine
	Platelet activating factor
	Serotonin
Endothelial cells	Arachidonic acid metabolites
	Interleukins
	Platelet activating factor
	Tissue thromboplastin (tissue factor)

platelets, mast cells, and fibroblasts. Although they play a major role in normal IIR and host protection, the cellular components are also the source of many of the circulating mediators[13] implicated in the damage present in sepsis and MSOF. As the various cells become activated and participate in specific functions, the mediators they are producing may "spill over" into the tissue and circulation, causing extension of the injury and systemic effects[11,15] (Table 2-3).

Biochemical mediators. As mentioned, biochemical mediators are produced primarily by immune cells. They may also be generated by damaged endothelium and the wound. Although the mediators serve a very physiologic, protective function in the "normal" IIR, uncontrolled activation and spillover may lead to pathogenic levels of these mediators. Detrimental changes then occur in circulating volume, oxygen supply and demand, and metabolism[11,16-24] (Table 2-4).

Levels of host defense

Host defense operates at three levels: external barriers against invasion and tissue injury, nonspecific systems against foreign pathogens, and antigen-specific responses to foreign pathogens. Integrating the major components of the IIR described above, these three levels work in concert to prevent invasion by foreign pathogens and promote healing of damaged tissue.[13]

External barriers. Just as the battle cry of today's health care is *prevention*, so too does the host defense system make a valiant attempt to prevent invasion rather than fight it. The body is equipped with various natural defenses or external barriers to prevent pathogenic invasion[13,25] (Table 2-5). These mechanisms of defense include (1) acidic pH, (2) normal flora compete with pathogenic species for nutrients and attachment sites and produce inhibitory substances, (3) flushing or mechanical removal, (4) cilia and mucus activity, (5) bactericidal secretions, and (6) the mechanical barrier provided by intact skin and epithelium.

Unfortunately for the patient in the ICU, many therapies directed at other disease processes, such as sepsis, alter the natural defenses. Antibiotics destroy the balance of normal flora; antacids and H_2-blockers raise gastric pH; sedatives depress respiratory depth and secretion removal as well as potentiating intestinal ileus; and endotracheal tubes bypass protective mechanisms of the respiratory system. The most dangerous interventions may be the numerous invasive devices and procedures that insult the external barrier of the skin and thus provide increased portals of entry for opportunistic and pathogenic organisms.

Nonspecific response. Although in theory the nonspecific and specific immune responses can be viewed separately, in vivo their activity is intricately interwoven, with each enhancing the activity

Table 2-4 Pathophysiologic Derangements with Associated Mediators and Contributing Factors

Derangement	Mediators/Factors
Systemic vasodilatation	Bradykinin
	Complement
	Endorphins
	Histamine
	Prostaglandins
	Serotonin
Microvascular permeability	Complement
	Bradykinin
	Histamine
	Leukotrienes
	Oxygen-derived free radicals
	Platelet activating factor
Coagulation/microvascular thrombi	Hageman factor activation
	Tissue thromboplastin
	Platelet aggregation
	WBC aggregation
	Endothelial damage
	Tissue trauma
	Arachidonic acid metabolites
	Tumor necrosis factor
	Endotoxin
	Interleukins
	Expression of tissue thromboplastin by immune cells and endothelium
Selective vasoconstriction	Renin/angiotensin
	Catecholamines
	Leukotrienes
	Prostaglandins
	Platelet activating factor
	Thromboxane
	Serotonin
Endothelial damage	Complement
	Endotoxin
	Histamine
	Interleukins
	Tumor necrosis factor
	Lysosomal enzymes
	Oxygen-derived free radicals
	Immune complexes
	Platelet aggregation
	WBC aggregation
	Hypoxia
	Acidosis
Myocardial depression	Myocardial depressant factor
	Complement
	Endorphins
	Histamine
	Acidosis
	Ischemia
	Impaired adrenergic responsiveness
Excessive cellular activity	Complement
	Proteases
	Kinins
	Interleukins
	Tumor necrosis factor
	Leukotrienes
	Platelet activating factor
	Platelets
	Prostaglandins
	Cell debris

Modified from Huddleston VB. Multisystem organ failure: A pathophysiologic approach, Boston, 1991;25.

Table 2-5 Natural Defenses and External Barriers[13,25]

Defense/barrier	System
Intact epithelium	Integument
	Respiratory
	Gastrointestinal
	Genitourinary
Acidic pH	Gastrointestinal
	Genitourinary
	Integument
Resident flora	Integument
	Respiratory
	Gastrointestinal
	Genitourinary
Mechanical removal/ flushing	Respiratory: cough, sneeze
	Gastrointestinal: peristalsis, defecation
	Genitourinary: urination
Cilia activity and mucus production	Respiratory
	Gastrointestinal
	Genitourinary
Bactericidal secretions	Gastric juices: acid, enzymes
	Milk: lactoperoxidase
	Tears, saliva, perspiration: lysozyme
	Sebum: fatty acids
	Semen: spermine
Secretory IgA	Respiratory
	Gastrointestinal
	Genitourinary

of the other. Classically, the nonspecific immune response involves the mechanisms of inflammation and phagocytosis. Inflammation is the body's initial response to insult or invasion and involves a nonspecific response to tissue injury triggered by mechanical, chemical, or microbial stimuli.[13] The goal of inflammation is to enhance the movement of nutrients and IIR cells and mediators to the injury site, thus preventing foreign invasion and extension of injury.

Following injury, the plasma enzyme cascades of complement, kinin, coagulation, and fibrinolysis as well as phagocytic cells such as neutrophils (in the circulation) and macrophages (in the tissue) are activated by microorganisms, cell debris, and endothelial damage. Both antigen/antibody complexes (classic pathway) and certain microorganisms (alternate pathway) activate the complement

cascade (see Fig. 3-3). Circulating complement proteins are cleaved, releasing active complement split products (for example, C3a, C3b, and C5a) that carry out numerous functions, such as cellular activation and opsonization (Table 2-2). These components acting in concert with other inflammatory mediators and white blood cells cause the signs and symptoms commonly associated with inflammation: rubor (erythema), tumor (edema), calor (heat), and dolor (pain). Fig. 2-1 summarizes this inflammatory response.[13,14,26] Although very beneficial as a local response, appropriate regulation of inflammation is necessary to keep the cells and mediators sequestered in the region of injury and prevent their spread to the systemic circulation and remote sites.

When a foreign pathogen enters the body, it usually comes into contact with tissue phagocytes and other antigen-presenting cells (APCs) (see Table 3-1). The macrophage is both a phagocyte and an APC, and it has nonspecific receptors for binding foreign pathogens. If the organism gains access to the blood, circulating neutrophils become activated and phagocytize foreign pathogens. The neutrophil can also migrate into the tissues and phagocytize debris at the wound or site of inflammation (Fig. 2-2). Phagocytic cells do not require previous exposure to the pathogen for phagocytosis to occur; however, phagocytosis is enhanced if the microorganism is opsonized by antibodies or complement.

Complement opsonization (coating) of the pathogen enhances phagocytosis because the phagocytes have receptors specific for complement. Therefore the phagocyte attaches to the pathogen by binding the complement coating the pathogen[13,14,27] (Fig. 2-3). Once engulfed, the pathogen is killed by lytic enzymes and oxygen-derived free radicals (ODFR).[28] The degraded microbial products are processed and returned to the surface of the APC (such as a macrophage) and presented to the T-cell residing in the peripheral lymphoid tissue. This antigen processing and presentation is a vital aspect of macrophage/T-cell interaction and stimulates the release of numerous cytokines (intercellular messengers) such as interleukins and gamma interferon, which are necessary for an effective specific response. Macrophage release of interleukin-1 stimulates the antigen-specific T lymphocyte to proliferate. Thus the macrophage/T-cell interaction is one of the major links

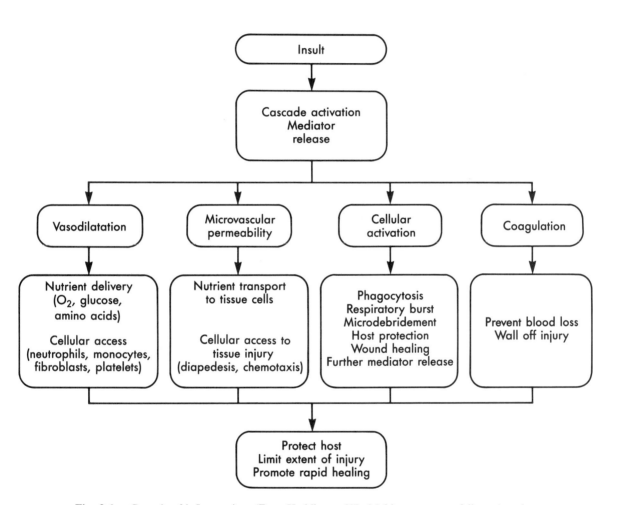

Fig. 2-1 Cascade of inflammation. (From Huddleston VB. Multisystem organ failure: A pathophysiologic approach, Boston, 1991;6.)

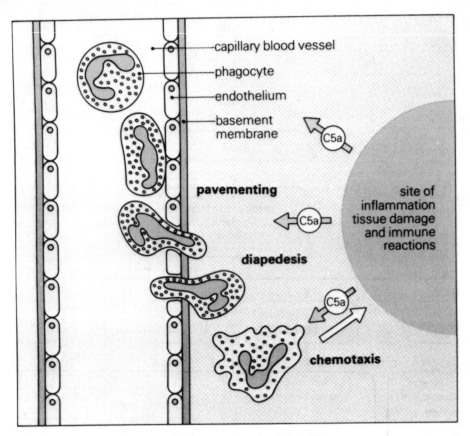

capillary blood vessel

phagocyte

endothelium

basement membrane

C5a

pavementing

C5a

site of inflammation tissue damage and immune reactions

diapedesis

C5a

chemotaxis

Fig. 2-2 Chemotaxis and migration of phagocytes from the blood to the tissue. (From Male D, Roitt I. Adaptive and innate immunity. In: Roitt I, Brostoff J, Male D, eds. Immunology, 2nd edition. London: Gower Medical Publishing, 1989;1.4.)

between the specific and nonspecific immune response.[13,29]

Specific response. In cell-mediated immunity (CMI), different T lymphocyte subsets orchestrate the IIR and regulate its function.* The subsets are distinguished by the presence of specific markers or receptors on their cell surfaces. Upon recognition of the presented antigen, T4 cells (helper T cells) proliferate and produce lymphokines (cyto-kines produced by lymphocytes) such as interleukin-2 that enhance B cell proliferation and antibody production, macrophage activation, and additional T-cell activity.[29,30] Without T-helper activity, the entire IIR becomes severely dysfunctional. The T8 cells participate in down regulation (suppressor T-cell activity) of the IIR and in cytotoxic (cytotoxic T cells) activities against intracellular infections, tumor cells, and foreign donor tissue.[31] The ratio of T4 cells to T8 cells reflects the balance between activation and suppression of the immune response and is approximately 2:1. Changes in both absolute counts as well as the T4 to T8 ratio occur in both healthy immune responses and dysfunction of the immune system.[32] The ratio is increased in infection, as the T4-helper cell population increases; it is decreased in AIDS secondary to T4 destruction

*White blood cells, particularly lymphocytes, express a large number of molecules on their cell surfaces. These surface molecules can be used to identify different cellular subsets. A nomenclature system known as the CD (cluster determinant) system has been developed to label cells based on the presence of these surface molecules. Thus T4 cells are referred to as CD4 T cells, and T8 cells are referred to as CD8 T cells. For simplicity, the terms T4 and T8 will be used in this text.

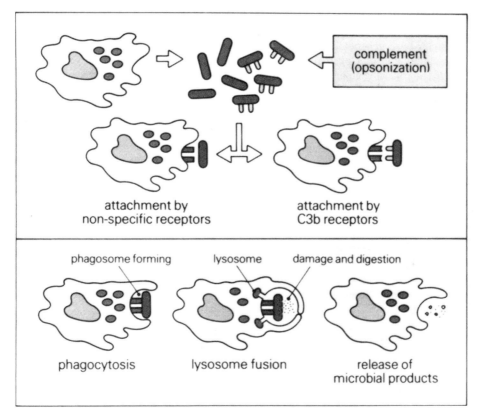

Fig. 2-3 Opsonization and phagocytosis of microorganisms. Opsonization may occur via binding with complement and/or antibody. (From Male D, Roitt I. Adaptive and innate immunity. In: Roitt I, Brostoff J, Male D, eds. Immunology, 2nd edition. London: Gower Medical Publishing, 1989;1.5.)

by the virus and possibly increased T8 proliferation.

In humoral immunity (HI), specific B cells recognize the antigen and differentiate into antibody-producing plasma cells. Antibodies bind with the antigen, yielding the antigen/antibody immune complex,[33-35] which is removed by phagocytic cells in the reticuloendothelial system. Recognition of antigen by B cells and B cell activation are highly complex and require precise cell-to-cell interaction with T-helper cells, although the exact mechanism of activation has not been defined.[28,29]

CMI and HI are distinguished from other levels of host defense by two important characteristics: memory and specificity. Following exposure to antigen, a small percentage of lymphocytes return to the secondary lymphoid tissue and reside there as

memory cells. The memory cells enable the host to mount a more rapid and vigorous response with repeated exposures.[13,35]

Primary lymphoid tissue. The lymphoid tissue is organized into either discretely capsulated organs (spleen or lymph nodes) or nonencapsulated accumulations of lymphoid tissue. Lymphoid organs are classified as either primary (central) or secondary (peripheral) organs. Lymphopoiesis (the differentiation and maturation of functional lymphocytes) occurs in the primary lymphoid organs of the thymus and bone marrow. During the fetal and neonatal periods, the lymphocytes develop, mature, and also acquire the ability to recognize specific antigens. In the thymus, the T lymphocytes learn to differentiate between self and nonself, a process known as thymic education. The recognition of self is based on the presence of specific molecules residing on the cell membrane surface of most body cells. These molecules (also known as surface antigens) are genetically coded by the major histocompatibility complex (MHC), which plays an important role in regulating interactions between cells of the immune response and in T-cell recognition of presented antigen.[36]

In humans, the MHC is the gene complex that determines the human leukocyte antigen (HLA) expression on body cells and is located on the short arm of the sixth chromosome. Although HLA typing is important in organ transplantation, the major role of the MHC is regulation of immune responsiveness and the distinction of self from nonself.

MHC gene products are divided into two classes: Class I and Class II. Class I antigens are found on the cell membrane of all nucleated cells and function as surface recognition molecules for T8-cytotoxic T cells. Class II antigens are not as widely distributed and are normally expressed on antigen presenting cells (see Table 3-1), lymphocytes, and endothelial cells. T4-helper cells only recognize presented antigen on the surface of APCs in the presence of specific Class II molecules; therefore MHC Class II surface antigens must be present on the cell surface of APCs such as macrophages for the T cell to recognize foreign antigen (Fig. 2-4).

This has clinical implications because much of the immunosuppression of trauma, stress, hemorrhage, surgery, and blood transfusions discussed in the following pages is related to macrophage/T-cell interaction. Decreased MHC Class II surface molecule expression may be partially responsible for poor interaction. Ertel et al have shown that the elevated intracellular calcium seen after ischemia induces a decrease in MHC Class II expression that can be attenuated with calcium channel blockers.[37] In summary, for effective lymphocyte activity, the lymphocytes must be able to differentiate self from nonself and must be able to interact with the presented antigen on the APC. The presence of MHC Class II molecules facilitates both of these activities.

Secondary lymphoid tissue. The secondary lymphoid tissue in the periphery provides the site where lymphocytes interact with each other, APCs, and the antigen. The white pulp of the spleen contains large numbers of lymphocytes, macrophages, and other APCs. As blood flows through the spleen, microorganisms are trapped by the splenic macrophages, processed, and presented to the surrounding lymphocytes. The lymphocytes are activated and begin proliferating. The active T cells produce lymphokines that stimulate other immune cells (Table 2-3). B cells differentiate into plasma cells that produce antibodies.

Similar activity occurs in the lymph nodes, which are common at branches of lymphatic vessels. Many APCs with large amounts of MHC antigen on their surfaces are present within the nodes. As lymph passes through the nodes, the APCs phagocytize, process, and present any antigen in the lymph fluid to the resident lymphocytes, and activation occurs. When presented antigen stimulates lymphocyte proliferation, the secondary lymphoid tissue (particularly lymph nodes) enlarges.

The nonencapsulated tissue of the lymphoid system (MALT: mucosa-associated lymphoid tissue) is commonly associated with mucosal surfaces of the gut, respiratory tract, and genital tract, which are common access sites for microorganisms to enter the body. Tonsils in the upper respiratory tract and the Peyer's patches in the gut are examples of MALT.

The lymphocytes not only migrate from primary to secondary lymphoid tissue during maturation, but constantly recirculate between the blood, lymph, and other secondary organs. Approximately 95% of total body lymphocytes are in the nodes and spleen at any given time, with only 5% actually circulating in the blood. Lymphocyte traffic shuts down following entry of an antigen into a node with lymphocytes sensitive to that antigen; therefore antigen-specific lymphocytes are retained in the nodes that drain the area of antigen invasion or accumulation.[36]

Specificity. Each T or B cell reacts only with the specific antigen that it recognizes. Genetically, the body has the potential to produce more than 10^6 different antibodies, each with its own specificity.[38] This concept of specificity coupled with the ability of investigators to produce monoclonal antibodies has become important in generating new immunomodulation techniques and treatment regimens for the MSOF patient.[39-43] See Chapter 16 for a discussion on immunotherapy.

Summary

The body's response to injury (accidental, ischemic, surgical, or microbial) involves inflammation, immunologic activity, and repair. Depending

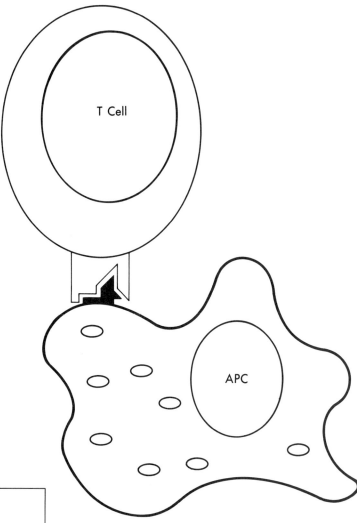

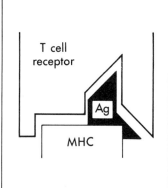

Fig. 2-4 Hypothetical macrophage/T-cell interaction requiring the presence of MHC surface antigen on the antigen presenting cell. Abbreviations: *APC*, Antigen presenting cell; *MHC*, major histocompatibility complex; *Ag*, presented antigen.

on the agent (bacterial, viral, fungal, or parasitic), one mode of response (phagocytic, CMI, or HI) may play a stronger role than the other two. CMI, specifically T8 cytotoxic cells, plays a major role in viral and parasitic infections, while HI and phagocytosis are the chief mechanisms used to combat bacterial infection.[28,44] In an uncomplicated scenario, the response is rapid, localized, and results in healing. Unfortunately in the critical care environment, a myriad of complications are common. Immunosuppression, dysregulation, and uncontrolled inflammatory activity often occur, resulting in tissue damage, organ dysfunction, and ultimately MSOF.[10,11,45-47] Chapter 3 and Appendix A provide further information on the cells and mediators of the IIR.

IMMUNE RESPONSE ABNORMALITIES AND CLINICAL IMPLICATIONS

The term *immunosuppression* is commonly used in the ICU. The patients can be immunosuppressed because they are stressed, malnourished, or suffering from a traumatic insult. But what exactly does the term mean? What impact does it have on the patient? On care and assessment? Is Mr. Smith's immunosuppression the same as Mr. Jones's? Probably not, at least not exactly. The intricacy of the IIR is overwhelming in its complexity, components, and interrelationships. Alterations can occur anywhere among the numerous pathways, cells, and mediators. Global interventions to prevent infection or stimulation of inflammation such as hand washing, aseptic technique, and nutrition are certainly helpful; however, they may not be enough to protect the critically ill patient exposed to alterations in the IIR, resistant environmental pathogens, and breakdown of natural defense barriers. As knowledge of immune mechanisms increases, future therapies may be more precisely targeted to specific malfunctions in the IIR.[11,48,49] Numerous risk factors have been implicated in the development and progression of immune dysfunction, including stress, trauma, hemorrhage, blood transfusions, surgery, anesthesia, and malnutrition (Table 2-1).

Stress

According to Webster, stress is a "physical, chemical, or emotional factor to which an individual fails to make a satisfactory adaptation, and which causes physiologic tensions that may be a

Table 2-6 Clinical Conditions with Associated Immune Alterations/Dysfunction

Condition	Alteration in immune activity
Stress[53,56,59]	↑ neutrophil counts
	↓ lymphocyte, monocyte, and basophil counts
	↓ chemotaxis
	↓ phagocytosis
	↓ mediator release
	↓ IL-1, IL-2
	↓ antibody production
	↓ IL-2 receptors on T cells
	↓ natural killer activity
Trauma[66-69]	↓ macrophage/T-cell interaction
	↓ antigen processing and presentation
	↓ T-helper cell proliferation and activity
	↑ PGE$_2$ (inhibitory) production by macrophages
	↓ antibody production
	↑ T-cell suppressor activity
	↓ neutrophil phagocytic activity
	↓ IL-1, IL-2
Hemorrhage[37,71,74]	↓ macrophage/T-cell interaction
	↓ antigen processing and presentation
	↓ T-cell proliferation and lymphokine production
	↓ natural killer cell activity
	↓ MHC Class II expression
Blood transfusions[72,81,82]	↓ antigen processing and presentation
	↓ T-cell proliferation
	↓ T4:T8 ratio
	↓ natural killer cell activity
Surgery/ anesthesia[69,85,86]	↓ macrophage/T-cell interaction
	↓ antigen processing and presentation
	↓ T-helper cell proliferation and activity
	↑ PGE$_2$ production by macrophages
	↑ T-cell suppressor activity
	↓ lymphocyte traffic out of lymph nodes
	↓ phagocytosis
Malnutrition[89,90]	↓ cell-mediated immunity
	↓ lymphocyte count
	↓ T4:T8 ratio
	↓ natural killer activity
	↓ humoral immunity

Abbreviations: *IL*, Interleukin; *MHC*, major histocompatibility complex; *PG*, prostaglandin.

contributory cause of disease."[50] Observations that stressful conditions contribute to immunosuppression have been in the literature for decades.[51-53] As our understanding of the IIR increases, our understanding of neuroendocrine system interaction with the IIR increases. Stressful conditions have been shown to affect many aspects of the IIR, including phagocytosis, lymphocyte cytotoxicity, and antibody production[53-55] (Table 2-6).

Corticosteroids have long been associated with the immunosuppressant effects of stress.[56,57] Circulating corticosteroids, both endogenous (cortisol) and exogenous (prednisone or methylprednisolone), have both antiinflammatory and antilymphocyte effects. Corticosteroids decrease lymphocyte, monocyte, and basophil counts in the blood.[56] Some of this effect may be due to the redistribution of lymphocytes from the circulating pool to the peripheral lymphoid tissue.[57,58]

Monocyte/macrophage activity is also hindered by corticosteroids; therefore chemotaxis, phagocytosis, and mediator release necessary for the inflammatory process may be inhibited. Although neutrophil counts increase, the cells have a decreased ability to adhere to the vessel wall and move through it to an injury site. Other effects seen with large doses of corticosteroids include de-creased production of IL-1, IL-2, IgG, decreased T-helper cell proliferation, and decreased arachidonic acid metabolism.[59]

Although the antiinflammatory effects of corticosteroids would seem to be helpful in sepsis and MSOF when overwhelming inflammation and "loss of control" are rampant, the potent immunosuppressant effects may be devastating to an immunocompromised patient exposed to numerous pathogenic organisms (Fig. 2-5). Recent research has shown that high-dose corticosteroid therapy does not have a place in the present treatment of sepsis and MSOF.[60-63]

Although circulating corticosteroids may have profound effects on immune activity, studies have shown that even when the release of circulating steroids is inhibited, immunosuppression still occurs in the stress state. Along with glucocorticoid receptors, many immune cells (especially lymphocytes) have receptors on their surfaces for catecholamines, acetylcholine, insulin, and other hormonal substances[53] that are released during the stress state and have the potential to affect specific aspects of the IIR. Also, the lymphoid organs are innervated by the autonomic nervous system,[53,54] and their function may also be affected by autonomic nervous system activity.

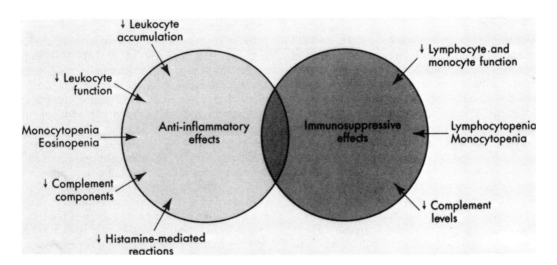

Fig. 2-5 The antiinflammatory and immunosuppressive effects of corticosteroids. (From Hooks MA. Immunosuppressive agents used in transplantation. In: Smith SL, ed. Tissue and organ transplantation: Implications for professional nursing practice. St. Louis: Mosby–Year Book, 1990;57.)

Several mechanisms have been proposed for the steroid-independent immunosuppression seen in stress. IL-2, which is necessary for T-cell proliferation, is decreased after stress. Investigators[55] have shown that T cells also have fewer IL-2 receptors to receive the IL-2 that is present. Without T-helper proliferation, other aspects of the IIR that depend on T-helper assistance are not effective, such as phagocytosis, antibody production, and natural killer cell (NK) activity. Weiss et al[55] hypothesize that a circulating protein factor is present during the stress state that suppresses the immune response.

Not only does the neuroendocrine system affect the immune response, but the immune response affects the neuroendocrine system. Some cytokines released during the IIR act as neurotransmitters. IL-1's ability to induce fever is one example. Also, IL-1 may activate the hypothalamus-pituitary-adrenal axis, leading to production of steroids during infection. This may be a protective mechanism to limit destructive immune mechanisms, such as overwhelming inflammation.[64]

Stress disturbs the homeostasis of the body's major regulatory systems: nervous, endocrine, and immune. The intricate balance between the various hormones required for the body to maintain equilibrium is lost during the stress state, and multiple derangements are observed at the bedside.[53]

Trauma

Research on the "immunosuppression of trauma" is expanding as advances in immune technique and trauma care increase the ability to study the phenomenon. Although more patients are surviving the initial injury, secondary complications remain a major source of morbidity and mortality in critical care units. Changes in humoral mediators, as well as cellular number and activity, have been noted.[65,66] Mediators most often implicated in posttraumatic immunosuppression are the prostaglandins and cytokines produced by activated immune cells.[67,68] Common cellular dysfunction includes altered macrophage function, decreased T-cell proliferation and activity, increased suppressor T-cell activity, and decreased neutrophil activity and killing.[67,68] Antibody synthesis is also decreased.

The clinical outcome of trauma-related immunosuppression is an increase in both opportunistic and pathogenic infection in the trauma population.

Progression into fulminant septic shock and MSOF may ensue. Therefore the critical care team should prevent infection, identify and treat it early when it does occur, and enhance the body's ability to respond to invasion. This enhancement requires knowledge of the immune alterations occurring after trauma and is an area of much interest and research at present.

The major problem occurring after trauma appears to be a depression of macrophage/T-cell interaction caused by increased production of the inhibitory prostaglandin PGE$_2$, decreased production of IL-1 by macrophages, and decreased production of IL-2 by T cells. Both IL-1 and IL-2 facilitate T-helper activity. Without proper macrophage/T-cell interaction, the body loses the effects of antigen processing, presentation, and T-helper stimulation; therefore further activation of macrophages and stimulation of antibody production are lost. Suppressor T-cell activity is also increased.[68,69] All these factors decrease the host's ability to fight invasion and multiplication of pathogenic organisms, thus setting the stage for infection, sepsis, and MSOF.

Hemorrhage. Not only does the trauma victim experience direct injury, but the patient is also exposed to stress, hemorrhage, surgery, anesthesia, and blood transfusions, all of which have immunosuppressant effects.[53,70-72] Hemorrhage causes major disturbances in organ systems and the immune response, even simple hemorrhage without massive tissue trauma.[71] Hepatocellular dysfunction has been shown to occur early after hemorrhage and persist despite aggressive fluid resuscitation.[73] Alterations in the immune response include decreased T-cell proliferation, lymphokine production, and NK activity.[37] In addition, macrophage activity, including antigen processing and presentation and MHC Class II expression (which is necessary for T-cell interaction and stimulation), is also depressed.[74] Because the liver plays a key role in overall immune activity and because macrophage/T-cell interaction is so crucial in activating the antigen-specific component of the IIR, increased susceptibility to infection is a major concern for trauma patients and others experiencing a hemorrhagic event.

Although the changes that occur in trauma and hemorrhage are well-documented, the mechanisms responsible for these changes have yet to be elucidated. Because calcium channel blockers have improved antigen presentation and IL-1 production by macrophages, some investigators believe that a toxic influx of calcium from the extracellular space into the macrophage may be partially responsible for the macrophage dysfunction[37] and concomitant T-cell depression seen in hemorrhage and ischemia.[75] One interesting note: it is thought that this calcium influx occurs during resuscitation at the time of reperfusion, not during the ischemic period.[76] This may be of clinical benefit because damage occurs not in the field but at the time of resuscitation; therefore preventive measures may be taken during the resuscitation. Investigators postulate that lipid peroxidation—caused by oxygen-derived free radicals formed through the xanthine oxidase pathway during reperfusion—alters membrane permeability and integrity and allows large amounts of calcium to enter the cell.[37] In addition to the direct immunosuppression of trauma, the patient is also at increased risk for septic complications because hemorrhagic shock induces bacterial translocation from the gut. Ischemia and loss of gut barrier function contribute to increased permeability of the gut wall and increased movement of bacteria into the lymph and portal circulation[77] (see Chapter 9).

Blood transfusions. Adding further insult to the compromised patient, blood transfusions are often used in trauma patients and others to combat hemorrhage. Numerous studies have implicated blood transfusions in immunosuppression. This was initially observed when donor graft survival was lengthened in transplant patients who had received transfusions before the transplantation. The question was raised that if blood transfusions suppressed immune rejection of the graft, maybe they were also suppressing the IIR to invasion by other foreign antigens, thus increasing the risk of infection or even malignancies.[78,79]

Changes seen after blood transfusion include decreased T4:T8 ratios, decreased NK activity, decreased macrophage processing and presentation, and decreased T-cell proliferation.[80,81] Decreased IL-2 ("good" cytokine) production and increased PGE$_2$ ("bad" prostaglandin) production that occur following blood transfusion may partially mediate this dysfunction. IL-2 is necessary for effective T-helper activity, and PGE$_2$ depresses macrophage/T-cell interaction. The question remains whether blood transfusion alone causes immunosuppression or whether the other factors involved in a traumatic or septic insult work together to produce immunosuppression. The IIR alterations seen in graft survival, which are specific responses, may be different than the alterations seen after trauma or sepsis, which are associated with nonspecific responses.[72,82]

Surgery/anesthesia

Patients undergoing surgical procedures have long been known to have impaired immunologic reactivity.[83,84] Because the surgical procedure is accompanied by anesthesia, trauma to the body, possible blood transfusion, and an overall stress response, it is difficult to isolate which events cause which alterations in the IIR. Most likely, the interactions of these events operate synergistically to mediate overall host immunosuppression and thus increased susceptibility to infection.[70,85,86]

Alterations noted in the surgical patient include ineffective T4-helper cell proliferation, increased supressor activity of T8 cells, and dysfunctional activity in monocytes and macrophages.[87] Anesthesia alone is associated with decreased immunoresponsiveness,[83,84] with both decreased phagocytosis and lymphocyte proliferation noted in the anesthetized patient. Recent studies demonstrate a decrease in lymphocyte traffic out of lymph nodes, accompanied by a decrease in antibody production in the surgical patient.[85] In addition, PGE$_2$ is increased in anesthesia and trauma, both surgical and accidental.[68,85] As mentioned above, appropriate macrophage/T-cell interaction is crucial for all aspects of the immune response to function effectively: macrophage phagocytic ability, T-cell helper functions, and B-cell differentiation and antibody formation. Without this interaction, the host is unable to mount an effective IIR, and the likelihood of sepsis increases.[67,68,86]

Malnutrition and substance abuse

Malnutrition, both starvation and protein deficient, causes or exacerbates a variety of systemic functions: most profoundly the immune system and wound healing. These two are closely related because effective immune system function is necessary for wound microdebridement and protection. Malnutrition also deprives the patient of protein, glucose, oxygen, and other nutrients needed for stable tissue formation and wound repair. T-cell proliferation and helper ability are impaired in the malnourished patient but can often be restored following protein/calorie supplementation.[88]

Malnutrition is often associated with and may be secondary to chronic drug and alcohol abuse. Excessive substance abuse leads to decreased food intake and alters nutrient digestion, absorption, storage, and utilization. All aspects of metabolism are affected.[89] Alcohol may also increase the breakdown and turnover of many vitamins and minerals, further increasing demand on an already decreased supply.[90]

Summary

There are six strikes against the trauma patient—trauma, stress, hemorrhage, blood transfusions, surgery, and anesthesia—even before arriving in the unit, where he will then be bombarded with antibiotics, invasive procedures, and, commonly, iatrogenic malnutrition (Table 2-1). Surgical patients and other critically ill individuals also have several of these strikes against them. The risk therefore is great for septic complications and MSOF in the critically ill patient (Table 2-6). This is confirmed in the literature, which continues to report major morbidity and mortality in the trauma patient secondary to septic and inflammatory complications and MSOF.[7-9,11,16,19] Destruction of surface barriers, overload of tissue debris, and activation of coagulation all contribute to the already complicated clinical scenario.

ASSESSMENT AND LABORATORY FINDINGS

With the advent of new laboratory equipment and more sophisticated techniques, the clinician is no longer solely dependent on the simple WBC count with differential to assess the immune response. Not only can total cell counts be performed, but mediator levels and activity, effectiveness of both humoral and cell-mediated immunity, and counts of specific cellular subsets can be determined.[91] Although some of these "high-powered" techniques are only available to investigators for study purposes, many are beginning to make their way to the bedside for clinical use and diagnosis.

As always, for intelligent interpretation of laboratory data and assessment of therapeutic effectiveness, knowledge of a test's significance and implications is vital to the clinician's ability to provide thorough, rationale-based care. Although sophisticated laboratory techniques are very helpful, status of the patient's immune system and defense capabilities is also apparent from data obtained during a routine physical assessment.

Natural defenses

Assessing the status of natural defenses or external barriers to invasion is the initial step in assessment of host defense.[92] Is the skin intact? Is it fragile? Is it edematous? Are there numerous invasive lines and devices in place that would allow for the invasion of microorganisms? Table 2-7 details organ-specific assessment parameters and their effect on immune function.[25,92]

Cells and tissues of the immune system

The complete blood count (CBC) and CBC with differential are two of the most commonly drawn laboratory studies in the ICU. Not only do they provide information concerning absolute cell counts, such as neutrophil, monocyte, and lymphocyte, but the percentage of count relative to the total is also reported, providing the clinician with information necessary to assess the status and activity of the IIR (Table 2-8). The ability of other organs such as the bone marrow and lymphoid organs to meet the peripheral demand is also reflected in the cell counts.

Neutrophils. In bacterial infection, the neutrophil differential is increased and in viral infections, the lymphocyte differential is increased. It must be remembered that cell counts measure only those cells actually circulating in the blood. Neutrophils marginated along vessel walls and lymphocytes sequestered in the lymph nodes and the lymphatic circulation are not reflected in the count. Actually, 90% to 95% of the body's lymphocytes reside in the secondary lymphoid tissue of the spleen, lymph nodes, and mucosa-associated lymphoid tissue.[93] In addition to inflammation or infection, other factors can also increase WBC counts. By increasing cardiac output and blood flow, exercise and catecholamine release can increase neutrophil count (neutrophilia, leukocytosis) because marginated cells are flushed off the vessel wall and into the circulation.

If inflammation and infection continue, more immature neutrophils (known as bands) are released by the bone marrow as it attempts to meet the

Table 2-7 Systems Assessment with Potential IIR Impact and Complications[24,92]

System	Risk factors	Impact on IIR	Potential complications	Assessment
Central nervous system	Invasive drains, ICP monitoring, Incision line, Cranial nerve impairment, Spinal cord injury	Increased microbial access, IIR activation, Impaired natural defenses (gag, cough, blink)	Inflammation/infection, Aspiration, Corneal abrasions, Immobility → skin breakdown	↓ LOC, ↓ CPP, inflammation at wound site, respiratory depression, ↑ ↓ temperature, ↑ ↓ BP, ↑ ↓ heart rate, ↓ Glasgow Coma Score, ↑ ↓ respiratory rate, ↑ ↓ tidal volume, skin breakdown
Pulmonary	Artificial airway, Mechanical ventilation, Barotrauma, High FiO_2 levels	Bypass of natural defenses (humidity, mucociliary escalator), Increased microbial access (ETT, oral secretions), Activation of alveolar macrophages with toxic mediator release, Altered surfactant production	Aspiration, Atelectasis, Pneumonia, ARDS, Oxygen toxicity and alveolocapillary damage	↑ respiratory rate, ↓ depth, ↑ SOB, dyspnea, diaphoresis, use of accessory muscles, ↓ SEC, ↑ PIP, thick and greenish-yellow sputum, ↑ V/Q mismatching, intrapulmonary shunt > 20%, wheezes, crackles, infiltrates on CXR, ventilatory dependence, ↓ pH, ↓ SaO_2, ↓ SvO_2, ↓ PaO_2, ↑ $PaCO_2$, ↑ lactate
Cardiovascular	Invasive monitoring, Poor perfusion	Increased microbial access, Tissue ischemia → IIR activation with third spacing and edema, Cellular activation and mediator release	Reperfusion injury, Cellulitis, Bacteremia/septicemia, Endothelial damage and clotting abnormalities	↑ CO, ↓ ↑ SVR, ↑ ↓ heart rate, ↓ BP, ↓ ejection fraction, ↑ PAP, ↑ PCWP, ↓ ↑ CVP, cold and pale skin, inflammation at access sites, weak pulses, narrow pulse pressure, ectopy, MI, ↑ isoenzymes, ↑ lactate
Gastrointestinal	Nasogastric tube, Antacid therapy, H_2-blocker therapy, Stress ulceration, Antibiotics, Ileus	↑ pH → ↑ bacterial colonization, IIR activation, Inhibition of normal flora's protective functions, Inability to clear bacterial load	Colonization of esophagus and tracheobronchial tree, Pneumonia, Overgrowth of pathogenic organisms in the GI tract, Translocation of bacteria to the lymph and blood	↓ bowel sounds, upper/lower GI bleeding, abdominal distention, diarrhea, impaction, ileus, stress ulceration/erosion, mucosal atrophy, guaiac + stool, enteric organisms on blood culture, jaundice, ascites, ↓ drug clearance, bleeding, ↑ liver function tests, ↓ plasma proteins, ↑ ammonia, ↓ clotting factors, hepatomegaly, splenomegaly
Genitourinary	Bladder catheter, Antibiotics, Hyperglycemia	Increased microbial access, Altered normal flora in vagina, Promotion of yeast growth	Urinary tract infection, Septicemia, *Candida* infections	↑ urine output, malodorous discharge, ↑ weight, ↑ PCWP, ↑ CVP, ↑ weight, peripheral edema, ↑ BUN, ↑ creatinine, ↑ potassium, ↑ magnesium, ↓ pH, ↓ bicarbonate

Abbreviations: *ICP*, intracranial pressure; *IIR*, inflammatory/immune response; *FiO₂*, fraction of inspired oxygen; *ETT*, endotracheal tube; *ARDS*, adult respiratory distress syndrome; *H₂*, histamine type 2 receptor; *LOC*, level of consciousness; *CPP*, cerebral perfusion pressure; *BP*, blood pressure; *SOB*, shortness of breath; *PIP*, peak inspiratory pressure; *SEC*, static effective compliance; *V/Q*, ventilation/perfusion ratio; *CO*, cardiac output; *SVR*, systemic vascular resistance; *PAP*, pulmonary artery pressure; *PCWP*, pulmonary capillary wedge pressure; *MI*, myocardial infarction; *CVP*, central venous pressure; *BUN*, blood urea nitrogen; *SaO₂*, arterial oxygen saturation; *SvO₂*, venous oxygen saturation; *PaO₂*, partial pressure of oxygen in arterial blood; *PaCO₂*, partial pressure of carbon dioxide in arterial blood.

Table 2-8 Normal White Blood Cell Values

Cell type	Absolute number (mm³)	Differential (%)	Function/change
Granulocytes			
Neutrophils	3000-7000	60-70	↑ with inflammation or infection ↓ with bone marrow suppression or exhaustion
Segmented	2800-5600	56	↑ value-right shift
Bands (immature)	150-600	3-6	↑ value-left shift
Eosinophils	50-500	1-4	↑ in allergy and parasitic infections
Basophils	25-100	0.5-1	Involved in Type I hypersensitivity reactions (anaphylactoid) ? role in infection
Mononuclear cells			
Monocytes	100-800	2-8	↑ with chronic infection, TB, malaria, some viruses
Lymphocytes (total)	1000-4000	20-45	↑ in viral infections ↓ in HIV disease
T cells	800-3200	80% of TLC	
B cells	100-600	10%-15% of TLC	
NK cells	50-400	5%-10% of TLC	

Abbreviations: *WBC*, white blood count; *TB*, tuberculosis; *NK*, natural killer; *HIV*, human immunodeficiency virus; *TLC*, total lymphocyte count. Modified from Tribett D. Immune system function: Implications for critical care nursing practice. Crit Care Nurs Clin North Am 1989;1:727.

increased demand in the periphery. The appearance of circulating bands and other immature cells is referred to as a "shift to the left" because the immature cells are traditionally drawn on the left side of the page in maturation diagrams (Fig. 2-6). The bone marrow eventually becomes exhausted and can no longer match the demands in the periphery. Low neutrophil counts (neutropenia) are not uncommon at the end stage of sepsis and MSOF, and infection can still be present even when the WBC count decreases. Chemotherapy, radiation therapy, and hematologic malignancies also contribute to neutropenia. Because neutrophils are necessary for the development of pus, a severely neutropenic patient can have an infection without the presence of purulent drainage. The loss of neutrophils also contributes to the body's inability to remove bacteria and other foreign debris.[13]

Lymphocytes. In assessing humoral immunity, both B cell counts and specific antibody assays can be performed. In cell-mediated immunity, absolute T cell counts as well as subset ratios are examined. A low T4:T8 ratio reflects a decrease in T4-helper cells or an increase in the T8 cytotoxic/suppressor cells; therefore the ratios must be interpreted concurrently with absolute counts and the patient's clinical picture.[32] The low ratio signifies an imbalance of immune regulation toward down-regulation of the specific immune response. The T4:T8 ratio has been shown to be generally decreased in sepsis[94] and AIDS.[95] Conversely, a high ratio signifies an increase in T4-helper activity or a decrease in T8 suppressor activity. Increased T4 activity is greatly increased as a normal response to bacterial invasion, and the ratio may increase to 20:1 in *Staphylococcus* and *Klebsiella* infections.[32] A decrease in T8 cell counts is often present in autoimmune diseases. One interesting subset of

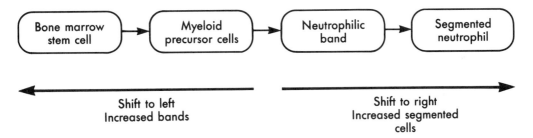

Fig. 2-6 Maturational diagram of the neutrophil.

septic nonsurvivors in the study by Dahn et al[94] demonstrated a high ratio secondary to decreased T8 cells. Without the regulatory controlling effect of suppressor T8-cell activity, the IIR is not limited, and an exaggerated and magnified immune and metabolic response might overwhelm the host.[94] These data provide further support to the hypothesis that MSOF may be a result of overwhelming inflammation and activation of the IIR. The use of the T4:T8 ratio will become more clinically significant as the activity of the various subsets is more precisely defined.

Lymphoid tissue. Because the liver, spleen, and lymph nodes play a major role in host defense, knowledge of previous alterations in these organs aids in assessment of immune function. If the patient has a history of cirrhosis or other hepatic disease, the Kupffer cells (liver macrophages) may not adequately clear foreign matter in the circulation or bacteria translocating from the gut.[5,96] Congestive heart failure accompanied by hepatic congestion may also decrease the liver's phagocytic capabilities.

A previous splenectomy may predispose the patient to infectious complications, especially in children and young adults. Recent research has shown an increased incidence of sepsis and thromboembolic complications 10 to 15 years after a splenectomy.[97-99] The spleen is a major lymphoid organ with a large population of T and B cells. Following the spleen's removal, the other lymphoid organs usually "make up the difference," but this compensatory activity may be stressed in times of overwhelming infection.[97-99]

Enlarged lymph nodes signify the proliferation of T and B cells in the nodal tissue secondary to antigen exposure. Although their enlargement signifies the presence of infection, it also demonstrates the lymphocytes' ability to respond and prolifer-

ate.[36] Resection of nodal tissue in the past should be noted on the patient's history.

Circulating mediators of the inflammatory/immune response

Because many of the mediators in sepsis and MSOF are unstable, have short half-lives, or occur in minute concentrations, the level of specific mediators may be difficult to measure directly. The presence of a mediator may have to be extrapolated from the existence of its metabolites, levels of precursor molecules, or presence of activity that is attributable to the mediator in question.[91,100] Two common techniques used to measure mediator or mediator metabolite concentrations are the radioimmunoassay (RIA) and enzyme-linked immunosorbent assay (ELISA). The ELISA technique may be preferable because it does not involve the handling and disposal restrictions associated with the use of radioactive materials[101]; however, the RIA is generally more sensitive for mediators present at low concentrations.

Several mediators that can currently be measured include activated complement proteins (split products), endotoxin, arachidonic acid metabolites, prothrombin, and certain cytokines. Such cytokines as TNF, IL-1, and IL-2 have been measured with these techniques in concentrations as low as 10 pg/mL.[102,103] More attention is now being given to making these tests more clinically feasible and timely.[102] Activated macrophages release neopterin, and increased levels have been shown to correlate with the development of sepsis and MSOF.[104-107]

Immunologic responsiveness

Cell counts and mediator concentrations give the bedside clinician clues concerning the availability of IIR components, but the assessment can be taken one step further by measuring the cells' actual responsiveness to specific mediators. The mediator levels are insignificant if the cell has no receptor and thus no responsiveness to the mediator's presence. Changes in receptor number and type have been noted in the septic state.[108] The ability of T and B cells to proliferate in response to antigenic exposure can be measured in the laboratory, along with circulating antibody levels. The neutrophils' participation in chemotaxis, phagocytosis, and bactericidal activity can also be determined.

The intradermal injection of antigens to which most people have been previously exposed (streptococcus, diphtheria, tetanus, and *Candida*) is used to evaluate overall immune responsiveness. Skin testing involves a delayed type hypersensitivity (DTH) reaction in which sensitized lymphocytes are drawn to the local area of injection.[109] On arrival, the T cells release lymphokines that attract macrophages to the area, setting up a local inflammatory reaction (erythema, induration, or warmth). If lymphocytes and macrophages are nonresponsive to the antigen, no inflammation is seen and the patient is considered anergic. Anergy is associated with increased incidence of sepsis and greater mortality.[110,111]

CONCLUSION

With knowledge of mediator concentrations and immune responsiveness, patient management can focus on restoring and controlling the immune response. Known as immunotherapeutics or immunomodulation, these therapies are aimed at enhancing IIR, restoring control, and removing excessive levels of potentially harmful mediators. Levels can (1) provide information concerning the nature and extent of the process, (2) predict patients at risk for further complications, especially if underlying problems are not responsive to present therapy, and (3) monitor effectiveness of therapeutic regimens. Several studies have noted that even in the presence of various initiating events, the basic feature common to all patients with MSOF is inflammation.[8,9,11,112-114] By monitoring the mediators of this inflammation and modifying their presence and activity, the health care team may have the potential to upset the fatal course many of these patients travel. Chapter 3 discusses specific cells and mediators, their physiologic role, and their impact on the overall MSOF process.

REFERENCES

1. Roitt I, Brostoff J, Male D. Immunology. 2nd ed. London: Gower Medical Publishing; 1989.
2. Sell S. Immunology, immunopathology and immunity. 4th ed. New York: Elsevier; 1987.
3. Byram DA. Future expectations for critical care nurses: Competence in immunotherapy. Crit Care Nurs Clin North Am 1989;1:797-806.
4. Brogley JL, Sharp EJ. Nursing care of patients receiving activated lymphocytes. Oncol Nurs Forum 1990;17:187-193.
5. Baue AE. Multiple organ failure: Patient Care and Prevention. St. Louis: Mosby–Year Book; 1990.
6. Dorinsky PM, Gadek JE. Mechanisms of multiple nonpulmonary organ failure in ARDS. Chest 1989;96:885-892.
7. Goris RJ. Multiple organ failure: Whole body inflammation? Schweiz Med Wochenschr 1989;119:347-353.
8. Goris RJ et al. Multiple organ failure: Generalized autodestructive inflammation. Arch Surg 1985;120:1109-1115.
9. Goris RJ et al. Multiple organ failure and sepsis without bacteria. Arch Surg 1986;121:897-901.
10. Pinsky MR. Multiple systems organ failure: Malignant intravascular inflammation. Crit Care Clin 1989;5:195-198.
11. Pinsky MR, Matuschak GM. Multiple systems organ failure: Failure of host defense homeostasis. Crit Care Clin 1989;5:199-220.
12. Huddleston VB. Multisystem organ failure. In: Mims BC, ed. Case studies in critical care nursing. Baltimore: Williams & Wilkins; 1990:494-499.
13. Male D, Roitt I. Adaptive and innate immunity. In: Roitt I, Brostoff J, Male D, eds. Immunology. 2nd ed. London: Gower Medical Publishing; 1989:1.1-1.10.
14. Walport M. Complement. In: Roitt I, Brostoff J, Male D, eds. Immunology. 2nd ed. London: Gower Medical Publishing; 1989:13.1-13.16.
15. Hyers TM, Gee M, Andreadis NA. Cellular interactions in the multiple organ injury syndrome. Am Rev Respir Dis 1987;135:952-953.
16. DeCamp MM, Demling RH. Posttraumatic multisystem organ failure. JAMA 1988;260:530-534.
17. Cunnion RE, Parrillo JE. Myocardial dysfunction in sepsis. Crit Care Clin 1989;5:99-118.
18. Bersten A, Sibbald WJ. Circulatory disturbances in multiple systems organ failure. Crit Care Clin 1989;5:233-254.
19. Fry DE. Multiple system organ failure. Surg Clin North Am 1988;68:107-122.
20. Dantzker D. Oxygen delivery and utilization in sepsis. Crit Care Clin 1989;5:81-98.
21. Hotter AN. The pathophysiology of multi-system organ failure in the trauma patient. Clin Issues Crit Care Nurs 1990;1:465-478.
22. Gutierrez G, Lund N, Bryan-Brown CW. Cellular oxygen utilization during multiple organ failure. Crit Care Clin 1989;5:271-288.
23. Barton R, Cerra FB. The hypermetabolism multiple organ failure syndrome. Chest 1989;96:1153-1160.
24. Huddleston VB. Multisystem organ failure: A pathophysiologic approach. Boston, 1991.
25. Tribett D. Immune system function: Implications for critical care nursing practice. Crit Care Nurs Clin North Am 1989;1:725-740.
26. Brostoff J, Hale T. Hypersensitivity-Type I. In: Roitt I,

Brostoff J, Male D, eds. Immunology. 2nd ed. London: Gower Medical Publishing; 1989:19.1-19.20.

27. Hood LE et al. Immune effector mechanisms and the complement system. In: Hood LE et al, eds. Immunology. 2nd ed. Menlo Park, CA: Benjamin/Cummings Publishing Co; 1984:334-365.

28. Rook G. Immunity to viruses, bacteria and fungi. In: Roitt I, Brostoff J, Male D, eds. Immunology. 2nd ed. London: Gower Medical Publishing; 1989:16.1-16.16.

29. Feldmann M, Male D. Cell cooperation in the immune response. In: Roitt I, Brostoff J, Male D, eds. Immunology. 2nd ed. London: Gower Medical Publishing; 1989:8.1-8.12.

30. Rook G. Cell-mediated immune responses. In: Roitt I, Brostoff J, Male D, eds. Immunology. 2nd ed. London: Gower Medical Publishing; 1989:9.1-9.14.

31. Lydyard P, Grossi C. Cells involved in the immune response. In: Roitt I, Brostoff J, Male D, eds. Immunology. 2nd ed. London: Gower Medical Publishing; 1989:2.1-2.18.

32. Giorgi JV. Lymphocyte subset measurements: Significance in clinical medicine. In: Rose NR, Friedman H, Fahey JL, eds. Manual of clinical laboratory immunology, 3rd ed. Washington, D.C.: American Society for Microbiology; 1986:236-246.

33. Turner M. Molecules which recognize antigen. In: Roitt I, Brostoff J, Male D, eds. Immunology. 2nd ed. London: Gower Medical Publishing; 1989:5.1-5.12.

34. Steward M. Antigen recognition. In: Roitt I, Brostoff J, Male D, eds. Immunology. 2nd ed. London: Gower Medical Publishing; 1989:7.1-7.10.

35. Barrett JT. Textbook of immunology: An introduction to immunochemistry and immunobiology. 5th ed. St. Louis: Mosby–Year Book; 1988.

36. Lydyard P, Grossi C. The lymphoid system. In: Roitt I, Brostoff J, Male D, eds. Immunology. 2nd ed. London: Gower Medical Publishing; 1989:3.1-3.10.

37. Ertel W et al. Immunoprotective effect of a calcium channel blocker on macrophage antigen presentation function, major histocompatibility class II antigen expression, and interleukin-1 synthesis after hemorrhage. Surgery 1990;108:154-160.

38. Hay F. The generation of diversity. In: Roitt I, Brostoff J, Male D, eds. Immunology. 2nd ed. London: Gower Medical Publishing; 1989:6.1-6.12.

39. Boyd JL, Stanford GG, Chernow B. The pharmacotherapy of septic shock. Crit Care Clin 1989;5:151-156.

40. Priest BP et al. Treatment of experimental gram-negative bacterial sepsis with murine monoclonal antibodies directed against lipopolysaccharide. Surgery 1989;106:147-155.

41. Exley AR et al. Monoclonal antibody to TNF in severe septic shock. Lancet 1990;335:1275-1277.

42. Mayoral JL, Dunn DL. Cross-reactive murine monoclonal antibodies against the core/lipid A region of endotoxin inhibit production of tumor necrosis factor. J Surg Res 1990;49:287-292.

43. Ziegler EJ et al. Treatment of gram-negative bacteremia and septic shock with HA-1A human monoclonal antibody against endotoxin. N Engl J Med 1991;324:429-436.

44. Taverne J. Immunity to protozoa and worms. In: Roitt I, Brostoff J, Male D, eds. Immunology. 2nd ed. London: Gower Medical Publishing; 1989:17.1-17.21.

45. Balk RA, Bone RC. The septic syndrome: Definition and clinical implications. Crit Care Clin 1989;5:1-8.

46. Dorinsky PM, Gadek JE. Multiple organ failure. Clin Chest Med 1990;11:581-591.

47. Anderson BO, Harken AH. Multiple organ failure: Inflammatory priming and activation sequences promote autologous tissue injury. J Trauma 1990;30:S44-S49.

48. Sheagren JN. Mechanism-oriented therapy for multiple systems organ failure. Crit Care Clin 1989;5:393-410.

49. Petrak RA, Balk RA, Bone RC. Prostaglandins, cyclooxygenase inhibitors, and thromboxane synthetase inhibitors in the pathogenesis of multiple systems organ failure. Crit Care Clin 1989;5:302-314.

50. Webster's third new international dictionary. Unabridged. Springfield, MA: Merriam-Webster Inc; 1986.

51. Ishigami T. The influence of psychic acts on the progress of pulmonary tuberculosis. Am Rev Tubercul 1919;2:470-484.

52. Holmes TH, Rahe RH. The social readjustment rating scale. J Psychosom Res 1967;11:213-218.

53. Khansari DN, Murgo AJ, Faith RE. Effects of stress on the immune system. Immunol Today 1990;11:170-175.

54. Dunn AJ. Nervous system-immune system interactions: An overview. J Recept Res 1988;8:589-607.

55. Weiss JM et al. Behavioral and neural influences on cellular immune responses: Effects of stress and interleukin-1. J Clin Psych 1989;50(5 suppl):43-53.

56. Cupps TR, Fauci AS. Corticosteroid-mediated immunoregulation in man. Immunol Rev 1982;65:133-155.

57. Ogawa K, Sueda K, Matsui N. The effect of cortisol, progesterone and transcortin on phytohemagglutin-stimulated human blood mononuclear cells and their interplay. J Clin Endocrinol Metab 1983;56:121-126.

58. Fauci AS, Dale DC. Alternate-day prednisone therapy and human lymphocyte subpopulations. J Clin Invest 1975;55:22-32.

59. Hooks MA. Immunosuppressive agents used in transplantation. In: Smith SL, ed. Tissue and organ transplantation: Implications for professional nursing practice. St. Louis: Mosby–Year Book; 1990:48-80.

60. Bone RC et al. A controlled clinical trial of high-dose methylprednisolone in the treatment of severe sepsis and septic shock. N Engl J Med 1987;317:653-658.

61. Veterans Administration Systemic Sepsis Cooperative Study Group. Effect of high-dose glucocorticoid therapy on mortality in patients with clinical signs of systemic sepsis. N Engl J Med 1987;317:659-665.

62. Bernard GR et al. High-dose corticosteroids in patients with the adult respiratory distress syndrome. N Engl J Med 1987;317:1565-1570.

63. Nicholson DP. Review of corticosteroid treatment in sepsis and septic shock: Pro or con. Crit Care Clin 1989;5:151-155.

64. Besedovsky H et al. Immunoregulatory feedback between interleukin-1 and glucocorticoid hormones. Science 1986;233:652-654.

65. Holch MW et al. Graduation of immunosuppression after surgery or severe trauma. Prog Clin Biol Res: Second Vienna Shock Forum 1989;308:491-494.

66. Maghsudi M et al. Early deterioration of the immune system following multiple trauma. Prog Clin Biol Res: Second Vienna Shock Forum 1989;308:507-512.

67. Ertel W et al. Dynamics of immunoglobin synthesis after major trauma. Arch Surg 1989;124:1437-1442.

68. Faist E et al. Mediators and the trauma induced cascade of immunologic defects. Prog Clin Biol Res: Second Vienna Shock Forum 1989;308:495-506.

69. Faist E et al. Immunoprotective effects of cyclooxygenase

inhibition in patients with major surgical trauma. J Trauma 1990;30:8-18.

70. Waymack JP et al. Effect of blood transfusion and anesthesia on resistance to bacterial peritonitis. J Surg Res 1987;42:528-535.

71. Chaudry IH. Hemorrhage and resuscitation [editorial]. Am J Physiol 1990;259(4 Part 2):R663-R678.

72. Brunson ME, Alexander JW. Mechanisms of transfusion-induced immunosuppression. Transfusion 1990;30:651-658.

73. Wang P, Hauptman JG, Chaudry IH. Hepatocellular dysfunction occurs early after hemorrhage and persists despite fluid resuscitation. J Surg Res 1990;48:466-470.

74. Ayala A, Perrin MM, Chaudry IH. Defective antigen presentation following hemorrhage is associated with the loss of MHC class II (Ia) antigens. Immunology 1990;70:33-39.

75. Unanue ER, Allen PM. The basis of the immunoregulatory role of macrophages and other accessory cells. Science 1987;236:551-557.

76. Yano Y et al. Calcium-accented ischemic damage during reperfusion: The time course of the reperfusion injury in the isolated working rat heart model. J Surg Res 1987;42:51-55.

77. Baker JW et al. Hemorrhagic shock induces bacterial translocation from the gut. J Trauma 1988;28:896-906.

78. Gantt CL. Red blood cells for cancer patients [letter]. Lancet 1981;2:363.

79. Francis DMA, Sheaton BK. Blood transfusion and tumour growth: Evidence from laboratory animals [letter]. Lancet 1981;2:871.

80. Kaplan J et al. Diminished helper/suppressor lymphocyte ratios and natural killer activity in recipients of repeated blood transfusions. Blood 1984;64:308-310.

81. Stephan RN et al. Effect of blood transfusion on antigen presentation function and on interleukin-2 generation. Arch Surg 1988;123:235-240.

82. Brunson ME et al. Variable infection risk following allogeneic blood transfusions. J Surg Res 1990;48:308-312.

83. Graham EA. The influence of ether and ether anesthesia on bacteriolysis, agglutination, and phagocytosis. J Infect Dis 1911;8:147-175.

84. Moore TC. Anesthesia-associated depression in lymphocyte traffic and its modulation. Am J Surg 1984;147:807-812.

85. Spruck CH, Moore TC. Anesthesia-associated depression of peripheral node lymphocyte traffic and antibody production in sheep accompanied by elevations in arachidonic acid metabolites in efferent lymph. Transplant Proc 1988;20:1169-1174.

86. Browder W, Williams D. Immunosuppression in the surgical patient. J Natl Med Assoc 1988;80:531-536.

87. Costa A et al. Endocrine, hematological and immunological changes in surgical patients undergoing general anesthesia. Ital J Surg Sci 1989;19:41-49.

88. Pizzini RP et al. Dietary nucleotides reverse malnutrition and starvation-induced immunosuppression. Arch Surg 1990;125:86-90.

89. Leonard TK, Mohs ME, Watson RR. The cardiovascular effects of alcohol. I. In: Watson RR, ed. Nutrition and heart disease. Boca Raton: CRC Press; 1987:19-47.

90. Mohs ME, Watson RR. Ethanol induced malnutrition, a potential cause of immunosuppression during AIDS. Prog Clin Biol Res 1990;325:433-444.

91. Redl H, Schlag G. Biochemical analysis in posttraumatic and postoperative organ failure. Prog Clin Biol Res: Second Vienna Shock Forum 1989;308:649-672.

92. Hoyt NJ. Host defense mechanisms and compromises in

the trauma patient. Crit Care Nurs Clin North Am 1989;1:753-766.

93. Smith SL. Immunologic aspects of transplantation. In: Smith SL, ed. Tissue and organ transplantation: Implications for professional nursing practice. St. Louis: Mosby–Year Book; 1990:15-47.

94. Dahn MS et al. Altered T-lymphocyte subsets in severe sepsis. Am Surg 1988; 54:450-455.

95. Chachoua A et al. Prognostic factors and staging classification of patients with epidemic Kaposi's sarcoma. J Clin Oncol 1989;7:774-780.

96. Tinkoff G et al. Cirrhosis in the trauma victim: Effect on mortality rates. Ann Surg 1990;211:172-177.

97. Pimpl W et al. Incidence of septic and thromboembolic-related deaths after splenectomy in adults. Br J Surg 1989;76:517-521.

98. Shaw JHF, Print CG. Postsplenectomy sepsis. Br J Surg 1989;76:1074-1081.

99. Styrt B. Infection associated with asplenia: Risks, mechanisms, and prevention. Am J Med 1990;88(5):33n-42n.

100. Steward M, Male D. Immunological techniques. In: Roitt I, Brostoff J, Male D, eds. Immunology. 2nd ed. London: Gower Medical Publishing; 1989:25.1-25.3.

101. Lamche HR, Adolf GR. Highly sensitive enzyme immunoassays for antibodies to human tumor necrosis factor (TNF-alpha) and lymphotoxin (TNF-beta). J Immunol Meth 1990;131:283-289.

102. Liabakk NB, Nustad K, Espevik T. A rapid and sensitive immunoassay for tumor necrosis factor using magnetic monodisperse polymer particles. J Immunol Meth 1990;134:253-259.

103. McLaughlin PJ et al. Improvement in sensitivity of enzyme-linked immunosorbent assay for tumour necrosis factor. Immunol Cell Biol 1990;68(Pt 1):51-55.

104. Pacher R, Redl H, Woloszczuk W. Plasma levels of granulocyte elastase and neopterin in patients with MOF. Prog Clin Biol Res: Second Vienna Shock Forum 1989;308:683-688.

105. Pacher R et al. Relationship between neopterin and granulocyte elastase plasma levels and the severity of multiple organ failure. Crit Care Med 1989;17:221-226.

106. Jochum M et al. Posttraumatic plasma levels of mediators of organ failure. Prog Clin Biol Res: Second Vienna Shock Forum 1989;308:673-681.

107. Martich GD et al. Relation of serum neopterin to the hemodynamic and cytokine response following intravenous endotoxin administration to normal humans [abstract]. Crit Care Med 1991;19(4 suppl):S14.

108. Spitzer JA et al. Receptor changes in endotoxemia. Prog Clin Biol Res: Perspectives in Shock Research 1989;299:95-106.

109. Barnetson RSC, Gawkrodger D. Hypersensitivity-Type IV. In: Roitt I, Brostoff J, Male D, eds. Immunology. 2nd ed. London: Gower Medical Publishing; 1989:22.1-22.10.

110. Meakins JL et al. Delayed hypersensitivity and neutrophil chemotaxis. Effect of trauma. J Trauma 1978;18:240-247.

111. Christou NV et al. Estimating mortality risk in preoperative patients using immunologic, nutritional, and acute-phase response variables. Ann Surg 1989;210:69-77.

112. Nuytinck HKS et al. Whole-body inflammation in trauma patients. Arch Surg 1988;123:1519-1524.

113. Nerlich ML. The trigger for posttraumatic multiple organ failure: Surgical sepsis or inflammation? Prog Clin Biol Res: Second Vienna Shock Forum 1989;308:413-417.

114. Darling GE et al. Multiorgan failure in critically ill patients. Can J Surg 1988;31:172-176.

3 Inflammatory Mediators and Multisystem Organ Failure

Virginia Byrn Huddleston

From the initial discussions by Baue[1] and others in the mid-1970s to more recent research on multisystem organ failure (MSOF), investigators in both basic science and clinical research have attempted to identify a common link among patients succumbing to MSOF. Although shock, hypoperfusion, endotoxemia, and septic shock are common denominators in the development of MSOF, recent research increasingly points to overwhelming inflammatory activity as a primary underlying mechanism resulting in organ dysfunction and failure distant from the initial site of insult.[2-4]

The following discussion presents the physiologic and pathophysiologic roles of the major inflammatory mediators of sepsis and the MSOF process. Although most mediators initially serve a very protective, physiologic function, regulatory mechanisms can fail. Mediator activity then becomes exaggerated or uncontrolled, leading to the development and progression of MSOF.[2,3,5,6] An uncontrolled inflammatory/immune response (IIR) initiates maldistribution of circulating volume, oxygen supply and demand imbalances, and metabolic alterations.[7-11]

The mediators in the following discussion are not limited to soluble substances in the circulation, but they include structures such as the endothelium, cells such as white blood cells (WBCs) and platelets, and biochemical substances such as oxygen-derived free radicals. As Baue[12] states: "The mediators of inflammatory responses are numerous, fascinating, complex, and incompletely understood. . . . The biologic purpose of these cells and activities is sound: they are necessary for mounting an inflammatory response, for healing, and for survival. However, they may also run wild, becoming toxic to other cells." Although presented here in isolation, in the critically ill patient, these mediators are continuously affected by interactions among themselves, the physiologic environment, and treatment regimens. Failure of host defense homeostasis is related not only to overwhelming activation but to loss of inhibitory pathways as well.[13] Appendix A provides a quick reference of the major mediators, including function, mediator source, and action.

ENDOTHELIUM
Physiologic role

Once thought to function solely as an inert barrier between the fluid phase of blood and the solid phase of tissue, the endothelial layer is now recognized as a dynamic, metabolic site.[14] The endothelium is a unicellular layer of specialized cells that lines the entire vascular system from the aorta, arteries, and capillary beds, through the venules and veins, and back through the vena cava to the heart. In major vessels, subendothelial structures of collagen, smooth muscle fibers, and elastic tissue are present; however, in the capillary bed, only the endothelium remains. The endothelial cells are surrounded by a basement membrane on the tissue side of the vessel.[15,16]

The endothelial cells approximate at sites known as intercellular clefts or junctions (Fig. 3-1). In response to mediators such as complement, histamine, and kinin, endothelial cells retract and the junctions widen, leading to the increased capillary permeability and edema commonly seen in inflammation.[17] These widened junctions allow for the egress of plasma proteins and the diapedesis of WBCs from the blood to the tissue site of injury.[18]

The endothelium serves many purposes in addition to its barrier function between blood and tissue (see box on p. 38). One of the most important functions of the endothelium is to keep the blood fluid; thus it has many anticoagulant properties.[19]

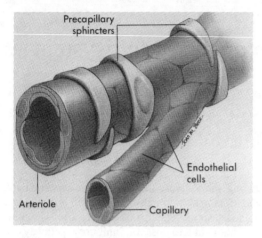

Fig. 3-1 Endothelial anatomy. (From Thibodeau GA, ed. Structure and function of the body. 9th ed. St. Louis: Mosby–Year Book, 1992.)

FACTORS IMPAIRING ENDOTHELIAL INTEGRITY AND FUNCTION

Mechanical disruption
Microorganisms and their toxins
Immune complexes
Shock
Hypoxemia
Acidosis
Platelet aggregation leading to microthrombi, mechanical obstruction, and decreased nutrition
Neutrophil aggregation leading to mechanical obstruction, oxygen-derived free radical formation, and protease release
Coagulation on the endothelial surface
Direct action of mediators such as TNF and IL-1

Abbreviations: *TNF*, tumor necrosis factor; *IL-1*, interleukin-1.

FUNCTIONS OF THE ENDOTHELIUM

Anticoagulation by maintaining smooth, nonadherent lining, forming tPA, generating prostacyclin, and generating other activators and inhibitors of platelet aggregation, coagulation, and fibrinolysis
Hydrolysis (inactivation) of vasoactive peptides such as bradykinin, angiotensin, and serotonin
Synthesis and release of growth factors
Endocytosis of small particles, including immune complexes, endotoxin, and bacteria
Antigen processing and presentation
Influence on carbohydrate and lipid metabolism through receptors for insulin, low-density lipoproteins, very low-density lipoproteins, and lipoprotein lipase
Synthesis and release of mediators: prostaglandins, thromboxanes, leukotrienes, and tissue factor (when injured)

The role of the endothelium in the homeostasis of coagulation includes:

1. Maintenance of a smooth, continuous blood vessel lining to prevent platelet adherence to subendothelial structures
2. Generation of prostacyclin, a prostaglandin that promotes vasodilatation and inhibits platelet aggregation
3. Synthesis and release of tissue plasminogen activator (tPA) to promote clot breakdown
4. Synthesis and release of antithrombin III and thrombomodulin

Therefore, if the function and integrity of the endothelium are disrupted, the hemostatic balance may be severely impaired. Procoagulant activity results, leading to thrombin formation and fibrin deposition.[20,21]

Unfortunately, many mediators and clinical conditions commonly seen in the critically ill patient damage the endothelium (see box above). Its extensive surface area, susceptibility to injury, and metabolic functions make it a key focus of research in sepsis, DIC, and MSOF.[20-22]

Impact on MSOF process

Although the endothelium has the potential to repair itself and maintain normal function, extensive damage overwhelms the endothelium's repair mechanisms, resulting in widespread permeability and coagulation abnormalities.[23,24] The increased capillary permeability, necessary in the initial stages of localized inflammation, extends to the systemic circulation and promotes fluid loss to the tissues. This third-spacing of fluid yields the generalized peripheral edema and organ edema commonly found in these patients. As tissues continue to swell, vascular flow is further obstructed, and tissue ischemia worsens. Proteins and other plasma elements are lost to the tissue, causing tissue damage, osmotic derangements, and lymph drainage system overload.[15]

As the endothelium suffers damage to its anticoagulant mechanisms, coagulation becomes accelerated, and large amounts of fibrin are deposited in the vasculature, further obstructing flow and potentiating ischemia, especially in the microvasculature. Damaged endothelium has actually been shown to express tissue factor (tissue thromboplastin), a potent activator of the extrinsic pathway of coagulation. This may actually be the most procoagulant stimulus for initiating disseminated intravascular coagulation (DIC).[20,21,25]

Endothelial damage also hinders other endothelial metabolic and receptor functions, leading to vasomotor abnormalities[26] and decreased detoxification of vasoactive substances, such as bradykinin, angiotensin, and serotonin. Damage to the endothelium further stimulates the IIR, making endothelial damage central to the self-propagation of the vicious cycle culminating in MSOF.[20,21]

HEMOSTASIS
Physiologic role

The mechanisms of coagulation and fibrinolysis are dependent on numerous anticoagulant and procoagulant factors operating in dynamic equilib-

rium. If the exquisite balance between these two systems is disrupted, systemic thrombosis or gross hemorrhage results, often developing simultaneously in one patient as DIC. Activation of hemostatic mechanisms accompanies injury, localized inflammation, and damage to the endothelium. Hemostasis is necessary to prevent excessive blood loss and isolate the injured site. Like the IIR, hemostasis is protective only if it remains localized to the site of injury. When coagulation is not contained or regulated, systemic abnormalities and coagulopathies such as DIC result. Chapter 4 presents a comprehensive discussion on DIC.

Impact on MSOF process

The combined effects of blood flow stagnation, tissue injury, and endothelial damage seen in shock, sepsis, and trauma may stimulate excessive coagulation. The close interrelationship between the IIR and coagulation triggers the activation of both systems when either is stimulated. The activity of the enzymatic plasma cascades is tightly interwoven, both in physiologic and pathophysiologic states. Hageman factor (factor XII) is the major link in this interdependency (Fig. 3-2). In the protective state, this interrelationship is very efficient because injury that requires hemostasis usually requires immune protection; however, in a poorly regulated situation, overwhelming inflammation, coagulation, and fibrinolysis ensue, with continual reactivation. Mediators then leave the local site of injury and move into the systemic circulation, causing alterations in organs remote from the site of injury.

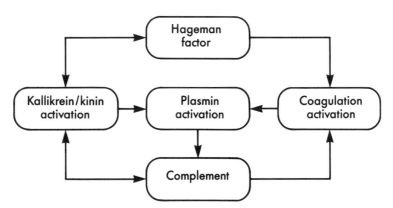

Fig. 3-2   Hageman factor as the link in the interlocking network of the plasma enzyme cascades.

Clotting abnormalities greatly increase the incidence of vascular obstruction, tissue ischemia, inflammation, and organ damage. Although there are many stimuli that trigger the hemostatic mechanism, damage to the vascular endothelium is currently thought to be the primary mechanism that induces the intravascular procoagulant state.[20,21,27] Certain mediators (lipopolysaccharide, tumor necrosis factor, interleukin-1, and immune complexes) induce the generation of tissue factor on the cell surface of endothelial cells[20,21] and macrophages (cells not normally thrombogenic), thus providing another link between inflammation and thrombosis.[28,29]

COMPLEMENT
Physiologic role

Complement is a triggered enzyme cascade composed of a complex series of approximately 20 circulating proteins. Although initially identified more than 100 years ago, the complement cascade still provides investigators with a large area of study. Its major role is to amplify the IIR, primarily in bacterial infections. The peptides splitting from the inactive "parent" molecules are biologically active, with C3a and C5a (also known as anaphylatoxins) being the best described. C3 is the major protein of the cascade.[30,31] Although complement is a major pathway in the process of inflammation and the nonspecific immune response, its actions are enhanced by activity in the specific immune response. Complement has a high avidity for the immunoglobulins IgG and IgM, and complement's classic pathway is triggered by antigen/antibody complexes formed during the specific immune response.[30] Complement may also bind directly with certain microbes and other substances, thus initiating the alternate pathway (Fig. 3-3).

The major physiologic function of complement is to initiate, enhance, or "complement" the inflammatory response. Activities include (1) induction of inflammation, (2) opsonization of foreign particles, (3) cellular activation of phagocytic cells (neutrophils, monocytes/macrophages), and (4) direct target-cell lysis.[30]

Induction of inflammation primarily results from the action of the anaphylatoxins. Not only do anaphylatoxins increase capillary permeability and vasodilatation directly, but they also cause the degranulation of mast cells and basophils, which leads to the release of histamine and other proinflammatory mediators that also increase vasodilatation, capillary permeability, and phagocytic activation[30] (see Fig. 2-1).

Opsonization facilitates phagocytosis by depositing (coating or binding) opsonins such as antibodies or C3b on to the antigen. The presence of opsonin on the antigen enhances binding with phagocytic cells such as neutrophils, monocytes, macrophages, and antigen-presenting cells, all of which have receptors for C3 or antibody (Fig. 3-4). Once bound, the phagocytes engulf the microbe and kill it. Complement enhances the binding with these phagocytes.

Complement assists in the *cellular activation* of the phagocytic cells of the IIR. The cells must be drawn to the injury site (chemotaxis) and activated to kill (respiratory burst). A concentration gradient of complement or other chemotactant substances develops near the injury site, and white blood cells move up the concentration gradient to the site of inflammation.[30] Once the pathogen is engulfed, the cell undergoes a respiratory burst and produces microbicidal mediators to use in combination with preformed mediators present within the granules and lysosomes of the phagocyte to kill the invader.[32]

Target-cell lysis occurs through the activity of the membrane-attack-complex (MAC), which is formed at the termination of the complement cascade. The MAC (C5b-C9) plugs into the target cell's membrane, leading to osmotic disequilibrium, cell lysis, and possibly increased arachidonic acid metabolism.[30] In this scenario, the pathogen is killed before phagocytosis. Phagocytosis is still necessary to degrade and remove cell debris; therefore the ultimate destruction of bacteria requires synergistic action with phagocytic cells.[32]

Impact on MSOF process

As with the other inflammatory mediators, complement's effects serve a very protective function, but only if production is regulated and localized to the site of injury. If large amounts of complement are activated and escape to the systemic circulation, its actions become detrimental. Overwhelming vasodilatation, capillary permeability, and phagocytic activation with concomitant release of toxic by-products serve to perpetuate the edema formation, cardiovascular instability, endothelial damage, clotting abnormalities, and other signs and symptoms seen in the MSOF patient.[33,34]

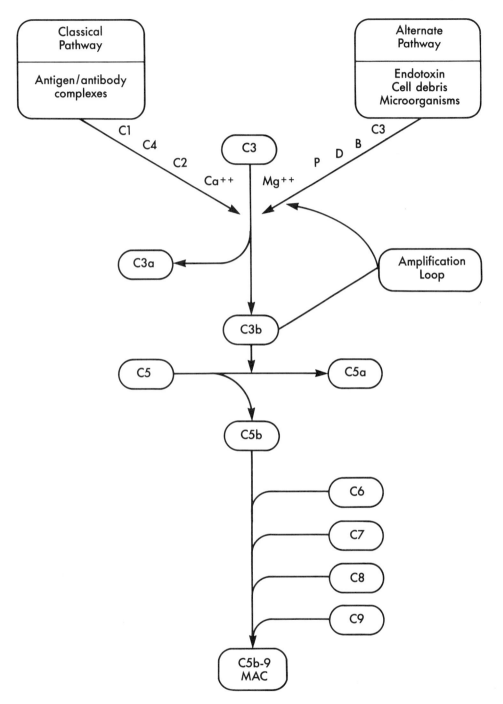

Fig. 3-3 Complement cascade. Abbreviations: *MAC*, Membrane attack complex; *P*, properdin; *B*, factor B; *D*, factor D; *C*, complement. (Modified from Hood LE, Weissman IL, Wood WB, Wilson JH, eds. Immunology. 2nd edition. Menlo Park, CA: Benjamin/Cummings Publishing, 1984;343.)

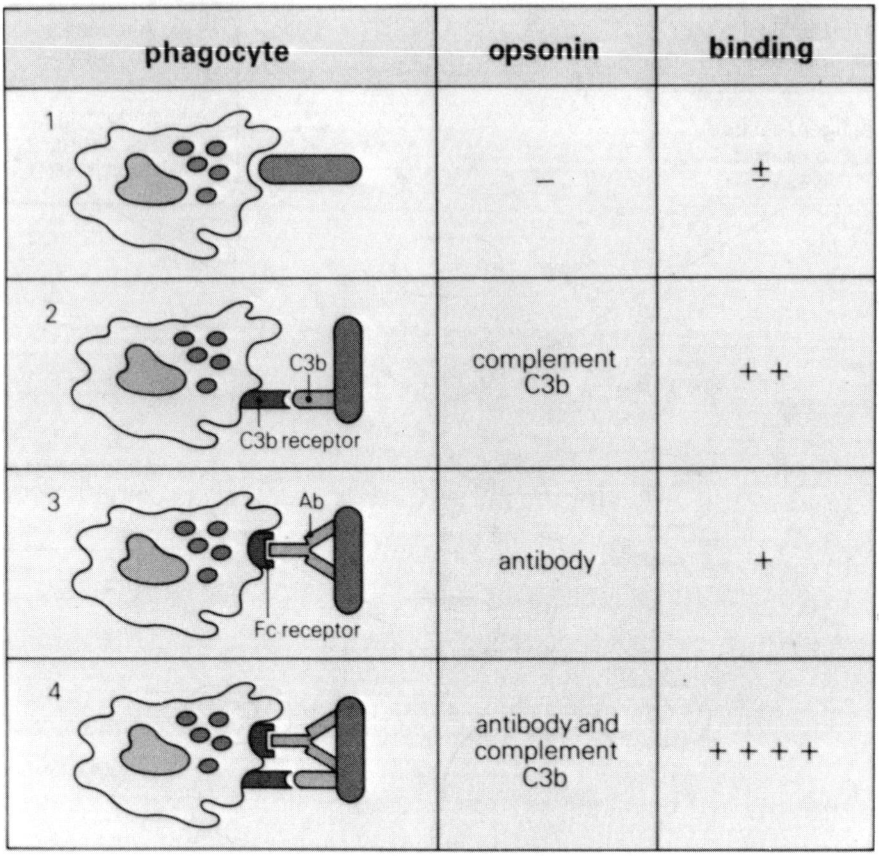

phagocyte	opsonin	binding
1	–	±
2 (C3b, C3b receptor)	complement C3b	+ +
3 (Ab, Fc receptor)	antibody	+
4	antibody and complement C3b	+ + + +

Fig. 3-4 Opsonization of microorganisms. Opsonization may occur via binding with complement and/or antibody. (From Male D, Roitt I. Adaptive and innate immunity. In: Roitt I, Brostoff J, Male D, eds. Immunology. 2nd edition. London: Gower Medical Publishing, 1989;1.6.)

Studies show that complement activation produces tissue and organ damage, particularly in the lungs and vasculature.[35,36] Hemodynamic changes and perfusion abnormalities in the liver and kidneys are also related to complement activation.[37,38] The point at which the cascade ceases to be protective and begins to damage the host has not been defined. Levels of circulating complement components can be assayed directly, or their functional capabilities can be determined.[39]

KALLIKREIN/KININ SYSTEM
Physiologic role

The kallikrein/kinin system is the fourth enzyme system (along with complement, coagulation, and fibrinolysis) of the interlocking plasma protein cascades. As mentioned before, these cascades work together after a physiologic insult to initiate hemostasis, inflammation, tissue repair, and host protection. The role of the kallikrein/kinin system has not been fully delineated. One of the major metabolites, bradykinin, is a potent vasodilator and has also been shown to increase capillary permeability in some tissue beds.[18,40] Its role in blood pressure regulation and renal blood flow is currently under investigation.[41] The kinins have been shown to stimulate neutrophil chemotaxis, phagocytosis, and respiratory burst activity. Kinin release also increases bronchoconstriction and microvascular permeability.[42]

Hageman factor provides the major link between the plasma enzyme cascades with its concomitant activation of the intrinsic coagulation cascade and kallikrein. Kallikrein then catalyzes the conversion of kininogen to kinin.[43] The kinins also indirectly activate complement,[18] further propagating the IIR (Fig. 3-2).

Impact on MSOF process

Severe infection is associated with increased activation of the kinin cascade.[44] Bradykinin has a very short half-life, so its presence and impact are inferred from the circulating levels of its precursors and activators. Previous research has implicated bradykinin in physiologic abnormalities seen in hemorrhagic shock, septic shock, endotoxemia, and tissue injury.[12] As a potent vasodilator, bradykinin potentiates problems of low systemic vascular resistance and hemodynamic instability seen in shock and MSOF. Increased capillary permeability and neutrophil stimulation also exacerbate the damage that occurs in a nonspecific, uncontrolled inflammatory response. Tissue edema and leukocyte aggregation lead to vascular compression and obstruction, further tissue ischemia, and maldistribution of circulating volume. Recent research has identified isoproterenol as a potential inhibitor of bradykinin-induced microvascular permeability.[40]

NEUTROPHILS
Physiologic role

The neutrophil is the major polymorphonuclear (PMN) granulocyte in the circulation. Along with eosinophils and basophils, the neutrophil differentiates from the hematopoietic stem cell in the bone marrow and matures through the myeloid lineage. Commonly referred to as a PMN, polymorph, granulocyte, or poly, its primary function is surveillance and phagocytosis of foreign pathogens. This can occur in the blood or following the neutrophil's migration into the tissue during the inflammatory response. Following a major insult, a significant number of neutrophils are also sequestered in the lung, where they adhere (marginate) to the lining of the pulmonary vasculature.

Once injury has occurred, neutrophils are drawn to the site by various chemotactant factors (complement, arachidonic acid metabolites, kinins) and activated by numerous cytokines (TNF, IL-1), bacterial wall fragments, prostaglandins, and cell debris (see Fig. 2-2). The infection is localized through the formation of an abscess. The neutrophil phagocytizes the pathogen and undergoes a respiratory burst as it converts to oxidative metabolism. These oxygen-dependent reactions produce highly reactive oxygen species, collectively referred to as oxygen-derived free radicals (ODFR) or simply free radicals.[32,45]

These free radicals (oxygen-dependent), along with the cytotoxic enzymes and substances (non-oxygen-dependent: lysozyme, myeloperoxidase, lactoferrin) in the neutrophil's granules and lysosomes, are then secreted into the phagolysosome, where they carry out their microbicidal activity and breakdown of cellular debris.[32,46] During the process of phagocytosis and intracellular killing, the neutrophil also releases these microbicidal substances into the extracellular environment. Although this increases the protective function and activity of the neutrophil, excessive activation and excretion may potentiate tissue damage and organ dysfunction.[45] Prostaglandin synthesis may also be increased with WBC–endothelial cell interactions.[47]

Impact on MSOF process

There is no question that mediators synthesized and released by activated neutrophils can damage vascular endothelium and parenchymal tissue (see box below). Neutrophil aggregation can also cause direct vascular obstruction or endothelial damage and thrombosis, further contributing to tissue ischemia and inflammation. At what point the neutrophil's activity ceases to be protective and becomes damaging, and to what extent that damage occurs, is still a matter of great debate.[48]

Proteases such as elastase can damage the extracellular matrix. Oxygen-derived free radicals lead to increased capillary permeability and cell membrane perturbation. Free radicals potentiate severe protease-induced damage because they dam-

---

MEDIATORS RELEASED BY NEUTROPHILS

Interleukins
Leukotrienes
Oxygen-derived free radicals
Platelet activating factor
Prostaglandins
Proteases (collagenase, elastase)
Tissue factor (tissue thromboplastin)

age enzymes normally responsible for breaking down and eliminating the harmful proteases.[45,49,50] Arachidonic acid metabolites such as prostaglandins and leukotrienes affect the smooth muscle of the vasculature and specific organs.

The majority of work done on neutrophil-related organ damage is found in the adult respiratory distress syndrome (ARDS) literature.[51-55] Although the neutrophil and its products are implicated in the pulmonary hypertension, abnormal lung mechanics (decreased compliance, increased resistance to air flow), and vascular permeability that are the hallmarks of ARDS, research has shown that ARDS can occur in the neutropenic patient as well.[56] However, other research has shown that the severity of damage is lessened if neutrophils are depleted.[57,58] This suggests that other factors working either independently or in concert with neutrophil activation and activity may be responsible for the pathogenesis of ARDS.[12]

Neutrophils provide a necessary element in the inflammation and protective actions of the nonspecific response, but if a persistent inflammatory focus (abscess, necrotic tissue, or occult infection) or improper down-regulation is present, neutrophil aggregation, activity, and mediator release may contribute to organ damage and host demise.[59]

OXYGEN-DERIVED FREE RADICALS
Physiologic role

Oxygen-derived free radicals and their role in homeostasis and pathogenesis are currently an exciting and expanding area of both basic science and clinical research. The myocardial infarction patient and reperfusion injury,[60] the vascular patient and restoration of flow,[61] the coronary artery bypass graft patient and the stunned myocardium,[62] mechanical ventilation and oxygen toxicity,[63] and neutrophil activation and ARDS[45,63] all provide settings in which oxygen-derived free radicals may develop and interact with surrounding tissue.

A radical (all are "free" by definition) is an atom or group of atoms carrying unpaired electrons in its outer orbits. Numerous sources of free radicals exist in the body: xanthine oxidase systems, activated phagocytes, mitochondria, and arachidonic acid pathways.[64] They are normally produced during oxidative metabolism in small concentrations and are highly reactive and very unstable.[65] Once produced, they do not diffuse very far, and reac-

tivity and toxicity vary with the particular species.[12] The body has numerous enzyme systems (superoxide dismutase and catalase) and membrane antioxidants (vitamin E, beta carotenes) to break down the free radicals into nontoxic species, usually H_2O and O_2.[45,66]

Impact on MSOF process

The increased presence of free radicals can cause significant damage to cell membranes of both vascular endothelial cells and tissue. Lipid peroxidation occurs as free radicals react with polyunsaturated fatty acid in the cell membrane. This alters the membrane's fluidity, secretory function, and ionic gradients.[12,67] Endothelial damage, increased capillary permeability, altered cell receptor function, and denaturation of protein may also occur, further stimulating the IIR.[12,66] If the endothelium is damaged, procoagulant factors induce development of thrombi in the microcirculation.

During postischemic reperfusion or the respiratory burst of phagocytic cells, free radicals can be formed at toxic levels. In reperfusion injury, specific enzymes and substances in the tissue undergo transformations during ischemia (see Chapter 5). When blood and oxygen are returned to the tissue, the molecular oxygen (O_2) reacts with the "new" enzymes and substances to produce the superoxide radical (Fig. 3-5). The formation of hydrogen peroxide follows, and in the presence of iron, hydroxyl radical production can occur (Fig. 3-6).[45] In myocardial reperfusion, the formation of free radicals irritates the myocardium, causing the increased ectopy often seen following reperfusion during thrombolytic therapy.[66]

The increased permeability, edema, and inflammation that accompany free radical damage may lead to vascular occlusion, either from edematous tissue compression or accelerated microthrombi formation. Tissue ischemia, extended infarcts, compartment syndrome, and loss of organ system integrity may all ensue. The "stunned" myocardium seen after the patient comes off bypass may also be related to production of free radicals in the revascularized myocardium.[62]

A patient experiencing a low-flow state (cardiopulmonary arrest, shock, or cross-clamp placement) followed by resuscitation may have increased production of free radicals as the tissues are reperfused in the postresuscitation period. As-

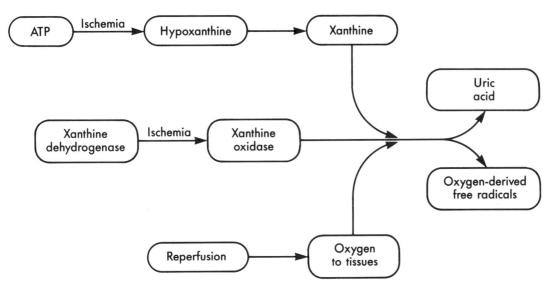

Fig. 3-5 Free radical formation in ischemia and reperfusion injury. (From Huddleston VB. Multisystem organ failure: A pathophysiologic approach. Boston; 1991:26.)

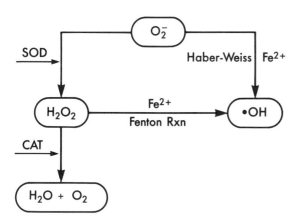

Fig. 3-6 Iron-dependent reactions in oxygen-derived free radical production. In the Haber-Weiss and Fenton reactions, iron is required for the production of hydroxyl radicals; therefore iron-chelating agents inhibit the reactions and thus hydroxyl radical production. Because the hydroxyl radical is more potent than the other radicals, inhibiting their formation may attenuate free radical injury. Abbreviations: *CAT*, Catalase; *SOD*, superoxide dismutase; *rxn*, reaction.

sessment of edema, capillary refill, pulses, and skin temperature is necessary to assess the adequacy of limb perfusion. Unfortunately, measuring regional perfusion in various vital organs is not possible at the bedside on a routine basis. Indirect measures such as urine output, level of consciousness, liver enzymes, and other laboratory values have to be used to assess adequacy of organ perfusion.

Free radical production also increases during the respiratory burst of phagocytic cells. The mechanism involves the activation of NADPH oxidase. Radicals are used for their bactericidal activity, but may escape from the cell and cause damage to the surrounding tissue and vasculature. Intracellular damage may also occur if production is excessive.[68] Because of the leukocytosis and margination of neutrophils in septic shock and MSOF and the increased production of free radicals when these cells are activated, it is highly plausible that free radicals are playing a definitive role in the organ damage that occurs in MSOF.[45,63,69,70] Ibuprofen has recently been shown to inhibit not only the cyclooxygenase pathway but free radical generation as well. Because iron is required in the production of hydroxyl radicals, iron-chelating agents such as ibuprofen and deferoxamine decrease hydroxyl radical production and may decrease tissue damage and lipid peroxidation associated with free radical activity.[71,72]

MAST CELL
Physiologic role

Mast cells are found in almost all tissues of the body, especially near blood vessels and the external environment. At least two types of morphologically distinct mast cells exist. One is found predominantly in the connective tissue of the peritoneal and pleural spaces and the skin. The majority of its granules contain heparin sulfates, histamine, and a chymotrypsin-like enzyme. The other type resides in the gastrointestinal mucosa and contains chondroitin sulfates, a trypsinlike enzyme, and less histamine. The mast cell originates in the bone marrow and is very similar in both structure and function to the blood basophil. Their relationship is not completely defined.[73]

The mast cell plays a key role in the acute response to injury (primarily inflammation) but may affect the microenvironment in latter responses as well.[13] The mast cell releases both preformed and newly generated mediators when it is stimulated or directly injured by mechanical factors (crush or burn), endotoxin, complement, or bradykinin. Preformed substances released include histamine, proteases, heparin, and chemotactic factors. Generated substances include prostaglandins and leukotrienes. Platelet activating factor (PAF) and TNF may also be released. Not only is the immediate environment affected (local response), but mediators released by mast cells can enter the circulation and cause systemic disturbances such as anaphylaxis.[74]

Impact on MSOF process

The mast cell as a major source of mediator release may play a role in the development of MSOF, although definitive documentation is not yet available. The major mediators released by mast cells are histamine, proteases, and arachidonic acid metabolites.[74] Histamine's inflammatory effects include vasodilatation, increased capillary permeability, and chemokinesis (increases WBC movement, but not necessarily toward the specific site). It can also cause urticaria, bronchoconstriction, and increased gastric acid secretion, all of which are detrimental in a critically ill patient.[74]

The arachidonic acid metabolites contribute to the bronchoconstriction, platelet aggregation, and vasodilatation already mentioned. Once again, initially protective physiologic functions in host defense are augmenting activity that is detrimental to the host. This scenario occurs repeatedly with many of the components of the IIR.

RETICULOENDOTHELIAL SYSTEM AND THE MACROPHAGE
Physiologic role

Classically, the reticuloendothelial system (RES) is viewed as a network of phagocytic tissue macrophages including both the resident macrophages of the liver, spleen, and bone marrow as well as the more mobile tissue macrophages that are present in many organs and tissues throughout the body. Macrophages differentiate from circulating blood monocytes that have emigrated from blood vessels into the tissues. The tissue to which the monocyte migrates modifies the differentiation process, which leads to variations in morphology between different tissue macrophages. Thus the tissue macrophages are assigned specific names

Table 3-1 Tissue Macrophages and Antigen-Presenting Cells

Cell	Organ/Location
Alveolar macrophages	Lungs
Splenic macrophages	Spleen
Monocytes	Blood
Synovial A cells	Synovia
Intraglomerular mesangial cells	Kidney
Kupffer cells	Liver
Microglial cells	Brain
Langerhans' cells	Skin
Interdigitating dendritic cells	Lymphoid tissue
Follicular dendritic cells	Lymphoid tissue
Follicular cells	Thyroid
Astrocytes	Brain
Endothelial cells	Vasculature
Fibroblasts	Connective tissue
B lymphocytes	Lymphoid tissue

Modified from Feldmann M, Male D. Cell cooperation in the immune response. In: Roitt I, Brostoff J, Male D, eds. Immunology. 2nd ed. London: Gower Medical Publishing; 1989:8.1-8.12.

(Table 3-1). The macrophages may be tissue-fixed, such as the microglia of the CNS; wandering, such as alveolar macrophages of the lung; or endothelial cell–fixed, such as liver Kupffer cells.[73] A newer term, *mononuclear phagocytic system,* is currently used to classify not only tissue macrophages and circulating monocytes of the RES but other antigen-presenting cells (APC) as well. APCs such as follicular dendritic cells of the lymph node and spleen, Langerhans cells of the skin, and interdigitating cells of the thymus are cells involved in antigen processing and presentation[46,73] (Table 3-1).

The major function of the monocytes and macrophages is the antigen processing and presentation that follow the nonspecific phagocytosis and removal of soluble and particulate antigen and debris from the circulation, tissue, and body cavities. The antigens and debris include bacteria, endotoxin, denatured protein, collagen, damaged RBCs, platelet aggregates, tissue debris, and other microaggregates. The macrophage can engulf pure antigen or opsonized antigen; however, phagocytosis is enhanced by opsonization because the macrophage has receptors on its cell surface for complement and antibodies (Fig. 3-4).

Once the macrophage has phagocytized the antigen, the antigen is processed into fragments that are then presented to lymphocytes to induce their activation and proliferation.[75] During processing and presentation, the macrophage releases IL-1, which activates T cells, B cells, and surrounding macrophages.[76,77] Although the macrophage can phagocytize antigen without previous T-cell activation and interaction, T-cell activation and mediator release (IL-2, gamma-IFN) increase macrophage phagocytic capabilities (Fig. 3-7). Thus the macrophage provides a major link between the nonspecific and specific immune response.[46]

Macrophages are also involved in the generation and secretion of various inflammatory mediators (complement components, proteases, and lysozyme) and cytokines (TNF and IL-1)[78] (see box on p. 48). Cytokines produced by monocytes and macrophages are referred to as monokines. Each monokine may have several functions, act on several different target tissues, or have functions that overlap with other cytokines. The monokines are thought to play a central role in the complications associated with septic shock, DIC, and MSOF, although alterations in activation or inhibition of phagocytosis and antigen processing and presentation may also affect the process.

Impact on MSOF process

Increased attention is being given to the macrophage and its role in the development and potentiation of MSOF. Many of the mediators thought to play a central role in this syndrome are released by activated macrophages.[79,80] Although macrophage activation and phagocytic activity are necessary to prevent systemic invasion by bacteria and other foreign agents, extensive macrophage activation also leads to increased release of potentially harmful mediators such as TNF, IL-1, prostaglandins, and oxygen-derived free radicals.[78,81]

Bacteria may enter the circulation from numerous sources: wound abscesses, infection at remote organs (lungs, kidneys, and bladder), or translocation from the gut. As the tissue macrophages (especially liver Kupffer cells) attempt to fight this pathogenic onslaught, they begin to release both preformed and newly synthesized mediators.[78,80,81] These mediators not only cause direct damage such as capillary permeability and vasodilatation, but they also increase activation

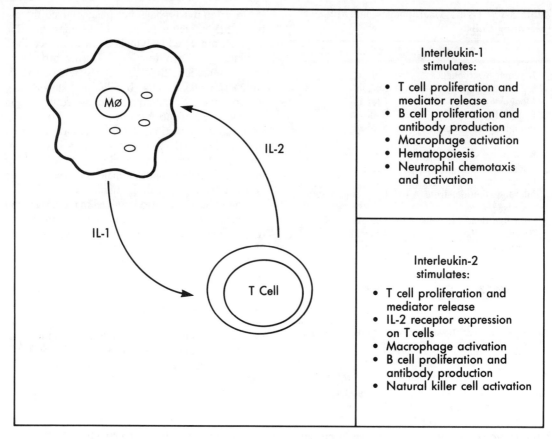

Fig. 3-7   Macrophage/T-cell interaction via cytokine production. Abbreviations: *IL*, Interleukin; *MØ*, macrophage.

MEDIATORS RELEASED BY MACROPHAGES

Coagulation factors
Colony stimulating factors
Complement proteins
Interferon
Interleukins
Leukotrienes
Oxygen-derived free radicals
Plasminogen activators
Platelet activating factor
Prostaglandins
Proteases
Tumor necrosis factor

or degranulation of other cells. Mast cells, basophils, other macrophages, lymphocytes, and neutrophils then amplify the process with release of their own mediators.[13] A mushroom effect occurs in which the system literally "feeds" off itself. Once a certain level of activation is reached, minimal stimulation is required from outside sources to keep the process active. In other words, even if the initial stimulus is treated by antibiotics, surgical debridement, or other appropriate treatment, the process may not reverse. Accelerated coagulation, DIC, tissue ischemia, and organ damage continue unabated.[82,83]

Macrophages play a major role in wound repair and defense, and the wound itself is a major source of macrophage accumulation, activation, and mediator release.[84] Macrophages aid in ridding the injured site of foreign material, cell debris, and dying leukocytes, providing "micro-debridement" in the wound. Macrophages also enhance wound granulation by producing locally acting growth factors.[78,85] Baue[12] even views the wound as an organ in itself, which calls upon the circulation, lungs, liver, and kidneys to support it. It communicates with the host and may make demands the host cannot keep, especially if the wound becomes infected. The septic wound "may initiate or activate processes that directly damage other organs,"[12] such as WBC aggregation and free radical release, complement activation, and immune complex formation. Newer research implicates the macrophage as a source of increased PGE$_2$ after injury, which has been shown to depress antigen processing and presentation.[86]

TUMOR NECROSIS FACTOR
Physiologic role

Tumor necrosis factor (TNF) is a monokine produced primarily by activated macrophages, particularly in response to microbial exposure. Also known as cachectin, TNF's isolation and characterization resulted from two distinct lines of investigation.[12] One group of investigators was attempting to characterize the substance that caused hemorrhagic necrosis of tumors when the patient was also septic (TNF); the other group was attempting to define the substance responsible for the wasting and cachexia commonly seen in patients with cancer or sepsis (cachectin). Beutler et al purified the substance in 1985.[87]

Although TNF is now considered to be the "major mediator of sepsis and MSOF," it does serve physiologic functions in the normal IIR. It enhances the phagocytic and killing activity of both neutrophils and macrophages, and may render tissue cells such as hepatocytes resistant to invasion, especially in parasitic infections.[88,89] TNF has also been shown to enhance lymphocyte activity and stimulate IL-1, PAF, and gamma-IFN release from various cells involved in the immune response. TNF induces fever and stimulates collagenase production, which leads to the tissue remodeling necessary for growth and repair of injured tissue. Because TNF suppresses lipoprotein lipase activity, fat uptake and storage are decreased and cachexia results.[87]

Impact on MSOF process

TNF mediates many of the toxic effects of endotoxin.[90,91] When isolated TNF is injected into *noninfected* laboratory animals, the animals exhibit many of the same signs and symptoms commonly found in sepsis and MSOF: hypotension, tachycardia, tachypnea, hyperglycemia, metabolic acidosis, fluid shifts, GI ischemia, and alveolar thickening.[92-94] Pharmacologic agents that inhibit TNF activity have been shown to attenuate some of these signs and symptoms.[95,96]

When the macrophage is activated by substances such as endotoxin, the macrophage releases TNF. The TNF not only affects local cells, but may enter the circulation and effect changes on distant organs and tissues not normally associated with a classic immune response.[83,93] Direct activities of TNF that contribute to organ dysfunction include stimulation of free radical release from neutrophils, endothelial damage, decreased vascular responsiveness to catecholamines, severe anorexia, increased capillary permeability, and other signs listed above.[97] Therefore endotoxin and other clinical conditions cause indirect damage by stimulating the macrophage to release TNF, which then causes the actual direct damage. Clinical research on sepsis has shown that patients with a positive TNF level have increased "Sepsis Severity Scores"[98] and a mortality rate twice that of TNF-negative patients.[99]

The discovery of more than 100 mediators (many of which initially serve a protective function) in the blood of patients with MSOF makes it very difficult to understand the intricate relationship between the various factors and also to know which factors to alter therapeutically.[100-102] At this point, TNF appears to be one of the primary mediators in initiating organ dysfunction and damage, either alone or in concert with other mediators such as interleukin-1.[12,103,104] Monoclonal antibodies specific for TNF and TNF receptors are currently under investigation and have been shown to decrease the incidence of shock in the septic state in laboratory animals.[95,105-107]

INTERLEUKIN-1
Physiologic role

Interleukins (IL) are another class of substances involved in signaling between cells of the immune response. They are numbered consecutively, and at the time of printing, 12 interleukins have been identified. IL-1 and IL-2 are the most well-known and documented in relation to MSOF pathology and clinical presentation.[108-111] Many functions of IL-1 and TNF overlap. Like TNF, IL-1 produces many beneficial effects in the IIR, but it has also been implicated in organ damage and failure.[103,110]

Macrophages and blood monocytes are a major source of IL-1, along with fibroblasts, natural killer (NK) cells, and damaged endothelium. The presence of thrombi or simple hemorrhage can also increase IL-1 release from the damaged endothelium. IL-1's protective effects include stimulation of both B-cell and T-cell activity (antibody production, mediator release) and proliferation and activation of macrophage and NK cells, and stimulation of hematopoiesis.[76,77] Production of acute phase reactants and an increase in adhesion of circulating WBCs to vascular endothelium are also seen.[75,110] IL-1 is necessary for fibroblast proliferation and wound healing and may play a role in linking the immune response to the neuroendocrine system.[112]

Impact on MSOF process

Increased cellular activation and release of IL-1 can lead to detrimental effects in the body. Isolated IL-1 inflicts cellular and tissue injury,[110] but more recent research focuses on its amplification of TNF activity and damage. Working in concert, TNF and IL-1 synergistically interact with numerous target cells and tissues.[76] Induction of procoagulant activity on the endothelium, decreased vascular responsiveness to catecholamines, increased muscle proteolysis,[113,114] and negative nitrogen balance have all been associated with IL-1 activity.[108,110,111,115] Once known as endogenous pyrogen, IL-1 also induces fever, which may or may not be helpful depending on the patient scenario. TNF and IL-1 may indirectly exacerbate vascular to tissue damage by causing increased neutrophil adhesion to the endothelium.[110,111] By-products of the neutrophil's respiratory burst and mediator release, such as free radicals and proteases, may then cause direct vascular damage or tissue damage.[45]

ARACHIDONIC ACID METABOLITES
Physiologic role

Arachidonic acid (eicosatetraenoic acid) is a fatty acid present in the phospholipid of most cell membranes except RBCs. Following stimulation

by catecholamines, neuroendocrine hormones, tissue injury, ischemia, hypoxemia, or endotoxin, phospholipase A_2 or C hydrolytically cleaves or liberates arachidonic acid (AA), which then enters the cyclooxygenase or lipoxygenase pathway within the cell (Fig. 3-8). The resulting metabolites of these two pathways are collectively known as eicosanoids, and they participate in many biologic activities (see box on p. 51). The three major eicosanoid classes are the prostaglandins and thromboxanes from the cyclooxygenase pathway and the leukotrienes from the lipoxygenase pathway.[116,117] The eicosanoids function in provision and regulation of the inflammatory response and have also been implicated in regulation of renal blood flow, initiation of labor, fever, and shock.[118]

Different eicosanoids are produced by the various tissues, and their actions are often antagonistic. PGI_2 (prostacyclin) causes vasodilatation and decreased platelet aggregation, while thromboxane A_2 causes vasoconstriction and increased platelet aggregation.[118] Eicosanoid functions overlap: PGE_1 and PGI_2 both cause vasodilatation; $PGF_{2\alpha}$ and TXA_2 both cause pulmonary hypertension. The specific eicosanoid generated is most likely determined by the cell type producing it, but other factors may lead to one or more being favored at a particular site.[117,119]

Impact on MSOF process

The eicosanoids have been implicated in many of the signs and symptoms of the septic state and MSOF, both systemically and in individual organs. Investigations into inhibition of the two pathways have shown attenuation of signs and symptoms associated with these two syndromes.[116,117,120] The most promising agents appear to be the nonsteroidal antiinflammatory agents such as ibuprofen and indomethacin, which inhibit the cyclooxygenase pathway.[121-123] Although the exact mechanism of action is yet to be established, improvements include decreased eicosanoid synthesis, inhibition of WBCs, and inhibition of free radical production.[124] Some of the vasodilatory prostaglandins (PGI_2 and PGE_1) have actually been infused to counteract pulmonary hypertension.[125,126] Along with pulmonary vasodilatation, an improvement in microcirculatory flow, inhibition of platelet aggregation, and improved oxygen delivery (DO_2) and oxygen consumption (VO_2) also occur.[126,127] Whether these effects will decrease the overall

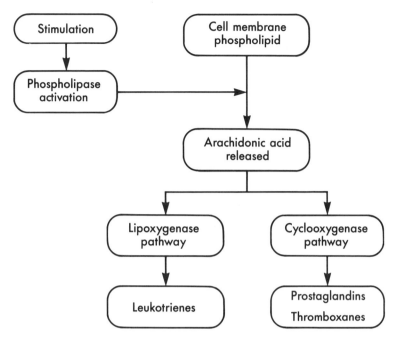

Fig. 3-8 Arachidonic acid metabolism.

BIOLOGIC TARGETS OF ARACHIDONIC ACID METABOLITES

Vasomotor tone
Microvascular permeability
Platelet aggregation
Macrophage/T-cell interaction
Temperature regulation
Cellular activation and mediator release
Bronchial smooth muscle tone

---

morbidity and mortality in ARDS and MSOF is yet to be seen.[128]

Eicosanoids play a role in shock, ischemia, ARDS, burn edema, reperfusion injury, and the redistribution of flow seen in the septic state.[117,129,130] Both cyclooxygenase and lipoxygenase products have been strongly implicated in the hemodynamic alterations and changes in lung mechanics that occur in ARDS.[116,131,132] Another interesting finding in lung injury shows a shift in the ratio of "good" eicosanoid to "bad" eicosanoid.

In ARDS, there is a decrease in prostacyclin and an increase in thromboxane A_2, leading to vasoconstriction and platelet aggregation.[133] Eicosanoids have also been implicated in dysfunction in other organs such as the kidneys. See specific organ chapters in Section Three for further information. Through their proplatelet activity, eicosanoids can enhance platelet aggregation, microembolization, and endothelial damage. Concomitant vasoconstriction can potentiate ischemia, further hindering blood flow to the organ bed.

PROTEOLYTIC ENZYMES
Physiologic role

Following activation, many phagocytic cells release proteolytic enzymes (proteases). The enzymes' ability to digest bacteria and other foreign protein matter makes them a necessary part of the IIR and wound healing.[15] Proteases also serve as enzymatic catalysts in the four enzyme cascades: complement, kallikrein/kinin, coagulation, and fibrinolysis.[45,134] Two common proteases under investigation are collagenase and elastase.

Impact on MSOF process

Collagenase and elastase degrade the collagen and elastin found in blood vessels, leading to vascular damage and remodeling. Free radicals enhance the destructive capabilities of the proteases, because the free radicals damage enzymes (such as alpha$_1$-protease inhibitor) that normally inactivate the proteases.[45,134] Vascular permeability increases with resultant tissue edema.

The proteases not only attack vascular structures but extracellular tissue matrix as well.[100,135] Direct parenchymal damage occurs to the organs (in addition to the existing ischemia and altered microvascular perfusion) as the proteases actually digest tissue walls.[45] Further inflammation is incited, and the vicious cycle continues. One severe example of this concerns the premature activation of proteolytic enzymes in the pancreas, which are ultimately formed for digestion. Premature activation leads to extensive tissue damage in the body of the pancreas itself, setting up the intense inflammation seen in pancreatitis (see Chapter 14). It is important to note that inflammation can occur without the presence of microorganisms.[136] Proteases play a significant role in this "aseptic inflammation" secondary to their tissue-damaging capabilities.

PLATELET ACTIVATING FACTOR
Physiologic role

Platelet activating factor (PAF) is a lipid mediator produced from the cell membrane of many different cells of the IIR, including mast cells, basophils, monocytes, macrophages, neutrophils, and damaged endothelium following phospholipase A$_2$ activation.[137] Once in the circulation, PAF triggers platelet activation and morphologic changes that increase the platelet's ability to aggregate. PAF also promotes neutrophil adhesion and stimulates their respiratory burst and degranulation (release of free radicals and digestive enzymes). Increased vascular permeability and vasomotor changes have also been associated with PAF release.[138]

Impact on MSOF process

Because excessive platelet activation leads to increased endothelial damage and clot formation, increased levels of PAF are ultimately dangerous for the host, especially if the PAF leaves the localized area of injury and circulates further downstream. Microcirculatory abnormalities caused by platelet plugs and vasoconstriction contribute to further tissue ischemia and necrosis. PAF may exacerbate preexisting coagulopathies such as DIC.[138,139] PAF has also been shown to induce the release of leukotrienes and free radicals from neutrophils. The combination of PAF, TNF, and endothelial damage contributes to the tissue destruction seen in MSOF.[104,139] In animal studies, PAF has also induced hypotension, myocardial depression, decreased coronary artery flow, vascular changes, renal dysfunction, metabolic acidosis, bronchoconstriction, and thrombocytopenia.[137,140-144]

CONCLUSION
Intrinsic control: function and failure

It is painfully evident that numerous pathways are not only operating in MSOF, but their activities are interdependent and often synergistic in effect: vasodilatation, vasoconstriction, endothelial damage, microvascular permeability, tissue edema, fibrin deposition, leukocyte aggregation, vascular obstruction, and metabolic derangements. The pathways continually activate themselves and each other. Their synergistic effects contribute to the pathophysiology of MSOF and combine to initiate and maintain maldistribution of circulating volume, oxygen supply and demand imbalances, and metabolic abnormalities.[76,101,145,146]

Not only is activation overwhelming, but inhibitory pathways may not be effective, leading to the uncontrolled, devastating responses of septic shock, tissue damage, and MSOF. This failure of inhibition is as significant as overwhelming activation.[13,45] Malignant intravascular inflammation is the term Pinsky and Matuschak[82,147] coined to describe what many now think to be the final common pathway in the journey to MSOF.[4,82,117,148]

When does the IIR cease to become protective and move to a malignant, uncontrolled state? What is protective in one clinical situation seems to be destructive in another setting. How can there be immunosuppression leading to sepsis and overwhelming inflammation leading to septic shock and MSOF in the same patient? Are they not antagonistic? Many research efforts are currently examining these questions, and a major focus of research is on modulating this uncontrolled response. The difficulty comes in suppressing the uncontrolled response without hindering the physiologic response necessary for protection and tissue repair.

REFERENCES

1. Baue AE. Multiple, progressive, or sequential systems failure: A syndrome of the 1970s. Arch Surg 1975;110:779-781.
2. DeCamp MM, Demling RH. Posttraumatic multisystem organ failure. JAMA 1988;260:530-534.
3. Fry DE. Multiple system organ failure. Surg Clin North Am 1988;68:107-122.
4. Goris RJ. Multiple organ failure: Whole body inflammation? Schweiz Med Wochenschr 1989;119:347-353.
5. Hotter AN. The pathophysiology of multi-system organ failure in the trauma patient. Clin Issues Crit Care Nurs 1990;1:465-478.
6. Huddleston VB. Multisystem organ failure. In: Mims BC, ed. Case studies in critical care nursing. Baltimore: Williams & Wilkins; 1990:494-499.
7. Cunnion RE, Parrillo JE. Myocardial dysfunction in sepsis. Crit Care Clin 1989;5:99-118.
8. Bersten A, Sibbald WJ. Circulatory disturbances in multiple systems organ failure. Crit Care Clin 1989;5:233-254.
9. Dantzker D. Oxygen delivery and utilization in sepsis. Crit Care Clin 1989;5:81-98.
10. Barton R, Cerra FB. The hypermetabolism multiple organ failure syndrome. Chest 1989;96:1153-1160.
11. Gutierrez G, Lund N, Bryan-Brown CW. Cellular oxygen utilization during multiple organ failure. Crit Care Clin 1989;5:271-288.
12. Baue AE. Multiple organ failure: patient care and prevention. St. Louis: Mosby–Year Book; 1990.
13. Yurt RW, Lowry SF. Role of the macrophage and endogenous mediators in multiple organ failure. In: Deitch EA, ed. Multiple organ failure: Pathophysiology and basic concepts of therapy. New York: Thieme Medical Publishers; 1990:60-71.
14. Ryan US, ed. Pulmonary endothelium in health and disease. New York: Marcel Dekker; 1987.
15. Guyton AC. Textbook of medical physiology. 8th ed. Philadelphia: WB Saunders; 1991.
16. Thibodeau GA. The circulatory system: Cardiovascular and lymphatic subdivisions. In: Thibodeau GA ed. Structure and function of the body. 9th ed. St. Louis: Mosby–Year Book; 1992.
17. Majno G, Shea S, Leventhal M. Endothelial contraction induced by histamine type mediators: An electron microscopic study. J Cell Biol 1969;42:647-672.
18. Male D, Roitt I. Adaptive and innate immunity. In: Roitt I, Brostoff J, Male D, eds. Immunology. 2nd ed. London: Gower Medical Publishing; 1989:1.1-1.10.
19. Gimbrone MA, ed. Vascular endothelium in hemostasis and thrombosis. New York: Churchill Livingstone; 1986.
20. Müller-Berghaus G. Septicemia and the vessel wall. In: Verstraete M, Vermylen J, Lijnen R, Arnout J, eds. Thrombosis and haemostasis. Leuven, Belgium: Leuven University Press; 1987:619-671.
21. Müller-Berghaus G. Pathophysiologic and biochemical events in disseminated intravascular coagulation: Dysregulation of procoagulant and anticoagulant pathways. Semin Thromb Hemost 1989;15:58-87.
22. Meyrick B, Johnson JE, Brigham KL. Endotoxin-induced pulmonary endothelial injury. Prog Clin Biol Res: Second Vienna Shock Forum 1989;308:91-100.
23. Freudenberg N. Reaction of the vascular intima to endotoxin shock. Prog Clin Biol Res: Second Vienna Shock Forum 1989;308:77-89.
24. Del Vecchio PJ, Malik AB. Thrombin-induced neutrophil adhesion. Prog Clin Biol Res: Second Vienna Shock Forum 1989;308:101-112.
25. Bevilacqua MP, Gimbrone MA. Inducible endothelial functions in inflammation and coagulation. Semin Thromb Hemost 1988;13:425-433.
26. Gidlof A, Lewis DH. Do endotoxinemia and sepsis impair the regulatory functions of capillary endothelial cells. Prog Clin Biol Res: Second Vienna Shock Forum 1989;308:157-162.
27. Bach RR. Initiation of coagulation by tissue factor. Crit Rev Biochem 1988;23:339-368.
28. McGee MP et al. Tissue factor and factor VII messenger RNAs in human alveolar macrophages: Effects of breathing ozone. Blood 1990;75:122-127.
29. Lyberg T et al. Procoagulant (thromboplastin) activity in human bronchoalveolar lavage fluids is derived from alveolar macrophages. Eur Respir J 1990;3:61-67.
30. Walport M. Complement. In: Roitt I, Brostoff J, Male D, eds. Immunology. 2nd ed. London: Gower Medical Publishing; 1989:13.1-13.16.
31. Hood LE et al. Immune effector mechanisms and the complement system. In: Hood LE, Weissman IL, Wood WB, Wilson JH. Immunology. 2nd ed. Menlo Park, CA: Benjamin/Cummings Publishing Co; 1984:334-365.
32. Rook G. Immunity to viruses, bacteria and fungi. In: Roitt I, Brostoff J, Male D, eds. Immunology. 2nd ed. London: Gower Medical Publishing; 1989:16.1-16.16.
33. Zimmerman T et al. The role of the complement system in the pathogenesis of multiple organ failure in shock. Prog Clin Biol Res: Second Vienna Shock Forum 1989;308:291-298.
34. Roxvall L, Bengtson A, Heideman M. Anaphylatoxin generation and multisystem organ failure in acute pancreatitis. J Surg Res 1989;47:138-143.
35. Bengtson A, Heideman M. Anaphylatoxin formation in sepsis. Arch Surg 1988;123:645-649.
36. Langlois PF et al. Accentuated complement activation in patient plasma during the adult respiratory distress syndrome: A potential mechanism for pulmonary inflammation. Heart Lung 1989;18:71-84.
37. Schirmer WJ et al. Complement activation in peritonitis: Association with hepatic and renal perfusion abnormalities. Am Surg 1987;53:683-687.
38. Schirmer WJ et al. Systemic complement activation produces hemodynamic changes characteristic of sepsis. Arch Surg 1988;123:316-321.
39. Steward M, Male D. Immunological techniques. In: Roitt I, Brostoff J, Male D, eds. Immunology. 2nd ed. London: Gower Medical Publishing; 1989:25.1-25.3.
40. Mullins RJ, Malias MA, Hudgens RW. Isoproterenol inhibits the increase in microvascular membrane permeability produced by bradykinin. J Trauma 1989;29:1053-1063.
41. Carmines PK, Fleming JT. Control of the renal microvasculature by vasoactive peptides. FASEB J 1990;4:3300-3309.
42. Ichinose M, Barnes PJ. Bradykinin-induced airway microvascular leakage and bronchoconstriction are mediated via a bradykinin B2 receptor. Am Rev Respir Dis 1990;142:1104-1107.
43. Kaplan AP, Silverberg M. The coagulation-kinin pathway of human plasma. Blood 1987;70:1-15.
44. Hesselvik JF et al. Coagulation, fibrinolysis, and kallikrein systems in sepsis: Relation to outcome. Crit Care Med 1989;17:724-733.

45. Weiss SJ. Tissue destruction by neutrophils. N Engl J Med 1989;320:365-376.

46. Barrett JT. Textbook of immunology: An introduction to immunochemistry and immunobiology. 5th ed. St. Louis: Mosby–Year Book; 1988.

47. Southern PA, Powis G. Free radicals in medicine. II. Involvement in human disease. Mayo Clin Proc 1988;63:390-408.

48. Vedder NB et al. Neutrophil-mediated vascular injury in shock and multiple organ failure. Prog Clin Biol Res: Persp Shock Res 1989;299:181-192.

49. Wasil M et al. The antioxidant action of human extracellular fluids: Effect of human serum and its protein components on the inactivation of alpha-1-antiproteinase by hypochlorous acid and by hydrogen peroxide. Biochem J 1987;243:219-223.

50. Hubbard RC et al. Oxidants spontaneously released by alveolar macrophages of cigarette smokers can inactivate the active site of alpha 1-antitrypsin, rendering it ineffective as an inhibitor of neutrophil elastase. J Clin Invest 1987;80:1289-1295.

51. Brigham KL, Meyrick B. Interactions of granulocytes with lungs. Circ Res 1984;54:623-635.

52. Heflin C, Brigham KL. Granulocyte depletion prevents increased lung vascular permeability after endotoxemia in sheep. Clin Res 1979;27:399A.

53. Tate RM et al. Oxygen radical-induced pulmonary edema: A mechanism for the production of non-cardiogenic pulmonary edema by neutrophils. Chest 1982;81:57S-59S.

54. Burchardi H et al. Neutrophil stimulation by PMA increases alveolar permeability in rabbits. Prog Clin Biol Res: Second Vienna Shock Forum 1989;308:323-330.

55. Rivkind AI et al. Sequential patterns of eicosanoid, platelet, and neutrophil interactions in the evolution of the fulminant post-traumatic adult respiratory distress syndrome. Ann Surg 1989;201:355-372.

56. Ognibene FP et al. Adult respiratory distress syndrome in patients with severe neutropenia. N Engl J Med 1986;315:547-551.

57. Mallick AA et al. Multiple organ damage caused by tumor necrosis factor and prevented by prior neutrophil depletion. Chest 1989;95:1114-1120.

58. Perkett EA, Brigham KL, Meyrick B. Granulocyte depletion attenuates sustained pulmonary hypertension and increased pulmonary vasoreactivity caused by continuous air embolization in sheep. Am Rev Respir Dis 1990;141:456-465.

59. Bersten A, Sibbald WJ. Acute lung injury in septic shock. Crit Care Clin 1989;5:49-80.

60. Black L, Coombs VJ, Townsend SN. Reperfusion and reperfusion injury in acute myocardial infarction. Heart Lung 1990;19:274-286.

61. Nelson K, Herndon B, Reisz G. Pulmonary effects of ischemic limb reperfusion: Evidence for a role of oxygen-derived radicals. Crit Care Med 1991;19:360-363.

62. Kloner RA, Przyklenk K, Patel B. Altered myocardial states: The stunned and hibernating myocardium. Am J Med 1989;86(suppl 1A):14-22.

63. Brigham KL. Role of free radicals in lung injury. Chest 1986;89:859-863.

64. Mullane KM, Salmon JA, Kraemer R. Leukocyte-derived metabolites of arachidonic acid in ischemia-induced myocardial injury. Fed Proc 1987;46:2422-2433.

65. Dormandy TL. Free-radical pathology and medicine. J R Coll Physicians Lond 1989;23:221-227.

66. van der Kraaij AMM et al. Lipid peroxidation and its significance for postischemic cardiovascular injury. Prog Clin Biol Res 1989;301:61-72.

67. Machiedo GW et al. The incidence of decreased red blood cell deformability in sepsis and the association with oxygen free radical damage and multiple-system organ failure. Arch Surg 1989;124:1386-1389.

68. Brigham KL. Oxidant stress and adult respiratory distress syndrome. Eur Respir J 1990;3(suppl 11):482s-484s.

69. Werns SW, Lucchesi BR. Leukocytes, oxygen radicals, and myocardial injury due to ischemia and reperfusion. Free Rad Biol Med 1988;4:31-37.

70. Kloner RA, Przyklenk K, Whittaker P. Deleterious effects of oxygen radicals in ischemia/reperfusion: Resolved and unresolved issues. Circulation 1989;80:1115-1127.

71. Demling RH, LaLonde C. Identification and modifications of the pulmonary and systemic inflammatory and biochemical changes caused by skin burn. J Trauma 1990;30(12 suppl):S57-S62.

72. Demling RH, LaLonde C. Early postburn lipid peroxidation: Effect of ibuprofen and allopurinol. Surgery 1990;107:85-93.

73. Lydyard P, Grossi C. Cells involved in the immune response. In: Roitt I, Brostoff J, Male D, eds. Immunology. 2nd ed. London: Gower Medical Publishing; 1989:2.1-2.18.

74. Brostoff J, Hale T. Hypersensitivity-Type I. In: Roitt I, Brostoff J, Male D, eds. Immunology. 2nd ed. London: Gower Medical Publishing; 1989:19.1-19.20.

75. Feldmann M, Male D. Cell cooperation in the immune response. In: Roitt I, Brostoff J, Male D, eds. Immunology. 2nd ed. London: Gower Medical Publishing; 1989:8.1-8.12.

76. Tracey KJ, Lowry SF. The role of cytokine mediators in septic shock. Adv Surg 1990;23:21-56.

77. Jelinek DF, Lipsky PE. Enhancement of human B cell proliferation and differentiation by tumor necrosis factor-alpha and interleukin 1. J Immunol 1987;139:2970-2976.

78. Ford HR et al. Characterization of wound cytokines in the sponge matrix model. Arch Surg 1989;124:1422-1428.

79. Cerra FB et al. Hypermetabolism/organ failure: The role of the activated macrophage as a metabolic regulator. Prog Clin Biol Res 1988;264:27-42.

80. Border JR. Hypothesis: Sepsis, multiple systems organ failure, and the macrophage. Arch Surg 1988;123:285-286.

81. Lazarou SA et al. The wound is a possible source of post-traumatic immunosuppression. Arch Surg 1989;124:1429-1431.

82. Pinsky MR, Matuschak GM. Multiple systems organ failure: Failure of host defense homeostasis. Crit Care Clin 1989;5:199-220.

83. Simpson SQ, Casey LC. Role of tumor necrosis factor in sepsis and acute lung injury. Crit Care Clin 1989;5:27-48.

84. Demling RH. Wound inflammatory mediators and multisystem organ failure. Prog Clin Biol Res 1987;236A:525-537.

85. Knighton DR, Riegel VD. The macrophages: Effector cell in wound repair. Prog Clin Biol Res: Perspectives in Shock Research 1989;299:217-226.

86. Faist E et al. Mediators and the trauma induced cascade of immunologic defects. Prog Clin Biol Res: Second Vienna Shock Forum 1989;308:495-506.

87. Beutler B et al. Purification of cachectin, a lipoprotein lipase-suppressing hormone secreted by endotoxin-induced RAW 264.7 cells. J Exp Med 1985;161:984-995.
88. Taverne J. Immunity to protozoa and worms. In: Roitt I, Brostoff J, Male D, eds. Immunology. 2nd ed. London: Gower Medical Publishing; 1989:17.1-17.21.
89. Beutler B, Cerami A. Cachectin (tumor necrosis factor): A macrophage hormone governing cellular metabolism and inflammatory response. Endocr Rev 1988;9:57-66.
90. Cerami A, Beutler B. The role of cachectin/TNF in endotoxic shock and cachexia. Immunol Today 1988;9:28-31.
91. Beutler B. Cachectin in tissue injury, shock, and related states. Crit Care Clin 1989;5:353-368.
92. Tracey KJ et al. Shock and tissue injury induced by recombinant human cachectin. Science 1986;234:470-474.
93. Schirmer WJ, Schirmer JM, Fry DE. Recombinant human tumor necrosis factor produces hemodynamic changes characteristic of sepsis and endotoxemia. Arch Surg 1989;124:445-448.
94. Johnson J et al. Human recombinant tumor necrosis factor alpha infusion mimics endotoxemia in awake sheep. J Appl Physiol 1989;66:1448-1454.
95. Tracey KJ et al. Anticachectin/TNF monoclonal antibodies prevent shock during lethal bacteraemia. Nature 1987;330:662-665.
96. Evans DA et al. The effects of tumor necrosis factor and their selective inhibition by ibuprofen. Ann Surg 1989;209:312-321.
97. Stephens KE et al. Tumor necrosis factor causes increased pulmonary permeability and edema. Comparison to septic acute lung injury. Am Rev Respir Dis 1988;137:1364-1370.
98. Damas P et al. Tumor necrosis factor and interleukin-1 serum levels during severe sepsis in humans. Crit Care Med 1989;17:975-978.
99. Debets JM et al. Plama tumor necrosis factor and mortality in critically ill septic patients. Crit Care Med 1989;17:489-494.
100. Jochum M et al. Posttraumatic plasma levels of mediators of organ failure. Prog Clin Biol Res: Second Vienna Shock Forum 1989;308:673-681.
101. Schlag G, Redl H, eds. Pathophysiologic role of mediators and mediator inhibitors in shock. Prog Clin Biol Res: First Vienna Shock Forum 1987;236A.
102. Neugebauer E et al. Mediators in septic shock: Strategies of securing them and assessment of their causal significance. Chirurg 1987;58:470-481.
103. Jacobs RF, Tabor DR. Immune cellular interactions during sepsis and septic injury. Crit Care Clin 1989;5:9-26.
104. Camussi G et al. Tumor necrosis factor/cachectin stimulates peritoneal macrophages, polymorphonuclear neutrophils, and vascular endothelial cells to synthesize and release platelet-activating factor. J Exp Med 1987;166:1390-1404.
105. Hinshaw LB et al. Survival of primates in LD100 septic shock following therapy with antibody to tumor necrosis factor (TNF alpha). Circ Shock 1990;30:279-292.
106. Shalaby MR et al. Binding and regulation of cellular functions by monoclonal antibodies against human tumor necrosis factor receptors. J Exp Med 1990;172:1517-1520.
107. Espevik T et al. Characterization of binding and biological effects of monoclonal antibodies against a human tumor necrosis factor receptor. J Exp Med 1990;171:415-426.
108. Dinarello CA. Interleukin-1. Rev Infect Dis 1984;6:55-95.
109. Dinarello CA. An update on human interleukin-1: From molecular biology to clinical relevance. J Clin Immunol 1985;5:287-297.
110. Dinarello CA. Biology of interleukin 1. FASEB J 1988;2:108-115.
111. Kampschmidt RF. The numerous postulated biological manifestations of interleukin-1. J Leuk Biol 1984;36:341-355.
112. Bernton EW et al. Release of multiple hormones by a direct action of interleukin-1 on pituitary cells. Science 1987;238:519-521.
113. Baracos V et al. Stimulation of muscle protein degradation and prostaglandin E2 release by leukocytic pyrogen (interleukin-1). N Engl J Med 1983;308:553-558.
114. Cozzolino F et al. Potential role of interleukin-1 as the trigger for diffuse intravascular coagulation in acute nonlymphoblastic leukemia. Am J Med 1988;84:240-250.
115. Dinarello CA et al. Multiple biological activities of human recombinant interleukin-1. J Clin Invest 1986;77:1734-1739.
116. Sprague RS et al. Proposed role for leukotrienes in the pathophysiology of multiple systems organ failure. Crit Care Clin 1989;5:315-330.
117. Petrak RA, Balk RA, Bone RC. Prostaglandins, cyclooxygenase inhibitors, and thromboxane synthetase inhibitors in the pathogenesis of multiple systems organ failure. Crit Care Clin 1989;5:302-314.
118. Ogletree ML. Overview of physiological and pathophysiological effects of thromboxane A2. Fed Proc 1987;46:133-138.
119. Ninnemann JL. Prostaglandins, leukotrienes, and the immune response. New York: Cambridge University Press; 1988.
120. Brigham KL. Conference summary: Lipid mediators in the pulmonary circulation. Am Rev Respir Dis 1987;136:785-788.
121. Byrne K et al. Increased survival time after delayed histamine and prostaglandin blockade in a porcine model of severe sepsis-induced lung injury. Crit Care Med 1990;18:303-308.
122. Waymack JP. The effect of ibuprofen on postburn metabolic and immunologic function. J Surg Res 1989;46:172-176.
123. Bernard GR et al. Prostacyclin and thromboxane A2 formation is increased in human sepsis syndrome: Effects of cyclooxygenase inhibition. Am Rev Respir Dis 1991;144:1095-1101.
124. Rockwell WB, Ehrlich HP. Ibuprofen in acute-care therapy. Ann Surg 1990;211:78-83.
125. Demling RH et al. The effect of prostacyclin infusion on endotoxin-induced lung injury. Surgery 1981;89:257-263.
126. Bihari DJ, Tinker J. The therapeutic value of vasodilatory prostaglandins in multiple organ failure associated with sepsis. Intens Care Med 1988;15:2-7.
127. Silverman HJ et al. Effects of prostaglandin E1 on oxygen delivery and consumption in patients with the adult respiratory distress syndrome: Results from the prostaglandin E1 multicenter trial. Chest 1990;98:405-410.
128. Russell JA, Ronco JJ, Dodek PM. Physiologic effects and side-effects of prostaglandin E1 in adult respiratory distress syndrome. Chest 1990;97:684-692.
129. Mullane K et al. Myocardial salvage induced by REV-5901: An inhibitor and antagonist of the leukotrienes. J Cardiovasc Pharmacol 1987;10:398-406.
130. Brigham KL, Sheller JR. Leukotrienes and ARDS. Intens Care Med 1989;15:422-423.
131. Bernard GR et al. Sulfidopeptide leukotrienes in ARDS. Am Rev Respir Dis 1991;144:263-267.

132. Snapper JR et al. Effects of cyclooxygenase inhibitors on the alterations in lung mechanics caused by endotoxemia in the unanesthetized sheep. J Clin Invest 1983;72:63-76.

133. Yellin SA et al. Prostacyclin and thromboxane A2 in septic shock: Species differences. Circ Shock 1986;20:291-297.

134. Neuhof H et al. Proteases as mediators of pulmonary vascular permeability. Prog Clin Biol Res: Second Vienna Shock Forum 1989;308:305-314.

135. Lang H, Fritz H. The role of phagocytic proteinases in the pathobiochemistry of inflammation. Adv Clin Enzymol 1986;3:168-178.

136. van Bebber IPT et al. Endotoxin does not play a key role in the pathogenesis of multiple organ failure: An experimental study. Prog Clin Biol Res: Second Vienna Shock Forum 1989;308:419-423.

137. Lefer AM. Induction of tissue injury and altered cardiovascular performance by platelet-activating factor: Relevance to multiple systems organ failure. Crit Care Clin 1989;5:331-352.

138. Braquet P, Hosford D. The potential role of platelet-activating factor (PAF) in shock, sepsis and adult respiratory distress syndrome (ARDS). Prog Clin Biol Res: Second Vienna Shock Forum 1989;308:425-439.

139. Bonavida B et al. The involvement of platelet-activating factor (PAF)-induced monocyte activation and tumor necrosis factor (TNF) production in shock. Prog Clin Biol Res: Second Vienna Shock Forum 1989;308:485-489.

140. Vargaftig BB et al. Platelet-activating factor induces a platelet-dependent bronchoconstriction unrelated to the formation of prostaglandin derivatives. Eur J Pharmacol 1980;65:185-192.

141. Kenzora JL et al. Effects of acetyl glyceryl ether phosphorylcholine (platelet-activating factor) on ventricular preload, afterload and contractility in dogs. J Clin Invest 1984;74:1193-1203.

142. Bessin P et al. Acute circulatory collapse caused by platelet-activating factor (PAF) in dogs. Eur J Pharmacol 1983;86:403-413.

143. Handley DA et al. Evaluation of dose and route effects of platelet activating factor–induced extravasation in the guinea-pig. Thromb Haemost 1984;52:34-46.

144. Sybertz EJ et al. Cardiac, coronary and peripheral vascular effects of acetyl glyceryl ether phosphorylcholine in anesthetized dogs. J Pharmacol Exp Ther 1985;232:156-162.

145. Huddleston VB. Multisystem organ failure: A pathophysiologic approach. Boston, 1991.

146. Schlag G, Redl H. Mediators in trauma. Acta Anaesthesiolog Belg 1987;38:281-291.

147. Pinsky MR. Multiple systems organ failure: Malignant intravascular inflammation. Crit Care Clin 1989;5:195-198.

148. Darling GE et al. Multiorgan failure in critically ill patients. Can J Surg 1988;31:172-176.

4 Coagulation and Disseminated Intravascular Coagulation

Tally N. Bell

MSOF is a significant threat to maintaining normal hemostatic function in the critically ill. Although hemostatic alterations commonly occur in severe disease or injury, they further insult the already compromised MSOF patient. The appearance of disseminated intravascular coagulation (DIC) is a potentially life-threatening condition that results from the physiologic disequilibrium in MSOF as it affects the hematologic system. Although end-organ failure of the hematologic system can manifest as DIC, more likely the development of DIC can be attributed to dysfunction of the complex physiologic interactions occurring among organ systems and the inflammatory/immune response. The purpose of this chapter is to review normal hemostatic mechanisms and the alterations that occur in these mechanisms during DIC, to explore the relationship of DIC and MSOF, to examine diagnostic and clinical assessment parameters, and to identify current therapeutic interventions and management of the critically ill MSOF patient with DIC.

DIC is an acquired coagulopathy that has been previously described in the literature by a variety of names, including defibrination syndrome, diffuse intravascular clotting, consumptive coagulopathy, and intravascular clotting syndrome.[1-3] It never occurs as a primary disorder, but arises as an intermediary mechanism of disease in numerous underlying conditions.[4,5] DIC is reported to occur in one of every 900 to 2400 adult admissions in large urban hospitals.[6] Depending on the patient's primary disorder, the mortality rate in DIC is estimated at 50% to 80%.[7] In patients with shock and infection as precipitating factors, the mortality rate can approach 90%.[7]

Feinstein defines DIC as "a dynamic pathologic process triggered by activation of the clotting cascade with the resultant activation of excess thrombin within the vascular system that leads to further activation of the coagulation system, shortened survival of certain hemostatic elements, deposition of fibrin in the microcirculation, and activation of the fibrinolytic system."[8] Paradoxically, this pathologic overstimulation of normal hemostasis produces a unique clinical situation where the patient simultaneously develops microvascular thrombi and hemorrhage.

Clinically, DIC can occur as an acute or chronic, generalized or localized process that is triggered by acute or chronic underlying disease states. DIC is "disseminated" in that it involves all aspects of coagulation. Because coagulation is a systemic phenomenon, DIC can potentially affect all organ systems and produce multiple organ failures. Acute, generalized DIC occurs more frequently in the critical care setting and is the focus of this chapter.

NORMAL HEMOSTATIC MECHANISMS

Hemostasis is defined as the arrest of hemorrhage at the site of injury.[9] Normal hemostasis represents the outcome of integrated interactions among blood vessels, platelets, coagulation proteins, and the fibrinolytic system. When physical and/or chemical derangements occur in these interactions, the stage is set for untoward bleeding and/or inappropriate clotting.

The vascular endothelium plays a significant role in hemostasis. In its normal, intact state, the endothelial lining of the blood vessels provides a nonthrombogenic, nonadherent surface that prevents coagulation and maintains blood fluidity[10,11]; however, damaged or excited endothelial cells exhibit properties that are thrombogenic.[1,12] The endothelium is important in both normal physiologic and pathophysiologic processes, and its dynamic role is integrated throughout this section.

Vasoconstriction

When the integrity of a blood vessel is interrupted by rupture or incision, the blood vessel immediately goes into vasospasm, and adjacent blood vessels constrict as a result of sympathetic nervous system activation.[13] The initiation of this response is not well understood; however, it appears that multiple factors including serotonin, the alpha-adrenergic system, thromboxane A_2 (TXA_2), and endothelin may contribute to the vasoconstrictive response.[9,12] Vasoconstriction promotes hemostasis by narrowing the blood vessel lumen and mechanically limiting blood flow at the site of injury.

The greater the extent of vessel trauma, the greater the extent of vasospasm. A crushing injury to a blood vessel produces more vascular spasm in that vessel than in one that has been cut.[14] Vasoconstriction contributes to hemostasis in the capillary bed, but alone it is insufficient to stop bleeding in larger vessels.[12,15] However, when larger blood vessels, particularly arteries, are traumatized, vasoconstriction is a critical event to prevent exsanguination.[1]

Platelet plug formation

Platelets do not adhere to intact endothelium. Endothelial cells secrete the prostaglandin called prostacyclin (PGI_2), a potent vasodilator that strongly inhibits platelet function.[9,11,16] However, when the endothelial lining of the blood vessel is disrupted and the subendothelial collagen of the basement membrane is exposed, the platelet reaction begins within seconds. This reaction initiates the formation of a platelet plug, an important step in hemostasis. When large vessels are damaged and vasoconstriction alone is ineffective to achieve hemostasis, platelet plug formation provides an essential element to slow blood loss.[15] As with vasoconstriction, platelet plug formation, in isolation, is insufficient to stop bleeding from major vessels.[16]

Shape change. Normal platelets at rest are disk-shaped and show little affinity toward one another

or normal endothelial cells.[16] However, when platelet activation is triggered by endothelial disruption, drastic platelet shape changes occur. Stimulated platelets rapidly become swollen and develop a spherical shape with numerous hairline projections, known as pseudopods or filopodia, protruding from their surfaces. The shape change serves two important functions in the hemostatic process: it increases the surface area for adhesion, and it increases the likelihood of platelet aggregation.[17,18]

Platelet release reaction. During the shape change, the alpha-granules and dense-granules become centrally located within the platelet.[16,18] In the platelet release reaction that follows, the contents of the alpha-granules and dense-granules are discharged outside the platelet for use in coagulation and blood vessel repair. Adenosine diphosphate (ADP) is released from the dense-granules and initiates platelet aggregation.[7,15] The alpha-granules release fibrinogen, factor V, factor VIII/von Willebrand factor, and thrombospondin.[18,19] During the release reaction, TXA_2 is extruded, as well as a platelet surface procoagulant that stimulates formation of a fibrin clot.[16] TXA_2 has potent vasoconstrictive properties and promotes platelet aggregation.[7,18]

Platelet aggregation. Platelet aggregation is essential for platelet plug formation. As platelet activation occurs, the platelets become sticky and, in the presence of von Willebrand factor, begin to adhere to one another and to the exposed collagen that underlies the damaged endothelium. Endothelial cells synthesize and secrete von Willebrand factor, thrombospondin, and fibronectin, all of which act as adhesion proteins for platelets.[10] Fibrinogen also must be present for platelet aggregation to occur.[16]

The liberated ADP and TXA_2 from the release reaction activate more platelets, which undergo the same shape and chemical changes. These platelets recruit more platelets until the platelet aggregate grows large enough to effectively plug the damaged blood vessel.[16,20] Investigators postulate that the balance between the opposing actions of PGI_2 and TXA_2 regulates the growth of the platelet plug.[18]

The resultant platelet plug is unstable and loosely formed, but it is usually successful in sealing small vascular disruptions to prevent blood loss. Over the next few hours, the aggregated platelets consolidate and lose their individual identities. Primary hemostasis concludes with the formation of the platelet plug. As the hemostatic process continues, a solid, nonsoluble fibrin clot enmeshes itself in the foundation of the platelet plug.

Role in fibrin formation. Although platelets are important in hemostatic plug formation, they are also critical in subsequent steps of the coagulation cascade. Within their cytoplasm, platelets contain an important protein, known as fibrin-stabilizing factor, which is essential for forming a stable fibrin clot. Platelet factor 3 (PF3), secreted by activated platelets during the aggregation phase, participates in reactions of the intrinsic clotting cascade. Additionally, platelets that have undergone the release reaction are more potent than dormant platelets and demonstrate greater effectiveness in clotting cascade reactions.[16]

Clotting cascade

Secondary hemostasis begins with activation of the clotting cascade. The clotting cascade involves the sequential release and activation of clotting factors. As each reaction occurs, it produces a subsequent reaction in a cascade effect. Clotting cascade activation leads to the formation of thrombin and eventually to fibrin clot formation. Clotting factors are essential components of the clotting cascade and are consumed during the process of coagulation (Table 4-1).

The liver is the primary site for biosynthesis of the plasma clotting factors with the probable exception of factor VIII.[1,16] Factor VIII is synthesized from hepatic sinusoidal endothelial cells and megakaryocytes, as well as from mononuclear cells in the spleen, kidney, lungs, and lymph nodes.[16,18] The biosynthesis of factors II, VII, IX, and X requires vitamin K. Although production of these factors continues in the absence of vitamin K, the final step in biosynthesis cannot proceed in its absence, thus rendering these factors nonfunctional.[16,21] Vitamin K also is required for the production of two anticoagulant proteins—protein C and protein S.[16,21]

When clotting cascade activation occurs, coagulation can proceed along two different pathways—the intrinsic pathway and the extrinsic pathway. Depending on the trigger that initiates the coagulation activity, one or both of the pathways can be involved. Although these pathways are stimulated differently and proceed differently, throm-

Table 4-1   Clotting Factors

Clotting factor	Name(s)
I	Fibrinogen
II	Prothrombin
III	Tissue factor, thromboplastin
IV	Calcium
V	Proaccelerin, labile factor, accelerator globulin (AcG)
VI	Not assigned
VII	Proconvertin, serum prothrombin conversion accelerator (SPCA), autoprothrombin I
VIII	Antihemophilic factor (AHF), antihemophilic globulin (AHG)
IX	Christmas factor, plasma thromboplastin component, autoprothrombin II
X	Stuart factor, Stuart-Prower factor, Prower factor
XI	Plasma thromboplastin antecedent (PTA)
XII	Hageman factor, contact factor
XIII	Fibrin stabilizing factor
—	Prekallikrein, Fletcher factor, and high-molecular-weight kininogen

From Bell TN. Disseminated intravascular coagulation and shock: multisystem crisis in the critically ill. Crit Care Nurs Clin North Am 1990; 2:256.

bin production and fibrin clot formation are the similar ultimate outcomes. Both pathways are essential to ensure normal hemostasis.

Fig. 4-1 diagrams a simplified schema of the intrinsic and extrinsic pathways of the clotting cascade. The concept of two separate and distinct pathways helps unravel the complex series of events that occur in coagulation and facilitates discussion of the pathophysiologic alterations that occur in DIC; however, recent evidence suggests that many links between the intrinsic and extrinsic pathways occur.[7,9] More recently, two plasma proteins essential in the intrinsic pathway have been recognized but are currently not reflected in most conventional clotting factor schemas. These proteins are prekallikrein and high-molecular-weight kininogen (HMWK).

Intrinsic pathway. The intrinsic pathway is stimulated by direct damage to the red blood cells or platelets or by blood coming into contact with negatively charged particles, such as exposed collagen occurring in endothelial damage.[22] Any of these

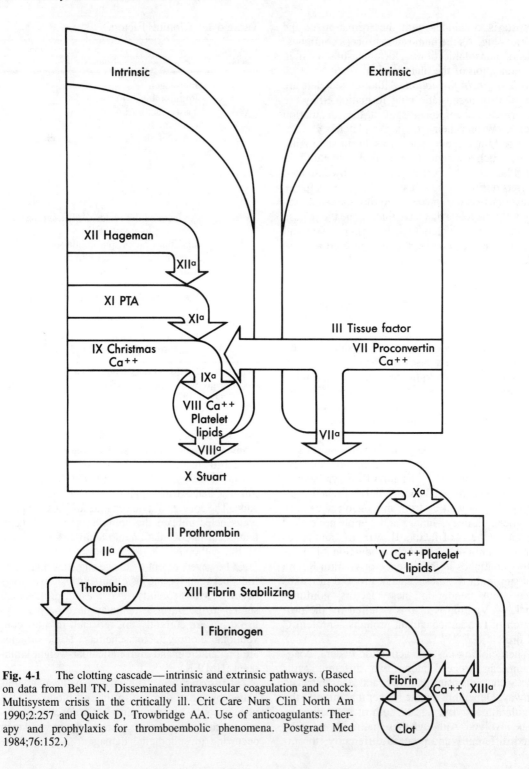

Fig. 4-1   The clotting cascade—intrinsic and extrinsic pathways. (Based on data from Bell TN. Disseminated intravascular coagulation and shock: Multisystem crisis in the critically ill. Crit Care Nurs Clin North Am 1990;2:257 and Quick D, Trowbridge AA. Use of anticoagulants: Therapy and prophylaxis for thromboembolic phenomena. Postgrad Med 1984;76:152.)

inciting events begins the contact phase of the intrinsic cascade.[9] Endothelial disruption and subsequent exposure of the basement membrane promotes several procoagulant activities. Although endothelial cells normally have little or no tissue factor production, when exposed to thrombin their tissue factor production dramatically increases. Endothelial cells synthesize factor V and possess binding sites for factors IX and X, all of which are involved in the coagulation cascade.

Additionally, the negatively charged surface attracts the circulating contact factors, factor XII and HMWK, which attach at the site of endothelial damage. HMWK is contained within endothelial cells and on their surface.[23] HMWK also exists in the plasma complexed with prekallikrein and factor XI.

After factor XII binds to the negatively charged surface, it develops weak but highly specific activity that converts prekallikrein to kallikrein. Kallikrein then converts factor XII into activated factor XII (factor XIIa) and activates the fibrinolytic system (NOTE: letter "a" denotes "activated").

Factor XIIa activates both kallikrein and factor XI. The activation of kallikrein involves HMWK as a cofactor in the conversion of precursor (prekallikrein) to the active kallikrein. A positive feedback loop exists as kallikrein cycles back to convert more factor XII to factor XIIa, and factor XIIa produces more kallikrein to accelerate the contact phase of coagulation[9,16,24] (Fig. 4-2).

The major consequence of activated factor XII is the subsequent activation of factor XI. Activated factor XI reciprocates by causing further production of factor XIIa. Factor XIa stimulates activation of factor IX in the presence of calcium. Factor IXa alone has no ability to continue the cascade. However, when factor IXa is complexed with factor VIII that has been converted to factor VIIIa in the presence of calcium and platelet phospholipids (PF-3), it becomes a potent activator of factor X.

At this point, the intrinsic pathway enters the final common pathway of both the intrinsic and extrinsic pathways. Factor X is converted to factor Xa. Factor Xa alone slowly activates prothrombin (factor II), but in the presence of factor V, calcium, and platelet phospholipids, it rapidly stimulates prothrombin's conversion to thrombin (factor IIa). Research demonstrates that this factor Xa complex is protected from inhibition by antithrombin III (AT

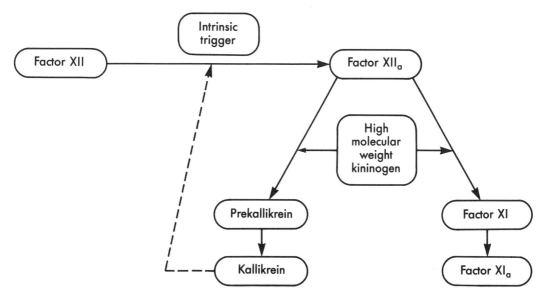

Fig. 4-2 Intrinsic system—factor XII reactions. (Based on data from Bell TN. Disseminated intravascular coagulation and shock: Multisystem crisis in the critically ill. Crit Care Nurs Clin North Am 1990;2:258 and Ravel R. Clinical laboratory medicine: Clinical application of laboratory data. St. Louis: Mosby–Year Book, 1989, 91.)

III).[9] Thrombin subsequently cleaves fibrinogen (factor I) to fibrin.

Cleavage of the fibrinogen molecule produces fibrin monomers. The fibrin monomers rapidly polymerize to produce a gelatinous mass of polymerized fibrin that adheres to the fused platelets. Initially the clot is held together by weak noncovalent bonds. Factor XIII, the fibrin stabilizing factor, is released and converted to factor XIIIa by thrombin. Through the action of factor XIIIa and in the presence of calcium, the fibrin strands are crosslinked to produce a strong, stable, insoluble clot that is hemostatically effective. The fibrin fibers create a matrix that entraps blood cells, plasma, and platelets. The resultant fibrin clot adheres to the damaged vascular endothelium and prevents further bleeding.

Two to six minutes is usually required for a clot to be produced through the intrinsic pathway. Within 1 hour following clot formation, the clot retracts, releasing serum from the clot and further closing the traumatized blood vessel.[25]

Extrinsic pathway. The release of tissue factor (tissue thromboplastin) from traumatized tissues activates the extrinsic pathway of the clotting cascade. Tissue factor is a membrane glycoprotein contained on most cells,[22] and certain tissues have particularly high concentrations of tissue factor, including the lung, brain, bone marrow, liver, kidney, placenta, and mesenteral fat.[1,26,27] Most tissue factor also contains large amounts of platelet phospholipid.[21] When the extrinsic pathway is activated following severe tissue trauma, blood clots begin to form within 15 to 20 seconds and are limited only by the amount of tissue factor present.[14]

Tissue factor complexes with factor VII and slowly activates factors IX and X. Factor VII, when complexed with calcium, is converted to factor VIIa by factors IXa and Xa. Factor VIIa cascades to stimulate further activation of factor X, thereby joining the final common pathway.

Clotting cascade interactions. As mentioned above, interactions exist between the intrinsic and extrinsic pathways. The most important linkage is the ability of factor VIIa to activate factor IX.[7,18,28] Therefore factor VII release can activate factor X through the extrinsic pathway and/or can activate factor IX with subsequent activation of factor X through the intrinsic pathway.

Reactions also occur in the clotting cascade that cause it to further activate itself.[18] Trace amounts of factor Xa, in the presence of calcium and platelet phospholipid, cause rapid conversion of factor VII to factor VIIa. This cyclical reaction produces a dramatic increase in the activity of factor VII. Thrombin, in trace amounts, can activate factors V and VIII, as well as platelets. Thrombin also enhances factor VII activity.[21]

Thrombin. Thrombin serves several functions in the hemostatic process. It cleaves fibrinogen into fibrin, forming the matrix mesh for a nonsoluble clot.[9,16,29] Thrombin generation is localized to cell surfaces, but it diffuses from those surfaces where it acts on fibrinogen.[3,18] Thrombin also stimulates platelet aggregation during platelet plug formation.[1,9] Additionally, thrombin incites further platelet aggregation and fibrin formation around the platelet plug.[9] Finally, thrombin serves a vital role by activating the fibrinolytic system to begin clot breakdown.[29]

Normal coagulation cannot occur without thrombin; however, once thrombin is present, it has the ability to promote a vicious cycle of continued clot formation. In addition to its effect on fibrinogen, thrombin can convert prothrombin directly to more thrombin. Thrombin also accelerates the actions of factors VIII, IX, X, XI, and XIII and platelets,[14] and thrombin also converts factors V and VIII into forms that have a higher procoagulant activity.[9,16] In later stages of reaction, thrombin limits its own production by inactivating factor V.[9]

It quickly becomes evident that thrombin's positive feedback mechanism can dramatically affect the coagulation process. Critical levels of thrombin produce a repetitive cycle of increased clotting, increased thrombin formation, and increased platelet aggregation. This cycle is an important component in the pathophysiology of DIC.

Fibrinolytic system

When a stimulus activates the coagulation system and subsequent fibrin clot formation, the fibrinolytic system is simultaneously activated to control and break down the blood clot to reestablish blood flow. Fibrinolysis represents an important anticoagulant process to balance coagulation and restrict the fibrin clot to the site of vessel wall injury. The process of fibrinolysis involves integrated interactions among four components: (1) plasminogen, (2) tissue plasminogen activator, (3)

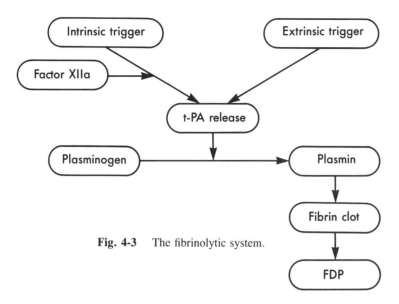

Fig. 4-3 The fibrinolytic system.

plasmin, and (4) fibrin (Fig. 4-3).

Fibrinolysis results in the enzymatic degradation of the fibrin clot by plasmin. As discussed previously, the fibrinolytic system is activated when factor XIIa activates kallikrein and when thrombin is produced. Factor XIIa initiates the release of two endogenous plasminogen activators—tissue plasminogen activator (t-PA) and urokinase.[30] Urokinase is responsible for keeping hollow organs clot-free,[16] and t-PA is the major physiologic activator of plasminogen.[3] Tissue plasminogen activator is present in a variety of body cells, particularly the endothelium in the microcirculation.[21]

Plasminogen exists in all fibrin clots, having been incorporated into the clot during its formation. The t-PA converts plasminogen, an inactive proenzyme, to the active dissolving enzyme plasmin. Tissue plasminogen activator has a high affinity for fibrin, and its adsorption to a fibrin clot greatly enhances the conversion of plasminogen to plasmin.[3,7,18] Because the plasmin activation mechanism depends on the presence of fibrin, lysis can occur only at the site of clot formation, thereby preventing systemic fibrinolysis.[22]

The fibrinolytic process continues when plasmin is released into the region of the clot, where it proteolytically degrades the fibrin strands. In the blood, plasmin also degrades other coagulation sys-

tem components, including factors V, VIII, and XIII, and fibrinogen, the same elements that thrombin activates.[16,31,32] Plasmin that enters the free circulation is rapidly destroyed by two primary plasmin inhibitors—alpha$_2$-antiplasmin and alpha$_2$-macroglobulin.[33] Plasmin inhibitors also ensure that plasmin's activity is limited to the area of fibrin deposition. Plasmin that is adsorbed onto fibrin appears to be protected from the effects of plasmin inhibitors.[3]

As plasmin dissolves the clot, it releases breakdown products known as fibrinogen/fibrin degradation products (FDP). As the crosslinked fibrin strands are proteolytically cleaved, they break off in fragments. The initial FDP fragment produced is fragment X. Fragment X then yields fragment Y and fragment D. Fragment Y is further degraded by plasmin to produce another D fragment and fragment E (Fig. 4-4). The identification of fragment D serves as the basis for a newer laboratory test to detect fibrin-specific degradation products.

FDPs exert an inhibitory effect on the coagulation system by interfering with fibrin polymerization and, in high concentrations, inhibiting platelet aggregation and the release reaction.[3,33] Normally, however, FDP concentration in the blood is too small to produce an anticoagulant effect because FDPs are efficiently removed from the circulation

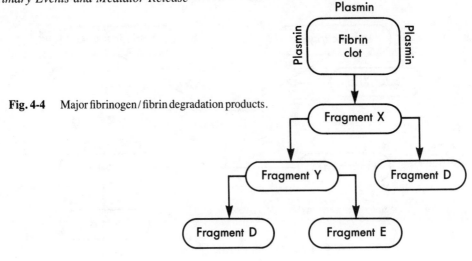

Fig. 4-4   Major fibrinogen/fibrin degradation products.

by reticuloendothelial cells of the liver and the spleen. Once fibrin fibers are removed, blood flow through the newly healed blood vessel resumes.

Hemostatic control mechanisms

Clearance. The body's procoagulant activities are counterbalanced by a number of hemostatic control mechanisms, many of which are poorly understood. These mechanisms are essential to maintain hemostatic homeostasis. An adequate blood flow rate is essential for eliminating activated clotting factors and clearing coagulation by-products. As blood moves through the circulatory network, activated coagulation factors and by-products are flushed from the site of injury and rapidly removed from the circulation by the hepatic system. The reticuloendothelial system, leukocytes, and the pulmonary circulation all assist in clearing activated coagulation factors, fibrin monomers, and small clots.

Coagulation inhibitors. Several systemic coagulation inhibitors exist in the circulation. These plasma proteins include (1) antithrombin III, (2) protein C and protein S, (3) alpha$_2$-antiplasmin, (4) alpha$_2$-macroglobulin, (5) alpha$_2$-antitrypsin, and (6) C-1 inactivator.[21] Of these anticoagulants, the best described are antithrombin III, the protein C/protein S systems, and alpha$_2$-antiplasmin.

Antithrombin III regulates the clotting cascade by chemically binding and slowly inactivating thrombin, as well as factors VIIa, IXa, Xa, XIa,

and XIIa, and plasmin and kallikrein.[7,27,34-36] Heparin, which is endogenously secreted in small quantities by liver and lung mast cells, is another naturally occurring antithrombin agent. The binding of heparin to AT III heightens the affinity of AT III for thrombin and can increase its antithrombin effectiveness a thousand-fold.[14] The speed at which AT III inactivates the clotting components depends on the amount of heparin present, but the degree of inactivation is solely dependent on the available amount of AT III.[36]

Protein C is a vitamin K–dependent coagulation inhibitor synthesized in the liver. Protein C exists in the circulation in an inactive form and is activated in the presence of thrombin. Thrombomodulin, the thrombin receptor of the endothelial cell, must complex with thrombin before protein C can exert any anticoagulant activity.[37] Activated protein C inactivates factors Va and VIIIa, thereby decreasing thrombin production.[15,16,18,30] Activated protein C also may enhance fibrinolytic activity by inactivating a t-PA inhibitor, thus increasing the rate of fibrin degradation.[18,33] Since protein C requires thrombin for conversion to its active form, its effects are limited to areas of active clotting. Protein C and antithrombin III have complementary effects because they each inactivate different coagulation factors.

Protein S functions as a cofactor for activated protein C and is required for activated protein C to bind to phospholipids on platelets and other cell surfaces. A vitamin K–dependent protein (protein S) exists in the circulation bound to a complement system protein.[18] The rate of inactivation of factor Va is increased in the presence of protein S.[30]

Alpha$_2$-antiplasmin is the major inhibitor of plasmin in the blood. Alpha$_2$-antiplasmin circulates in the plasma and is crosslinked with fibronectin into fibrin when fibrin is polymerized. Serving as a control for fibrinolysis, alpha$_2$-antiplasmin quickly binds and inactivates plasmin that detaches from the fibrin polymers.[38] Acute-phase reactions occurring in sepsis and trauma stimulate increased levels of alpha$_2$-antiplasmin.[39]

Thrombin. Thrombin's confinement to the fibrin fiber assists in maintaining some degree of hemostatic control. Approximately 85% to 90% of thrombin formed during clotting is adsorbed to the fibrin fiber[14]; thus fibrin is restrained from moving downstream away from the injury site. Thrombin is also partially inactivated when adsorbed to fibrin.

Endothelium. Although the endothelium's primary role in maintaining hemostatic homeostasis is anticoagulation, it has several other functions. Vascular endothelium provides surface binding sites for thrombomodulin and antithrombin III. The endothelium also synthesizes and releases prostacyclin, which decreases the platelet's responsiveness to activating stimuli. The synthesis and release of many activators as well as inhibitors of platelet aggregation, blood coagulation, and fibrinolysis occur from the vascular endothelium.

A delicate relationship must exist between procoagulant and anticoagulant activities to achieve hemostatic homeostasis. Without the body's integrated system of checks and balances, one can easily understand the potential risks of uncontrolled coagulation and hemorrhage.

ETIOLOGY OF DIC

A vast number of clinical conditions can precipitate DIC. Although DIC can occur with most any illness or injury, several clinical events with known procoagulant effects predispose the patient to develop DIC. These events include (1) arterial hypotension, often associated with shock; (2) hypoxemia; (3) acidemia; and (4) stasis of capillary blood flow.[23,40,41] These clinical events promote pathophysiologic alterations that incite activation of the clotting mechanism.

In general, three groups of pathologic processes

ETIOLOGY OF DIC

Endothelial damage

Sepsis, particularly gram-negative
Hypoxia
Cardiopulmonary arrest
Shock: hemorrhagic, septic, cardiogenic, and traumatic
Adult respiratory distress syndrome
Abdominal aortic aneurysm
Rocky Mountain spotted fever

Tissue factor release

Trauma
Burns
Head injury
Myocardial infarction
Surgical procedures
Dissecting aortic aneurysm
Malignant disease
Obstetric accidents

Direct activation of factor X

Acute pancreatitis
Snake venom
Hepatic disease

Miscellaneous

Massive blood transfusions
Hemolytic transfusion reactions
Anaphylaxis
Fresh-water near-drowning
Hypothermia
Renal disease
Diabetic ketoacidosis
Acute fatty liver of pregnancy
Malignant hyperthermia
Pulmonary embolus
Extracorporeal membrane oxygenation
Aspirin toxicity
Necrotizing enterocolitis

can promote the development of DIC. These include endothelial damage, release of tissue factor into the systemic circulation, and direct proteolytic activation of the clotting cascade at factor X. However, in many clinical situations where DIC is present, the pathologic processes that incite its development are often multiple and interrelated.[7] The box above gives a representative list of clinical disorders that can be complicated by DIC.

Endothelial damage

Endothelial damage results in the exposure of the negatively charged basement membrane, which when denuded is a hemostatically active vascular surface.[42] Many clinical situations, including sepsis, hypoxia, and low-flow states such as cardiopulmonary arrest and shock, can damage the vascular endothelium and cause intrinsic pathway activation.[43,44] Venous stasis resulting from prolonged bed rest can also disrupt the vascular endothelium.[45]

Any infectious process, including those caused by bacteria, viruses, rickettsiae, and fungi, can precipitate DIC. Gram-negative sepsis and septic shock are the most common causes of DIC* because endotoxin produces considerable activation of both the intrinsic and extrinsic pathways and overwhelming inflammation.

Most patients with meningococcal, pneumococcal, or staphylococcal septicemia experience acute DIC.[49] This is particularly true when the patient is asplenic or immunocompromised. Patients with meningococcemia may develop Waterhouse-Friderichsen syndrome, which is characterized by the rapid development of DIC with associated cutaneous and adrenal hemorrhage and shock.[5] The progressive organ system dysfunction that occurs in this syndrome corresponds to the severity of shock and associated intravascular coagulation.

Arterial aneurysm initiates DIC by activating the intrinsic pathway. Aortic aneurysm is most frequently associated with the development of DIC, although DIC with other aneurysm locations has been reported.[5] The exact mechanism of stimulation is unknown, but it is thought that injury to the subendothelial layer of the aortic wall produces the trigger for the pathophysiologic events in DIC. Abdominal aortic aneurysm (AAA) repair is considered an effective treatment modality when DIC is present in patients with AAA; however, the surgical repair can result in massive hemorrhage.

Release of tissue factor

The second group of pathologic processes that can incite DIC is the group that causes the release of the tissue factor into the circulation. Numerous conditions can activate the extrinsic pathway of the clotting cascade through the release of excessive

amounts of tissue factor, including trauma, certain surgeries, malignancies, and obstetric accidents.

Damage to body tissues from traumatic injury can cause excessive tissue factor release into the circulation and subsequent activation of the extrinsic pathway at factor VII. Fragments of damaged tissues and crushed cells enter the circulation and, in association with the circulatory stasis produced by hemorrhage, result in severe DIC.[5] Subsequent microthrombi development contributes to the appearance of multisystem dysfunction. Traumatic tissue injury from burns, blunt trauma, traumatic brain injury, and myocardial infarction are examples of conditions that initiate DIC through tissue factor release.

Some surgical procedures place the patient at risk for developing DIC by precipitating the release of procoagulant material into the circulation. DIC has been identified as a complication of transurethral prostatic resection,[18,50] as well as orthopedic procedures.[5] Surgical procedures that utilize cardiopulmonary bypass technology can precipitate DIC.[3] Use of an intraaortic balloon pump (IABP) to treat cardiogenic shock can contribute to low-grade DIC.[5] DIC can also occur in patients with dissecting aortic aneurysm and those experiencing transplantation and rejection crises.[46] DIC has been found to be a frequent complication in peritoneovenous shunt insertion for refractory ascites.[5]

Acute and chronic DIC often accompanies malignant disease. The appearance of DIC in acute promyelocytic leukemia (APL) is common.[18,42] Because the granules of the promyelocyte are high in tissue factor, an increased frequency of DIC occurs in APL, particularly when the cells are lysed with chemotherapy. Mucin-secreting carcinomas of the pancreas, prostate, stomach, bowel, and lung release procoagulant tumor products with tissue factor activity into the circulation to promote DIC. DIC has been noted in numerous types of leukemia, Hodgkin's disease, adenocarcinomas, sarcomas, and metastatic solid tumors.[3,5,18,51] Additionally, administering certain chemotherapeutic agents to treat leukemia and other malignancies can precipitate the development of DIC secondary to increased cell debris.[50]

Obstetric accidents are a common etiologic factor in the development of DIC. DIC can occur as a complication of placenta previa, abruptio placentae, retained dead fetus, missed abortion, and

---

*References 3, 7, 18, 23, and 46-48.

hypertonic saline abortion, and it is a predictable feature of amniotic fluid embolism.* The release of tissue factor into the bloodstream from these obstetric complications stimulates clotting cascade activity at factor VII.

Direct proteolytic activation

The third group of pathologic processes precipitates DIC through direct proteolytic activation of the clotting cascade at factor X. In acute pancreatitis, the introduction of pancreatic enzymes into the circulation can activate the clotting cascade at factor X.[3,49] The venom of snakebites also infuses proteolytic enzymes into the bloodstream, with the subsequent activation of factor X. Additionally, the numerous coagulation defects produced by hepatic disease can directly trigger the final common pathway at factor X.

Miscellaneous conditions. Numerous miscellaneous conditions exist that can be complicated by DIC. Complications arising from transfusion therapy can precipitate DIC in the critically ill patient. Massive blood transfusions dilute the clotting factors as well as the circulating naturally occurring antithrombins, thus placing the patient at risk for developing DIC. In hemolytic transfusion reactions, antigen-antibody complexes promote the release of procoagulant material from disrupted platelets and red blood cells contributing to diffuse bleeding and sudden hypotension in the patient.[16,46] Immune complexes are also responsible for initiating DIC following anaphylaxis.

PATHOPHYSIOLOGIC ALTERATIONS IN DIC

DIC is characterized by a pathologic overstimulation of the normal coagulation mechanism[29] resulting in disseminated coagulation and excessive fibrinolysis. The abnormality of hemostasis in DIC is the extent to which the normal coagulation mechanism is overstimulated and normal inhibitory mechanisms are overwhelmed when triggered by an underlying pathologic condition. The coagulation mechanism itself remains normal. Overstimulation and dissemination of blood coagulation in DIC produce both thrombotic and hemorrhagic events, the two primary pathophysiologic alterations in DIC. In association with the coagulation

system, fibrinolytic, kallikrein-kinin, and complement system activation further contribute to the thrombosis and hemorrhage produced in DIC.

Excessive clotting cascade activation

Primary pathologic conditions can trigger the coagulation mechanism and the onset of DIC through either the intrinsic or the extrinsic pathway, although the predominant pathway in DIC appears to be the extrinsic pathway.[23] DIC resulting from overstimulation of the extrinsic pathway occurs when damaged tissues and cells release the potent procoagulant tissue factor into the circulation. In gram-negative infection, a common primary condition precipitating DIC, endotoxin is produced that stimulates generation of tissue factor on the surface of monocytes. Experimental data indicate that tissue factor expressed on the surface of endothelial cells or monocytes and macrophages is the most decisive procoagulant material.[23] Tissue factor release stimulates factor VII and activates the coagulation mechanism through the extrinsic pathway. Endotoxin also damages the vascular endothelium, resulting in release of factor XII and subsequent activation of the intrinsic mechanism, platelets, and the complement cascade.

Factor XII activation stimulates the kallikrein-kinin system. Bradykinin, a potent vasodilator, is liberated, causing hypotension, increased vascular permeability, and shock.[9,52] Factor XII activation also stimulates the complement cascade, which contributes to the pathophysiologic events in DIC by producing anaphylatoxins. The cell lysis, increased vascular permeability, and platelet release reactions produced by complement activation all contribute more procoagulant material to further perpetuate the clotting cycle[52] and the inflammatory response.

The pathophysiologic alterations and clinical manifestations in DIC are reflective of the balance between the amounts of thrombin and plasmin generated by the overstimulated coagulation mechanism. The excessive thrombin produced in DIC contributes significantly to the physiologic derangements that occur. The amount of thrombin that enters the systemic circulation during DIC far exceeds the ability of the body's naturally occurring antithrombins, such as protein C and AT III, to control it. During the initial stages, 75% of DIC

---

*References 3, 16, 18, 42, and 46.

patients demonstrate a decrease in protein C, and almost all demonstrate a decreased level of protein C activity.[53] The reduction of AT III in severe hepatic disease may be a factor in determining this population's frequency of developing DIC.[54]

Thrombosis

Thrombin is initially generated in DIC when the clotting cascade is activated, resulting in platelet aggregation and clotting factor consumption. The fibrin monomer then polymerizes into nonsoluble fibrin clots. Because of the excessive thrombin present, an extensive number of fibrin clots are subsequently formed and deposited in the microcirculation. The circulatory obstruction that results from these intravascular microthrombi disrupts blood flow and creates widespread organ hypoperfusion, ischemia, infarction, and necrosis.[55]

Thrombin, in addition to converting fibrinogen to fibrin, promotes platelet aggregation.[9,50] In DIC,

when excessive amounts of circulating thrombin are present, numerous clumps of aggregated platelets develop and become trapped in the microvascular fibrin deposits. Progressive accumulation of activated clotting factors and platelets in this low flow state also contributes to the development of microvascular thrombi (Fig. 4-5).

In the critically ill patient, DIC can result as a complication of shock, or shock can result as a complication of DIC. Five aspects of shock that contribute to the development of DIC have been described. These include (1) sluggish blood flow caused by poor perfusion and capillary shunting, (2) metabolic acidosis, (3) release of ADP and phospholipids from traumatized cells, (4) hypoxemia of cells, and (5) endothelial damage.[13] These conditions create a physiologic imbalance, which results in an increased tendency to clot.

Shock is produced in DIC when massive intravascular fibrin deposits create microthrombi that

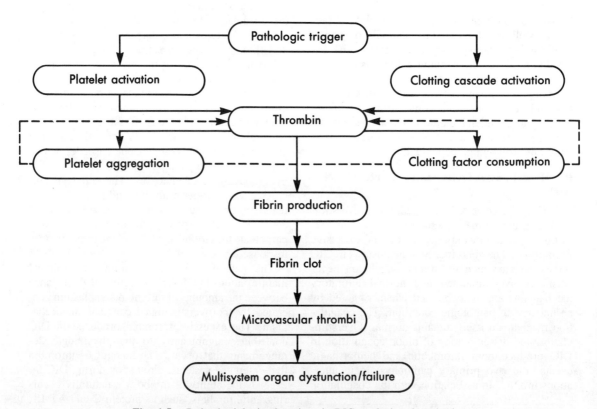

Fig. 4-5 Pathophysiologic alterations in DIC producing thrombosis.

obstruct the intravascular circulation. The resultant stagnation of blood flow produces lactic acidosis. Subsequent reactions increase clotting factor consumption and platelet aggregation. As the capillary blood flow progressively decreases, blood acidity rises, and cellular death occurs. Organ perfusion becomes increasingly compromised because of the increased blood acidity and cellular damage. As organ perfusion is impaired, manifestations of multisystem organ dysfunction and/or failure ultimately result.

The stasis of blood flow flow that occurs in shock potentiates the pathophysiologic processes in DIC, causing an accumulation of activated clotting factors in the circulation, in part as the result of impaired clearance by the mononuclear phagocyte system.[16] In shock syndromes, the combination of tissue hypoxia, endothelial injury, and blood stasis accelerates the development of thrombosis in acute DIC.[43,48]

Red blood cells can be mechanically damaged or destroyed by the thrombotic events in DIC as the cells travel through the fibrin matrix in the intravascular circulation and are sheared. The erythrocytes become fragmented, and microangiopathic hemolytic anemia occurs. The resultant hemolytic anemia, although produced by thrombotic events, subsequently contributes to the patient's hemorrhagic tendency.

Hemorrhage

In addition to the microvascular thrombi produced in DIC, hemorrhagic complications also occur. Continual, repeated stimulation of the clotting cascade results in the consumption of clotting factors, particularly fibrinogen, prothrombin, and factors V, VIII, and XIII, at a rate greater than the body can replenish them. Hemorrhage and the potential onset of shock result when the demand for clotting factors outweighs the supply.

Again, excessive amounts of thrombin play a significant role in the pathologic alterations that produce hemorrhage in DIC. The increased quantities of thrombin produced during the accelerated cascading of clotting factors feed back into the clotting cascade to convert prothrombin into more thrombin, thus perpetuating this repetitive cycle. Thrombin-induced platelet aggregation produces thrombocytopenia and increases the patient's risk of bleeding.[56,57] Platelet activation exposes a binding site on the platelet surface that serves as a positive feedback mechanism to further accelerate the clotting cascade.[16] Additionally, thrombin activates the fibrinolytic system, producing increased fibrinolysis that results in increased bleeding.[49]

Excessive plasmin is also produced when the coagulation mechanism is overstimulated. Accelerated plasmin activity begins to precipitously degrade fibrin before a stable clot has formed. In the absence of a stable clot, the potential for bleeding and/or hemorrhage is greatly increased. The intensified breakdown of fibrinogen into fibrin causes microvascular clots to randomly form in the capillary bed, where they are not needed, and prevents stable clots from forming at the site of trauma, where they are needed[20,50] (Fig. 4-6).

As fibrin is degraded by plasmin, FDPs are released. In DIC the normal hepatic, reticuloendothelial, and renal clearance mechanisms are saturated by increased FDPs, which contribute to the pathophysiologic events.[21] In particular, hepatic hypoperfusion resulting from hypostatic circulation impairs the clearance of hemostatic waste products.[42] DIC patients also have a decreased tissue macrophage clearing function that further aggravates the clearance process.[32] As a result, increased levels of FDPs remain in the circulation. In high concentrations, FDPs are very potent anticoagulants; therefore the bleeding diathesis in DIC is accelerated.[20,50]

It has been suggested that decreased tissue macrophage function may be due to a decrease in the circulating opsonin fibronectin.[50] Fibronectin is a large glycoprotein with adhesive properties. Fibronectin mediates the reticuloendothelial or macrophage clearance of particulate matter such as fibrin clumps and collagen debris. Decreased fibronectin levels in patients with DIC have been associated with a poor prognosis.[58]

Summary

By examining the repetitive nature of the pathophysiologic events in DIC, one can appreciate the paradoxical clinical situation produced by a patient simultaneously experiencing thrombosis and hemorrhage. Although hemorrhage is the predominate presenting sign, one must be cognizant of coexistent microvascular occlusion from thrombi. The formation of microthrombi in DIC is the more irreversible of the two events and contributes sig-

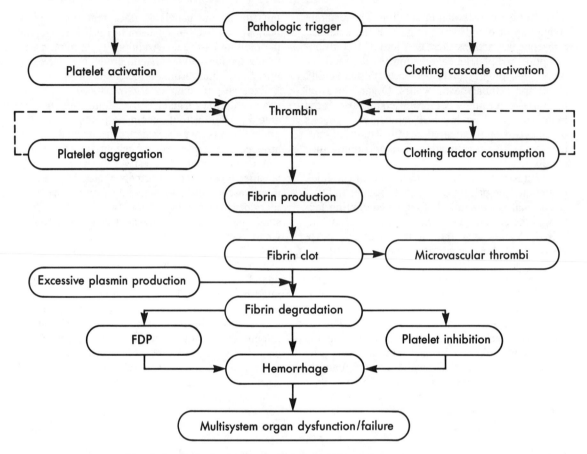

Fig. 4-6 Pathophysiologic alterations in DIC producing hemorrhage.

nificantly to the patient's morbidity and mortality through multiorgan dysfunction and possible death.[52] The self-perpetuating cycle of thrombosis and hemorrhage persists until the underlying pathologic process that triggered the DIC is removed or until appropriate therapeutic interventions halt the cycle.

RELATIONSHIP OF DIC AND MSOF

The interaction of the hematologic system with all other body systems contributes to the relationship of DIC and MSOF. Like shock, MSOF can precipitate DIC, or DIC can precipitate or exacerbate MSOF. DIC itself represents a functional failure of the hematologic system.[59] Although individual failure of the hematologic system (bone marrow exhaustion) can occur as MSOF sequentially progresses, hematologic failure expressed by conditions such as DIC more commonly occurs as the result of the earlier inflammatory response and pathophysiologic changes.

A rapidly emerging body of knowledge indicates that the vascular endothelium plays an integral, active role in the pathophysiologic derangements occurring in both DIC and MSOF. Intact vascular endothelium serves an important homeostatic function by balancing procoagulant and anticoagulant activities.[10] When perturbations of the endothelium occur through influences such as inflammation or injury, the endothelium can actively contribute to subsequent hematologic alterations, including DIC.

Regardless of its etiology, inflammation is often associated with a hypercoagulable state.[37] When the inflammatory/immune response is triggered, a number of humoral, cellular, and biochemical mediators common to both DIC and MSOF are released. The interrelated cascades of complement, kallikrein-kinin, coagulation, and fibrinolysis are intricately involved in both inflammation and coagulation. Activation of one usually stimulates activation of the other.

Cellular responses to inflammation contribute to DIC and MSOF. Activation of phagocytes, including macrophages and monocytes, leads to procoagulant activity and the deposition of fibrin at the site of the reaction.[46] Platelet activation from endothelial damage and clotting cascade activation is another contributing factor to the common pathophysiologic events in DIC and MSOF.

DIC and MSOF share common pathophysiologic and etiologic features; thus these two syndromes are commonly seen in the same patient. Although DIC can be precipitated by a number of pathologic conditions, shock, hypotension, hypoxemia, and inadequate tissue perfusion are commonly implicated in the development of both conditions. Uncontrolled inflammation and sepsis are major underlying conditions in DIC.[60] Likewise, uncontrolled inflammation or infection is viewed by many as the primary etiologic factor in MSOF.[59] When hematologic homeostatic mechanisms fail, the potential for DIC and MSOF heightens. In fact, MSOF may be the direct reflection of DIC, becoming the ultimate fatal complication.[5]

CLINICAL PRESENTATION AND ASSESSMENT PARAMETERS

The critically ill DIC patient displays a wide spectrum of signs and symptoms because of the diversity of primary conditions that can precipitate DIC. Subtle clinical signs can rapidly progress to fulminant DIC accompanied by significant hemorrhage and/or thrombosis. The patient's initial clinical manifestations are usually related to hemorrhagic involvement, although the initial pathologic events are thrombotic.[55] Careful systems assessments are needed to detect the life- and limb-threatening thromboses that can occur.

In examining the clinical manifestations of DIC and determining appropriate assessment parameters, the critical care practitioner must consider the patient's medical history as well as current medical problems. Organ systems that have been compromised by chronic or acute pathologic conditions may demonstrate pathophysiologic aberrations resulting from DIC. It is important to emphasize that all organ systems have the potential to experience dysfunction and/or failure in acute DIC. Underlying factors, such as alterations in tissue and/or organ perfusion, alterations in macrophage clearance functions, preexisting or coexisting organ dysfunction (particularly the hepatic system), and competency of the coagulation and fibrinolytic systems, can all influence the clinical presentation in DIC.

The classic acute, generalized DIC patient presents with rapid evolvement of bleeding at multiple sites. Ecchymoses, purpura, petechiae, hematomas, hemorrhagic bullae, and scleral and conjunctival hemorrhage can occur. Bleeding or oozing from past and present puncture or wound sites, tubes, drains, and body orifices can develop. Epistaxis and gingival bleeding are frequent occurrences. A decreased urine output results from dehydration, hypotension, or renal microvascular obstruction. Hematuria secondary to renal infarction and genitourinary, intracranial, pleural, and pericardial bleeding often complicates the clinical situation. Pulmonary hemorrhage is usually accompanied by hemoptysis, tachypnea, dyspnea, and chest pain.[49] Additionally, bleeding into closed compartments and body cavities can result from increased capillary fragility.

Cutaneous manifestations can result from the hemorrhagic events in DIC. Changes in skin color, such as pallor, cyanosis, and/or jaundice can occur. Jaundice suggests that excessive red cell hemolysis associated with the underlying coagulopathy has occurred.[61] Hemorrhagic necrosis of the adrenal glands and skin are characteristic of the life-threatening Waterhouse-Friderichsen syndrome that can complicate DIC.

Changes in level of consciousness, unexplained behavior changes, focal neurologic deficits, headache, pupillary changes, extremity paresis or paralysis, changes in mentation, confusion, and seizure activity can indicate cerebral hemorrhage, a serious neurologic complication of DIC. Frequent neurologic assessments should be incorporated into the plan of care.

Tarry, bloody stools and hematemesis can indicate gastrointestinal bleeding. Hyperactive bowel sounds, abdominal tenderness or pain, and abdominal distention can also be present. Retroperitoneal bleeding can cause nerve compression at L2 to L3, resulting in impaired lower extremity movement.[62]

The bleeding in DIC usually arises from multiple, unrelated sites. Bleeding in a critically ill patient who has no history of bleeding or who experiences prolonged bleeding should alert the critical care nurse to investigate further, particularly if the patient has any of the four predisposing conditions: arterial hypotension, hypoxemia, acidemia, and stasis of capillary blood flow.[63] Less overt signs of bleeding, such as restlessness and vital signs tending toward hypotension and tachycardia, can be significant.

The sudden appearance of shock in the critical care patient or the presence of shock that is refractory to traditional therapy can indicate the onset of DIC. In severe DIC, the shock may be out of proportion to the blood loss.[7] Changes in level of consciousness, hypotension, tachycardia, tachypnea, and restlessness are among the clinical findings that can occur. The series of events in DIC and shock continues in a cyclic manner until appropriate therapeutic interventions are implemented.

Manifestations of multisystem organ dysfunction and/or failure resulting from microvascular occlusion can occur in the DIC patient. The skin, lungs, and kidneys have the highest incidence of microvascular thrombi[52]; however, all organ systems are at risk. The patient's underlying disease and/or injury play a pivotal role in determining organ system dysfunction or failure from thrombosis. Although the clot deposition occurs primarily in the microcirculation, the macrocirculation can also be involved.[52]

Cutaneous microvascular thrombi cause focal areas of infarction in the fingers and toes and subsequent gangrene. More extensive thrombi cause cold, mottled fingers, toes, and extremities that can progress to acrocyanosis or skin necrosis. Pallor, cyanosis, coolness, and diaphoresis may be noted during circulatory checks when peripheral tissue hypoperfusion from thrombosis is present in DIC. Peripheral pulses can be obliterated when excess fibrin deposition produces microvascular thrombi in the peripheral circulation. Pain results when tissue ischemia and necrosis are present in DIC.

The critical care practitioner must observe for trends in neurologic assessment and vital sign data that indicate neurologic decompensation and increasing intracranial pressure. Cerebrovascular infarctions may produce significant neurologic findings, including focal deficits and CVA-like symptoms. Spinal artery thromboses producing quadriplegia and paraplegia can occur, but they are rare.[5]

Microvascular thrombi in the pulmonary system interfere with gas exchange at the alveolar level. Shortness of breath, hemoptysis, tachypnea, tachycardia, chest pain, cyanosis, hypoxemia, and acidosis may be present.[44]

Deposition of fibrin and thrombi in the renal microvasculature can produce oliguria, anuria, and hematuria. Ischemic renal cortical necrosis that develops can be complicated by concurrent acute tubular necrosis that develops secondary to hypotension, hypovolemia,[49] nephrotoxic inflammatory mediators, and therapeutic agents. Additionally, renal microvascular infarctions create fluid shifts that produce peripheral edema in the extremities.

DIAGNOSIS AND LABORATORY DATA

The diagnosis of DIC is based primarily on a high index of suspicion.[20] The abrupt onset of bleeding in a patient with no prior history of an underlying coagulation defect, sudden organ failure(s), and refractory shock should alert the critical care practitioner to suspect DIC. Changes in laboratory values can occur before clinical evidence of bleeding appears, and laboratory values can improve before the patient stops bleeding.[62]

Laboratory data serve as useful indices in the diagnosis and the related therapeutic management of DIC. Although laboratory data can be highly diagnostic of DIC, they can still be quite variable between patients, so it is important that the data are correlated carefully with the clinical situation.[64] The multiple abnormalities in the production and synthesis of coagulation factors when hepatic disease or failure is present make the subsequent diagnosis of DIC difficult. Diagnosis can also be difficult in the patient who has received multiple blood transfusions because of the dilution of clotting factors and platelets that occurs.[50]

Acute, generalized DIC is associated with a characteristic pattern of laboratory abnormalities, although no one test is pathognomonic for DIC. Different patterns of laboratory results can develop depending on the underlying pathology, the triggering mechanism for the DIC, and the balance between the patient's inherent coagulation activators and inhibitors.[3,65] Laboratory values presented may vary from laboratory to laboratory.

A decreased platelet count occurs in most cases of clinically apparent DIC.[6] A platelet count of less than $150,000/mm^3$ (normal is $150,000/mm^3$ to $450,000/mm^3$) usually occurs in acute DIC. The thrombocytopenia that occurs in DIC is the result of rapid platelet consumption during the clotting cascade coupled with the body's inability to replace them.

The activated partial thromboplastin time (APTT) and partial thromboplastin time (PTT) can be prolonged in DIC. The APTT and PTT both measure intrinsic pathway activity, but the APTT is currently the more widely used test for monitoring heparin therapy. In general, a normal APTT is 25 to 35 seconds. Traumatic venipuncture can affect the APTT results by contaminating the specimen with tissue factor, producing a falsely decreased value.[66]

The prothrombin time (PT) measures extrinsic pathway activity. The PT is prolonged when the triggering mechanism for DIC has activated the extrinsic pathway. PT values are usually prolonged when levels of factors II, V, VII, and X are less than 40% of normal.[66] A normal PT is in the 11- to 15-second range.

Thrombin time is long in DIC. This test measures a late phase of coagulation when fibrinogen is converted to fibrin in the presence of thrombin. Because thrombin itself is so rapidly inactivated by AT III, it cannot be measured directly.[33] The thrombin time test therefore allows the products of thrombin activity to be measured. Normal thrombin time is the time of control plus or minus 2 seconds when the control is 9 to 13 seconds.[66]

Since fibrinogen is consumed during activation of the clotting cascade, fibrinogen levels are less than 200 mg/dL. The normal range in the adult is 200 to 400 mg/dL.[66] Fibrinogen levels, however, can be normal even in cases of severe DIC. Because fibrinogen is an acute phase reactant, it is elevated in numerous conditions, including inflammation, infection, tissue necrosis, pregnancy, and some malignancies. This increased rate of fibrinogen production can then be offset by the increased consumption of fibrinogen in DIC; hence, the patient has a "normal" fibrinogen level.[7,16,32]

Fibrinogen/fibrin degradation products are pres-

ent in an increased amount because of the excessive fibrinolysis that occurs in DIC. The normal value for FDPs is less than 10 μg/mL. The usual test for FDPs does not distinguish between the breakdown products of fibrinogen and those of fibrin. Currently, FDPs are measured by a test that employs polyclonal antibodies; however, newer tests are being developed using monoclonal antibodies that do not cross-react with fibrinogen (see Chapter 16 for a description of monoclonal antibodies).

A recent test, D-dimer, uses monoclonal antibodies to measure the fibrin-specific degradation fragment, fragment D.[7,67,68] D-dimer does not detect fibrinogen or its degradation products; therefore it has a major advantage over current laboratory tests for FDPs.[68] In a series reported by Wilde et al ($n = 236$) that included 43 DIC patients, all 43 were found to have elevated D-dimer levels.[69] In the other patient groups studied, D-dimer was rarely found to be elevated when FDPs were normal. The finding of elevated FDPs confirmed by an elevated D-dimer test has high predictive value in the detection of DIC.[42,70]

Antithrombin III levels are low in DIC because AT III complexes with thrombin and factor Xa to block thrombin's activity.[3] Protein C and protein S are two other physiologic anticoagulants that can be decreased in DIC. The current utility of tests measuring protein C and protein S to diagnose DIC is not well documented.

The peripheral blood smear should be examined for the presence of schistocytes, helmet cells, burr cells, and fragmented red blood cells. Erythrocyte deformation occurs when the red blood cells are sheared as they travel through small blood vessels partially occluded by fibrin thrombi, resulting in microangiopathic hemolytic anemia.[16,32]

A clot tube should be drawn and examined in suspected cases of DIC. In DIC, the blood fails to clot in 1 hour or forms a small, poor clot that spontaneously lyses or breaks apart easily when the clot tube is shaken.

Investigators are examining the relative value of measuring thrombin/antithrombin III complex (TAT) and plasmin/alpha$_2$-antiplasmin complex (PAP) to aid in diagnosis and management of the DIC patient.[71] TAT is a sensitive parameter of coagulation system activation, whereas PAP is an indicator of fibrinolytic system activation. The potential of these two tests for diagnostic and management purposes has not yet been fully evaluated.

TAT/PAP has been found to be elevated in nearly all DIC patients,[72] although the ratio itself varies with different underlying pathologic conditions. However, it has also been reported that the TAT assay may be less effective than FDP in detecting hypercoagulable states even though it is a more direct method of measurement.[71] The utility of measuring serum levels of fibrinogen/fibrin degradation fragment E, the FgE assay, is being explored. One investigator reports the FgE assay to be 100% sensitive in detecting DIC.[71]

Carr recommends that measurement of platelets, PT, and fibrinogen be used as screening tests before the confirmatory tests of FDP and thrombin time are performed.[31] However, numerous other laboratory tests are used to detect DIC. The measurement of various clotting factors is possible, but is considered of little value in diagnosing DIC because of the variable factor behavior in DIC.[16] However, when hepatic disease is present, the measurement of factor VIII is necessary to accurately diagnose DIC. The euglobulin lysis time, the protamine sulfate paracoagulation test, the ethanol gelation test, and the plasma euglobulin test are other laboratory tests that can be used to diagnose DIC, although they are not generally recommended.

THERAPEUTIC MANAGEMENT

The critically ill patient with DIC and MSOF presents a true therapeutic management challenge for the health care team. The galaxy of underlying pathologic conditions precipitating DIC and the potentially life-threatening multisystem problems it produces demand knowledgeable assessment, intervention, and evaluation to decrease the high morbidity and mortality rates associated with this clinical situation.[63] No treatment regimen is definitive for DIC. Therapeutic management of DIC encompasses three aspects: (1) removal of the underlying pathologic condition, (2) restoration of an appropriate balance between coagulation and fibrinolysis, and (3) maintaining organ viability.

In addition to clinical assessment data, laboratory results should be continually monitored to evaluate the effectiveness of the therapeutic regimen in resolving the DIC process. The coagulation profile, hemoglobin, and hematocrit provide important information in the DIC patient who is bleeding. Particular attention should be given to fibrinogen levels, which when decreased indicate increased clotting.

Removal of underlying pathology

The primary goal of therapeutic management is removal of the underlying pathology.* Removing the primary pathologic trigger halts the procoagulant stimulus and allows the DIC process to resolve.[73] Once the underlying pathologic stimulus has been removed, the liver can replenish all plasma protein coagulation factors within 24 to 48 hours provided the patient has normal hepatic function.

As discussed in previous sections, numerous clinical situations cause the release of procoagulant material. Activation of factor XII by endotoxin perpetuates the clotting cascade and increases the patient's propensity to bleed. Conscientious aseptic technique and adherence to universal blood and body secretion protocols are necessary to prevent further infection that can seriously affect the DIC patient's prognosis. Frequent aseptic dressing changes and wound debridement, as necessary, help prevent a nidus of infection. When DIC results from underlying gram-negative infection, appropriate antimicrobial therapy, as well as management of concurrent septic shock, must be initiated. Monoclonal antibodies should be administered, as appropriate, particularly when DIC and gram-negative sepsis are present.

Surgical intervention may be warranted to remove the procoagulant stimulus resulting from neoplasms, trauma, and obstetric accidents when DIC is present. Aggressive therapy must be instituted to correct shock, hypoxia, acidosis, and capillary blood flow stasis, which precipitate DIC by contributing to clotting cascade activation. Methylprednisolone has been shown to decrease the incidence of DIC that occurs after traumatic tissue injury or shock,[5] although its use is contraindicated in sepsis and MSOF and remains controversial in many other conditions.

Restoration of balance

Replacement therapy. Replacement therapy to reestablish therapeutic levels of deficient coagulation components is considered an important treatment modality once the procoagulant stimulus has been treated. Replacement of clotting factors, platelets, and other coagulation elements becomes increasingly more important when clinically sig-

---

*References 3, 7, 16, 33, 45, 50, and 52.

nificant bleeding occurs as a result of DIC.[80] Replacement therapy, in conjunction with heparin therapy, interferes with thrombin activity and prolongs the half-life of the circulating clotting factors.[33] Even though the clotting components may not be completely normalized through replacement therapy, normal hemostasis can still be accomplished.

The use of replacement therapy in DIC has generated some debate. Central to the debate is concern that initiating replacement therapy "adds fuel to the fire"; increasing the availability of clotting factors and platelets to the repetitive cycles of coagulation and fibrinolysis in DIC intensifies thrombus formation. Although theoretically plausible, no clinical studies support the "fuel to the fire" debate surrounding replacement therapy, and some believe it is valuable in restoring hemostasis.[7,16,32,81]

Replacement of deficient clotting components can be achieved with a number of blood products. Fresh whole blood provides stable coagulation factors, but not the labile factors V and VIII.[80] Fresh whole blood can be used in cases of massive hemorrhage when volume replacement as well as clotting component replacement is necessary. In other clinical situations, replacement with fresh whole blood can place the patient at risk for circulatory overload. Fresh frozen plasma is valuable in DIC, because it provides all of the plasma coagulation proteins, platelets, and AT III. Each unit of fresh frozen plasma should raise the level of clotting factors by approximately 5%.[20] Fresh frozen plasma also aids in volume expansion.

Cryoprecipitated antihemophilic factor is an excellent replacement component for the hypofibrinogenemia associated with DIC, since it is rich in fibrinogen, factor VIII, AT III, protein C, fibronectin, and factor XIII.[3,56] Eight to ten bags supply 2 g of fibrinogen.[82] Because the proteins contained in cryoprecipitate can initiate an allergic reaction, side effects such as fever, itching, and hives can develop. Premedication with diphenhydramine (Benadryl), 25 to 50 mg, helps prevent such reactions.[83]

Thrombocytopenia in DIC can be controlled through the administration of platelet concentrates. One platelet pack should raise the platelet count of a 70-kg adult by 5000/mm^3.[82] Numerous factors diminish the patient's responsiveness to platelet replacement therapy, including active bleeding, infection with fever, and the presence of antiplatelet antibodies.[18]

Monitor the patient closely for signs of transfusion reaction. Appropriate measures must be taken to ensure that the patient's blood and the donor blood are properly matched. Although transfusion reactions can produce serious consequences in any patient, they are particularly problematic in the DIC patient because red cell hemolysis further intensifies bleeding episodes. Monitoring laboratory data provides valuable indices of replacement therapy effectiveness and the status of DIC resolution.

Heparin. When the underlying procoagulant stimulus cannot be removed or when hemorrhagic or thrombotic events continue despite removal of the inciting cause, additional interventions are attempted to restore an appropriate balance between coagulation and fibrinolysis. The use of heparin therapy may be considered in some clinical situations; however, anticoagulant therapy in DIC remains controversial. Its efficacy is difficult to document, and although no randomized clinical trials exist to document heparin's beneficial effects in decreasing the morbidity and mortality associated with DIC, numerous individual case studies exist in which heparin has dramatically improved the clinical picture.* However, another study reported that in at least 95% of DIC patients, heparin did not prove beneficial and could, in fact, be harmful.[7]

There is a general consensus that heparin is indicated in the management of DIC when intravascular microthrombi produce signs and symptoms of ischemic organ dysfunction or when potential loss of life or limb exists.[3,6,76] Heparin's effectiveness is established in some conditions (acute promyelocytic leukemia and retained dead fetus), but it is relatively contraindicated in other conditions (postoperative bleeding, peptic ulcer bleeding, central nervous system bleeding, and hepatic failure), and is the last recourse in others (refractory DIC).[6,24,52] In patients with DIC and septic shock, heparin is believed to be of no benefit.[77] Careful consideration is given to initiating heparin therapy in all DIC patients, particularly those with severe hepatic dysfunction, renal impairment, or vascular

---

*References 16, 31, 46, 49, 55, 74, and 75.

damage, because bleeding tendencies can be exacerbated.

Heparin produces two clinically important effects. In low doses, heparin markedly increases the activity of AT III, and together they neutralize free circulating thrombin with a resultant decrease in fibrin formation. The heparin/AT III complex also inhibits the activation of factors XIIa, IXa, Xa, and XIa. Since excessive thrombin generation stimulates the pathophysiologic alterations in DIC, heparin should theoretically interrupt the repetitive stimulation of the coagulation and fibrinolysis cycles. Additionally, heparin's anticoagulant activity prevents microvascular thrombi and subsequent capillary bed obstruction, as well as excessive platelet aggregation. Again, the effectiveness of heparin is greatly enhanced when adequate amounts of AT III exist. Exogenous heparin administration does not alter preexisting clots; however, by slowing the coagulation process it allows restoration of the clotting factors.[29]

The recommended dosage of heparin for DIC varies (500 u/hr[33], 5 to 10 u/kg every 4 hours[56], and 10 to 15 u/kg/hr).[78] The dosage must be adjusted when hepatic and/or renal dysfunction is present, and larger doses are necessary if the patient is febrile.[29] Careful monitoring of serial laboratory data is essential to evaluate the effects of heparin therapy.

Be alert for exacerbation of the bleeding diathesis, which can occur after heparin therapy is initiated. Any increase in bleeding must be reported immediately to the physician. A volume control device must always be used with intravenous heparin drips. Protamine sulfate should be readily available in the intensive care unit as an antidote for heparin overdose.

Fibrinolytic inhibitors. Fibrinolytic inhibitors, such as epsilon aminocaproic acid (EACA), generally have no value in the therapeutic management of DIC.[24,33,42,55] EACA slows the bleeding diathesis by preventing lysis of the intravascular microthrombi and the resultant release of FDPs. EACA acts to stabilize the microthrombi in DIC; however, it also impedes their clearance from the occluded microvasculature. EACA must never be administered to a DIC patient unless the patient concurrently receives heparin.[55] Administered in the absence of heparin therapy during DIC, EACA precipitates a catastrophic exacerbation of the thrombotic condition. The use of EACA has been reported to produce several cases of MSOF, perhaps related to EACA-induced microthrombi.[79]

Antithrombin III. The administration of antithrombin III concentrate is a newer, controversial treatment in DIC. A randomized series of 51 shock patients with DIC reported a distinct shortening of DIC when only antithrombin III was replaced.[84] In the same study, heparin therapy was found to be of no benefit, particularly when antithrombin III levels were decreased. When heparin and antithrombin III were administered simultaneously, thrombocytopenia and increased blood loss developed.

Another small study of intensive care patients (n = 15) with shock and DIC found that heparin therapy should be started only when antithrombin III activity was still within normal limits and that primary replacement of antithrombin III was indicated when antithrombin III activity was less than 70%.[36] This study found no benefits of simultaneous heparin and antithrombin III administration and reported a higher incidence of blood loss during concurrent therapy. In cases of irreversible shock with DIC, the investigator reported that antithrombin III administration may prove lifesaving. More randomized clinical trials with careful interpretation of the influence of other therapeutics need to be completed before the full value of antithrombin III therapy in DIC will be known.

Investigational agents. A number of experimental drugs are being explored for use in DIC. Gabexate mesylate (FOY [Japan]) is an experimental synthetic antithrombin agent that is currently unavailable in the United States. Gabexate mesylate exerts an inhibitory effect on thrombin's clotting activity and on other reactions in the clotting cascade. Gabexate mesylate may be of particular interest in DIC since its inhibitory effect on the clotting cascade occurs in the absence of antithrombin III.[85] Treatment with protein C and protein S is also being investigated. A small study of patients in Japan with DIC (n = 3) concluded that protein C or activated protein C administration significantly diminished the hypercoagulable state when therapeutic dosing with heparin was ineffective.[86] Nafamostat mesylate[87] and tranexamic acid[88] are other experimental drugs currently under study to prevent bleeding in DIC.

Hemostatic cofactor replacement. Hemostatic

deficiencies need to be corrected in the DIC patient. Folic acid deficiency results in thrombocytopenia and is corrected by administering exogenous folic acid. Vitamin K deficiency results in the hepatic system's inability to activate several important coagulation reactions involving the vitamin K–dependent clotting factors. The use of broad-spectrum antibiotics and lack of oral feedings in the critically ill patient potentiate a vitamin K deficiency.

Maintenance of organ viability

Impaired organ viability from microvascular thrombotic occlusion and hemorrhage is a major threat to the DIC patient. Impaired organ viability in DIC results from deposition of microvascular thrombi in the intravascular circulation from excessive fibrin production. Decreased circulating blood volume in the bleeding patient, producing hypovolemia and shock, also contributes to impaired organ function. Multisystem assessments are imperative to detect early signs of bleeding and thrombosis and to guide therapeutic management. It is imperative that the therapeutic regimen is individualized to support the presenting clinical problems and to minimize potential complications.

Thorough attention must be given to develop a plan of care that promotes organ viability and eliminates interventions that are deleterious to already compromised organ systems. The potential risks of therapeutic activities should be carefully weighed against the benefits of those activities for the patient.[63] In the critically ill DIC patient, the benefits may not outweigh the risks. Despite all precautions and gentle care, bleeding can occur.[29]

When DIC occurs, particularly in MSOF, aberrant bleeding can impair the viability of every organ system. The critical care practitioner must be cognizant that bleeding in DIC can be overt or covert, subtle or profuse. Although frank bleeding can occur, bleeding can also manifest as persistent oozing.

Adequate fluid replacement is imperative to restore sufficient circulating blood volume to optimize maximal tissue perfusion. Hypovolemia from hemorrhage and microvascular obstruction prevents adequate oxygen and nutrients from being delivered to the organ systems, resulting in hypoperfusion, potential cellular hypoxia, and acidosis.

Massive fluid resuscitation may be required to restore blood pressure, cardiac output, and urine output to normal limits. Because of the patient's depressed capillary circulation, be alert to signs of fluid overload during fluid resuscitation.

Vital signs must be carefully monitored for signs of hypovolemia and impending shock. Persistent hypotension, tachycardia, tachypnea, and orthopnea are significant findings in the DIC patient. Insertion of an arterial line is recommended to monitor and trend serial systolic and mean arterial blood pressure readings.[13] Although arterial line insertion is an invasive procedure that can cause the DIC patient increased bleeding at the site of insertion, it additionally provides direct access for blood sampling, thus eliminating trauma from repeated arterial and/or venous punctures. If an arterial line is present, cuff measurements of blood pressure should be avoided because the pressure from cuff inflation can produce capillary rupture and superficial bleeding.

Hemodynamic monitoring to evaluate the patient's fluid status can be achieved through CVP or pulmonary artery (PA) readings. Pressure determinations, including PAP, PCWP, and/or CVP, should be done every 2 hours, or more frequently as the patient's condition warrants. The data obtained from these measurements are vital to manage fluid replacement therapy. An abnormally high SVR reading, decreased CO, decreased PCWP, or decreased CI can indicate hypovolemia and potential hypoperfusion.[89] Hemodynamic support with dopamine and dobutamine may also be required.

The patient's medication profile must be evaluated to identify medications with anticoagulant and antiplatelet properties. Aspirin and aspirin-containing products interfere with platelet aggregation and inhibit coagulation. Many nonsteroidal antiinflammatory drugs also decrease platelet aggregation and intensify bleeding.[44] Other drugs known to interfere with platelet function include ethanol, tricyclic antidepressants, phenothiazines, furosemide, propranolol, and certain antibiotics.[46]

Other drugs intensify the DIC patient's bleeding tendency by counteracting, to some degree, the anticoagulant effect of heparin. These drugs include digitalis, nicotine, quinine, antihistamines, dextran, and tetracycline.[90] The effects, side effects, and possible drug interactions of the patient's

THERAPEUTIC MANAGEMENT IN DIC: ADDITIONAL NURSING INTERVENTIONS

The collaborative management of DIC focuses on three major goals: (1) removal of underlying pathologic conditions, (2) restoration of coagulation/fibrinolysis balance, and (3) maintenance of organ viability as discussed in the text. Additional nursing interventions that enhance the patient response to therapy are outlined below.

Altered renal, cerebral, cardiopulmonary, gastrointestinal, and/or tissue perfusion related to hemorrhage from clotting factor consumption, thrombocytopenia, excessive circulating FDPs, and secondary fibrinolysis; impaired circulating volume from excessive fibrin deposition in the microvasculature; and fluid shifts from increased capillary permeability.

Nursing interventions

Elevate lower extremities 15° to 20°

Measure calves every day

Avoid restrictive clothing

Evaluate for lower extremity bleeding if sequential compression hose ordered

Judiciously evaluate the need for and carefully perform turning and positioning

Use foam mattress pads, air mattresses, bed cradle, and therapeutic beds, as appropriate

Carefully inspect skin, particularly under extremity splinting devices

Use caution not to disrupt established clots

Minimize tape application to the skin. If necessary, use silk or paper tape. Use Montgomery straps (Johnson & Johnson) for frequent dressing changes

Measure abdominal girth as appropriate

Monitor for decreased urine output and increased specific gravity

Avoid limb restraints whenever possible

If invasive line not present, use small-gauge needles for venipuncture and venous cannulation unless replacement therapy requires a larger gauge

Apply local pressure for a minimum of 3 to 5 minutes for venipuncture and 10 minutes for arterial puncture

Apply cold compresses to bleeding sites as appropriate

Avoid IM injections

Perform care in a gentle manner

Ensure that all oxygen delivery is humidified

Use minimal amount of suction pressure for NT, ET, or oral suctioning

Prevent situations that produce a Valsalva maneuver, such as coughing, gagging, or straining

Use only electric razor

Gently use soft toothbrush, cotton or foam swabs and normal saline, diluted baking soda, or alcohol-free mouthwash for mouth care

Apply moisturizer frequently to lips

Adequately lubricate tubes before insertion

Apply antiembolism hose as ordered

Incorporate care of invasive lines and monitoring parameters into the plan of care

Evaluate continuous cardiac monitoring data for dysrhythmias or wave changes

Accurately document amounts of all oral, enteral, and/or parenteral intake and all output

Evaluate and Hematest all outputs as appropriate

Notify physician of abnormal systems assessments and of persistent hypotension, tachycardia, tachypnea, orthopnea, and significant blood loss.

Pain related to tissue ischemia or bleeding into closed spaces.

Nursing interventions

Assess for verbal and nonverbal indicators of pain

Assess and document character, intensity, location, and duration of any pain

Determine what activities contribute to or help relieve pain

Apply cold compresses to painful joints

Incorporate pharmacologic and nonpharmacologic interventions for pain control

Evaluate respiratory and circulatory status before administering narcotics

Document the effectiveness of pain control interventions

Notify the physician of significant or unrelieved pain

Anxiety related to critical illness, unfamiliar environment and events, and potential alteration in body image.

Nursing interventions

Help the patient and family adjust to the critical care environment

Evaluate the impact of the therapeutic interventions on the patient and family's emotional status

Evaluate patient and family resources to determine if outside assistance needed

Identify patient and family coping strategies and encourage adaptive coping styles

Validate the patient and family's knowledge base

Provide honest, careful answers to questions to maintain realistic hope

Allow family sufficient time to visit, particularly when patient's prognosis is poor

Create opportunities for family to assist in planning and participating in the patient's care, should they desire therapeutic regimen must be assessed on an ongoing basis.

Oxygen supply and transport must be maximized to promote organ viability in the DIC patient. The sudden onset of respiratory distress or ARDS is indicative of impaired lung perfusion. Supplemental oxygen or mechanical ventilation may be required to promote adequate tissue and organ oxygenation. Monitoring oxygen saturation with a pulse oximeter is a useful noninvasive measure.

Arterial blood gas data provide useful information about the existence or persistence of acidosis or hypoxia, two conditions that can trigger DIC. Pulmonary intravascular occlusion alters the pulmonary vascular dynamics, predisposing the patient to pulmonary shunting and subsequent compromised gas exchange.[61] Pulmonary hypertension, evidenced by increased PA pressures, suggests intrapulmonary vascular clotting.[62] Pulmonary embolism can occur from microvascular obstruction and produce an increased alveolar-arterial (A-a) oxygen gradient greater than 30 mm Hg.[89]

Critical illness requires additional calories and protein to meet the body's increased metabolic demands. Adequate nutrients are required, too, for production of new red blood cells to replace those lost through bleeding. Inadequate nutrition affects, and is affected by, the immune response, thus potentially increasing the occurrence and the severity of infection.[91] Additional nursing interventions to supplement the therapeutic management plan are found in the accompanying box on page 78.

CONCLUSION

Dysfunction in the complex physiologic interactions occurring among organ systems and the inflammatory/immune response in MSOF contributes to the pathophysiologic alterations in normal hemostatic function that produce the simultaneous thrombotic and hemorrhagic events in DIC. In the critically ill patient, DIC can also potentiate the development of MSOF. Although numerous clinical conditions can precipitate DIC and MSOF, uncontrolled inflammation and infection are commonly implicated in both conditions. Therapeutic management must focus on removing the underlying pathologic conditions, restoring an appropriate balance between coagulation and fibrinolysis, and maintaining organ viability. Intensive, knowledgeable assessment, planning, and intervention

are vital to minimizing the high morbidity and mortality rates associated with DIC and MSOF.

REFERENCES

1. Thompson AR, Harker LA. Manual of hemostasis and thrombosis. 3rd ed. Philadelphia: FA Davis, 1983.
2. Johanson BC et al. Standards for critical care. 3rd ed. St. Louis: Mosby–Year Book, 1988.
3. Lazarchick J, Krizer J. Interaction of fibrinolytic, coagulation, and kinin systems and related pathology. In: Pittiglio DH, Sacher RA, eds. Clinical hematology and fundamentals of hemostasis. Philadelphia: FA Davis, 1987.
4. Griffin JP. Be prepared for the bleeding patient. Nursing 1986; 16:34-40.
5. Baker WF. Clinical aspects of disseminated intravascular coagulation: A clinician's point of view. Semin Thromb Hemost 1989; 15:1-57.
6. Levitt LJ. Disseminated intravascular coagulation. In: Rippe JM, ed. Manual of intensive care medicine. Boston: Little Brown, 1989.
7. Logan LJ. Hemostasis and bleeding disorders. In: Mazza JJ, ed. Manual of clinical hematology. Boston: Little Brown, 1988.
8. Feinstein DI. Treatment of disseminated intravascular coagulation. Semin Thromb Hemost 1988; 14:351-362.
9. Saito H. Normal hemostatic mechanisms. In: Ratnoff OD, Forbes CD, eds. Disorders of hemostasis. Orlando: Grune and Stratton, 1984.
10. Bevilacqua MP, Gimbrone MA. Inducible endothelial functions in inflammation and coagulation. Semin Thromb Hemost 1987; 13:425-433.
11. Stemerman MB, Colton C, Morell E. Perturbations of the endothelium. In: Spaet TH, ed. Progress in hemostasis and thrombosis. Orlando: Grune and Stratton, 1987.
12. Jaffe EA. Endothelial cell structure and function. In: Hoffman R, Benz Jr EJ, Shattil SJ, Furie B, Cohen HJ, eds. Hematology: Basic principles and practice. New York: Churchill Livingstone, 1991.
13. Perry AG, Potter PA. Shock: Comprehensive nursing management. St. Louis: Mosby–Year Book, 1988.
14. Guyton AC. Textbook of medical physiology, 8th ed. Philadelphia: WB Saunders, 1991.
15. Van Dam-Meiras MCE, Muller AD. Blood coagulation as a part of the haemostatic system. In: Zwaal RFA, Hemker HC, eds. Blood coagulation. New York: Elsevier Science Publishers, 1986.
16. Babior BM, Stossel TP. Hematology: A pathophysiological approach. 2nd ed. New York: Churchill Livingstone, 1990.
17. Isenberg WM, Bainston DF. Megakaryocyte and platelet structure. In: Hoffman R, Benz Jr EJ, Shattil SJ, Furie B, Cohen HJ, eds. Hematology: Basic principles and practice. New York: Churchill Livingstone, 1991.
18. Rapaport SI. Introduction to hematology. 2nd ed. Philadelphia: JB Lippincott, 1987.
19. Zucker-Franklin B. Platelet morphology and function. In: Williams WJ, Beutler E, Erslev AJ, Lichtman MA, eds. Hematology. 4th ed. New York: McGraw-Hill, 1990.
20. Siegrist CW, Jones JA. Disseminated intravascular coagulopathy and nursing implications. Semin Oncol Nurs 1985; 1:237-243.

21. Bithell TC. Normal hemostasis and coagulation. In: Thorup OA, ed. Leavell and Thorup's fundamentals of clinical hematology. 5th ed. Philadelphia: WB Saunders, 1987.

22. Brandt JT. Current concepts of coagulation. Clin Obstet Gynecol 1985; 28:3-14.

23. Müller-Berghaus G. Pathophysiologic and biochemical events in disseminated intravascular coagulation: Dysregulation of procoagulant and anticoagulant pathways. Semin Thromb Hemost 1989; 15:58-87.

24. Nanfro JJ. Anticoagulants in critical care medicine. In: Chernow B, ed. The pharmacologic approach to the critically ill patient. 2nd ed. Baltimore: Williams and Wilkins, 1988.

25. Darovic G. Disseminated intravascular coagulation. Crit Care Nurs 1982; 2:36-46.

26. Osterud B. Initiation mechanisms: Activation induced by thromboplastin. In: Zwaal RFA, Hemker HC, eds. Blood coagulation. New York: Elsevier Science Publishers, 1986.

27. Griffith MJ. Inhibitors: Antithrombin III and heparin. In: Zwaal RFA, Hemker HC, eds. Blood coagulation. New York: Elsevier Science Publishers, 1986.

28. Bach RR. Initiation of coagulation by tissue factor. CRC Crit Rev Biochem 1988; 23:339-368.

29. Rooney A, Haviley C. Nursing management of disseminated intravascular coagulation. Oncol Nurs Forum 1985; 12:15-22.

30. Comp PC. Hereditary disorders predisposing to thrombosis. In: Coller BS, ed. Progress in hemostasis and thrombosis. Orlando: Grune and Stratton, 1986.

31. Carr ME. Disseminated intravascular coagulation: Pathogenesis, diagnosis, and therapy. J Emerg Med 1987; 5:311-322.

32. Colman RW, Rubin RN. Disseminated intravascular coagulation due to malignancy. Semin Oncol 1990; 17:172-186.

33. Fruchtman S, Aledort LM. Disseminated intravascular coagulation. Am J Cardiol 1986; 3:159B-167B.

34. Schwartz RS et al. Clinical experience with antithrombin III concentrate in the treatment of congenital and acquired deficiency of antithrombin. The antithrombin III study group. Am J Med 1989; 87:53S-60S.

35. Hauptman TG et al. Efficacy of antithrombin III in endotoxin-induced disseminated intravascular coagulation. Circ Shock 1988; 25:111-122.

36. Vinazzer H. Therapeutic use of antithrombin III in shock and disseminated intravascular coagulation. Semin Thromb Hemost 1989; 15:347-352.

37. Esmon NL. Thrombomodulin. In: Coller BS, ed. Progress in hemostasis and thrombosis. Philadelphia: WB Saunders, 1989.

38. Moake J. Hypercoagulable states: New knowledge about old problems. Hosp Pract 1991; 26:31-42.

39. Wolf P. The importance of alpha$_2$-antiplasmin in the defibrination syndrome. Arch Intern Med 1989; 149:1724-1725.

40. Vogelpohl RA. Disseminated intravascular coagulation. Crit Care Nurs 1981; 1:38-43.

41. Hudak CM, Gallo BM, Benz JJ, eds. Critical care nursing: A holistic approach. 5th ed. Philadelphia: JB Lippincott, 1990.

42. Bithell TC. Disorders of blood coagulation. In: Thorup OA, ed. Leavell and Thorup's fundamentals of clinical hematology. 5th ed. Philadelphia: WB Saunders, 1987.

43. Ratnoff OD. Disseminated intravascular coagulation. In: Ratnoff OD, Forbes CD, eds. Disorders of hemostasis. Orlando: Grune and Stratton, 1984.

44. Thelan LA, Davie JK, Urden LD. Textbook of critical care nursing: Diagnosis and management. St Louis: Mosby–Year Book, 1990.

45. Suchak BA, Barbon CB. Disseminated intravascular coagulation: A nursing challenge. Orthop Nurs 1989; 8:61-69.

46. Baue AE. Multiple organ failure: Patient care and prevention. St Louis: Mosby–Year Book, 1990.

47. Yurt RW, Lowry SF. Role of the macrophage and endogenous mediators in multiple organ failure. In: Deitch EA, ed. Multiple organ failure: Pathophysiology and basic concepts of therapy. New York: Thieme Medical Publishers, 1990.

48. Esparaz B, Green D. Disseminated intravascular coagulation. Crit Care Nurs Q 1990; 13:7-13.

49. Brozovic M. Disseminated intravascular coagulation. In: Bloom AL, Thomas DP, eds. Haemostasis and thrombosis. 2nd ed. New York: Churchill Livingstone, 1987.

50. Griffin JP. Hematology and immunology: Concepts for nursing. Norwalk CT: Appleton-Century-Crofts, 1986.

51. Young LM. DIC: The insidious killer. Crit Care Nurse 1990; 10:26-33.

52. Bick RL. Disseminated intravascular coagulation and related syndromes: A clinical review. Semin Thromb Hemost 1988; 14:299-338.

53. Turgeon ML. Clinical hematology: Theory and procedures. Boston: Little Brown, 1988.

54. Bolton FG. Disseminated intravascular coagulation. Int Anesth Clin 1985; 23:89-101.

55. Marder VJ. Consumptive thrombohemorrhagic disorders. In: Williams WJ, Beutler E, Erslev AJ, Lichtman MA, eds. Hematology. 4th ed. New York: McGraw-Hill, 1990.

56. Gregory SA et al. Hematologic emergencies. Med Clin North Am 1986; 70:1129-1149.

57. Lamb C. When you suspect DIC. Patient Care 1985; 19:84-87, 90, 93.

58. Hesselvik F et al. Fibronectin and other DIC-related variables in septic ICU patients receiving cryoprecipitate. Scand J Clin Lab Invest 1985; 45:67-74.

59. Fry DE. Diagnosis and epidemiology of multiple organ failure. In: Deitch EA, ed. Multiple organ failure: Pathophysiology and basic concepts of therapy. New York: Thieme Medical Publishers, 1990.

60. Tanaka T et al. Sepsis model with reproducible manifestations of multiple organ failure (MOF) and disseminated intravascular coagulation (DIC). Thromb Res 1989: 54:53-61.

61. Dolan JT. Critical care nursing: Management through the nursing process. Philadelphia: FA Davis, 1991.

62. Moorhouse MF, Geissler AC, Doenges ME. Critical care plans: Guidelines for patient care. Philadelphia: FA Davis, 1987.

63. Bell TN. Disseminated intravascular coagulation and shock: Multisystem crisis in the critically ill. Crit Care Nurs Clin North Am 1990; 2:255-268.

64. Nyman D. To the discussion on the definition of DIC and its treatment. Scand J Clin Lab Invest 1985; 45:31-33.

65. Blomback M et al. Blood coagulation and fibrinolytic factors as well as their inhibitors in trauma. Scand J Clin Lab Invest 1985; 45:15-23.

66. Tietz NW. Clinical guide to laboratory tests. 2nd ed. Philadelphia: WB Saunders, 1990.

67. Tomoaki T et al. Plasmin alpha$_2$-plasmin inhibitor-plasmin complex and FDP D-dimer in fulminant hepatic failure. Thromb Res 1989; 53:253-260.

68. Hafter R et al. Measurement of crosslinked fibrin derivatives in plasma and ascitic fluid with monoclonal antibodies against D-dimer using EIA and latex test. Scand J Clin Lab Invest 1985; 45:137-144.

69. Wilde JT et al. Plasma D-dimer levels and their relationship to serum fibrinogen/fibrin degradation products in hypercoagulable states. Br J Haematol 1989; 71:65-70.

70. Carr JM, McKinney M, McDonagh J. Diagnosis of disseminated intravascular coagulation: Role of D-dimer. Am J Clin Pathol 1989; 91:280-287.

71. Boisclair M et al. A comparative evaluation of assays for markers of activated coagulation and/or fibrinolysis: Thrombin-antithrombin complex, D-dimer, and fibrinogen/fibrin fragment E antigen. Br J Haematol 1990; 74:471-479.

72. Takahashi T et al. Thrombin vs. plasmin generation in disseminated intravascular coagulation associated with various underlying disorders. Am J Hematol 1990; 33:90-95.

73. Mayberry LJ, Forte AB. Pregnancy-related disseminated intravascular coagulation (DIC). MCN 1985; 10:168-173.

74. Karakusis PH. Considerations in the therapy of septic shock. Med Clin North Am 1986; 70:933-944.

75. Knuppel RA, Rao PS, Cavanaugh D. Septic shock in obstetrics. Clin Obstet Gynecol 1984; 27:3-10.

76. Cerra FB. Manual of critical care. St. Louis: Mosby–Year Book, 1987.

77. Luce JM. Septic shock: A threat to the threatened. Emerg Med 1987; 19:25-27, 31-33.

78. Wolfe DW. Hematologic complications of malignancy. Top Emerg Med 1986; 8:13-24.

79. Williams E. Plasma alpha$_2$-antiplasmin activity. Role in the evaluation and management of fibrinolytic states and other bleeding disorders. Arch Intern Med 1989; 149:1769-1772.

80. Pisciotto PT, Snyder EL. Use and administration of blood and components. In: Chernow B, ed. The pharmacologic approach to the critically ill patient. 2nd ed. Baltimore: Williams and Wilkins, 1985.

81. Newman RS. Excessive blood loss and its relationship to clotting system changes during and after major surgery. Crit Care Clin 1987; 3:417-427.

82. US Department of Health and Human Services, National Institutes of Health. Transfusion therapy guidelines for nurses. NIH publication no. 90-2668, 1990.

83. Hamilton GC. Hemostasis out of order. Emerg Med 1985; 17:82-88, 90, 92-93.

84. Blauhut B, Kramar H, Vinazzer H. Substitution of antithrombin III in shock and DIC: A randomized study. Thromb Res 1985; 39:81-89.

85. Umeki S et al. Gabexate mesylate as a therapy for disseminated intravascular coagulation. Arch Intern Med 1988; 148:1409-1412.

86. Okajima K et al. Treatment of patients with disseminated intravascular coagulation by protein C. Am J Hematol 1990; 33:277-278.

87. Takahashi H et al. Nafamostat mesylate (FUT-175) in the treatment of patients with disseminated intravascular coagulation. Thromb Haemost 1989; 62:90-95.

88. Takada A et al. Prevention of severe bleeding by tranexamic acid in a patient with disseminated intravascular coagulation. Thromb Res 1990; 58:101-108.

89. Swearingen PL, Hicks Keen J. Manual of critical care: applying nursing diagnosis to adult critical illness. 2nd ed. St Louis: Mosby–Year Book, 1991.

90. Kirchner CW, Reheis CE. Two complications of neoplasia: Sepsis and DIC. Nurs Clin North Am 1982; 17:595-606.

91. McFarland GK, McFarlane EA, eds. Nursing diagnosis and intervention: Planning for patient care. St Louis: Mosby–Year Book, 1989.

SECTION TWO

Pathophysiology

Following the primary events and overwhelming mediator activity, pathophysiologic changes occur at the systemic level. The exaggerated mediator response provokes maldistribution of circulating volume, imbalance of oxygen supply and demand, and alterations in metabolism. These three pathophysiologic changes incite ischemia, tissue damage, and organ failure.

5 Maldistribution of Circulating Volume

Elaine V. Robins

Maldistribution of circulating volume is a major component in the pathophysiology of multisystem organ failure (MSOF). Blood flow may be altered in the microvascular, organ, and regional circulations. These altered circulations are frequently triggered by a definable episode of shock that is followed by resuscitation. Risk factors identified by Cerra in the development of MSOF are sepsis; perfusion deficits, as with ruptured aneurysms; a persistent source of severe inflammation, such as pancreatitis; and a persistent source of dead or injured tissue, as with multiple trauma or severe burns.[1] Blood flow abnormalities occur with all of these risk factors.

Many clinical conditions may result in MSOF. Once the initial insult has occurred, common pathways are identifiable in the development and progression of MSOF. This chapter will focus on the pathophysiology and treatment of maldistribution of circulating volume to organs, tissues, and cells.

PATHOPHYSIOLOGY

Shock is the most common single cause of MSOF. Shock may be categorized as hypovolemic, cardiogenic, or distributive (septic, neurogenic, or anaphylactic). Hypovolemic shock (as seen with traumatic hemorrhage or ruptured aneurysms) and septic shock are most frequently implicated in the development of MSOF. Hypovolemia causes a tissue perfusion deficit initiated by the resistance vessels' response to the diminished blood volume. Septic shock is believed to directly cause a maldistribution of blood flow to the tissues secondary to the release of inflammatory mediators. These defects in blood flow occur primarily in the microcirculation and may be perpetuated at this level by the local processes that occur in response to the initial maldistributive defect.

The microcirculation consists of the arterioles, the capillaries, and the venules (Fig. 5-1). The arterioles are muscular structures with sympathetic innervation that provide about 80% of the total systemic vascular resistance in the normal state. From the arterioles, blood flows to the metarterioles and then to either the arteriovenous anastomoses or the true capillaries. A precapillary sphincter controls the point where the metarteriole branches into a capillary.

In response to hypovolemia, direct sympathetic vasoconstrictor activity increases arteriolar tone. Circulating factors such as catecholamines, angiotensin, vasopressin, and serotonin also increase arteriolar constriction. Other factors produce their effects only at the local level because of the short half-lives of these molecules. Factors known to constrict or dilate the arterioles are listed in Table 5-1.

The venules also have a smooth muscle coat but not as extensive as that of the arterioles. This smooth muscle gives the venule the ability to venoconstrict in response to catecholamines; therefore capillary pressure rises. This ability to venoconstrict remains intact even during tissue ischemia and hypoxia. Venoconstriction tends to increase capillary hydrostatic pressure; consequently, fluid shifts and edema formation occur.[2] Other factors that cause venoconstriction and venodilatation are listed in Table 5-1.[2-5]

The capillary bed, metarterioles, and precapillary sphincters have minimal innervation. The muscle fibers of the metarterioles and precapillary sphincters are controlled by local factors such as the concentrations of oxygen, carbon dioxide, hydrogen ions, and electrolytes rather than by sympathetic activity.[3] Dilatation of the capillary bed is affected by the humoral mediators histamine and

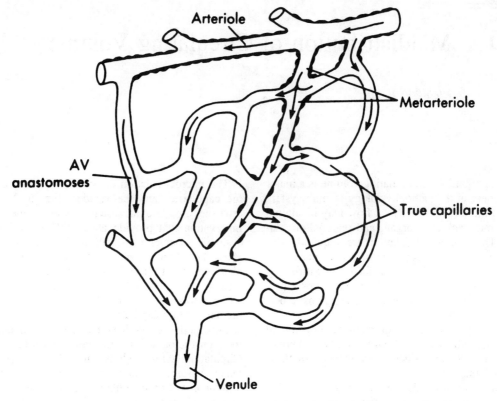

Fig. 5-1 Microcirculation. (From Perry AG, Potter PA, eds. Shock: Comprehensive Nursing Management. St. Louis: Mosby–Year Book, 1983:43.)

serotonin, which are released locally with tissue injury. As a passive exchange circuit, the capillary bed is vulnerable to extrinsic factors. Blood flow can be slowed or stopped by mechanical factors such as thrombi, cell aggregates, and increased blood viscosity. Interstitial edema will also retard flow through the capillary bed because edema compresses the capillaries.

Release of vasoactive mediators with injury or inflammation

Vasoactive mediators are released immediately with tissue injury or inflammation. These mediators are derived from humoral, cellular, or biochemical pathways and initiate changes in the distribution of the circulating volume at the systemic, regional, and local levels.[6-15] The humoral response includes the plasma enzyme cascades of complement, kallikrein/kinin, coagulation, and fibrinolysis (see Table 2-2).

The biochemical and cellular responses to sepsis, inflammation, and injury are intertwined with the humoral response. The humoral response and other factors activate numerous cells (neutrophils, macrophages, and lymphocytes), which in turn release many biochemical mediators that cause direct cell injury and maldistribution of circulating volume, such as tumor necrosis factor (TNF), interleukin-1 (IL-1), oxygen-derived free radicals (ODFR), platelet activating factor (PAF), proteases, and arachidonic acid metabolites (Fig. 5-2; Table 5-2).

Vasoactive mediators contribute to many of the vascular changes that occur with inflammation and injury.[6-15] Vasodilatation is stimulated by histamine, bradykinin, TNF, and select prostaglandins. Bradykinin's extremely powerful ability to increase blood flow and tissue edema in the area of its formation contributes to the disruption of the normal

Table 5-1 Vasoactive Mediators[2-5]

Mediator	Action	Site of action
Epinephrine	Dilatation at low doses	Arterioles and veins of skeletal and cardiac muscle
	Constriction at high doses (greater than 0.02 μg/kg/min)	Systemic arterioles and veins
Norepinephrine	Constriction (strong)	All arterioles and veins
Angiotensin	Constriction	All arterioles and veins
Vasopressin	Constriction	Systemic arterioles
Serotonin	Constriction	Systemic and pulmonary veins
	Dilatation	Precapillary sphincters
Bradykinin	Dilatation	Systemic arterioles
	Constriction	Systemic veins
Histamine	Dilatation	Systemic arterioles, veins, and precapillary sphincters
	Constriction	Pulmonary arterioles and veins
Endorphins	Dilatation	Systemic arterioles
Thromboxane A_2	Constriction	Peripheral, pulmonary, coronary, splanchnic, and renal arterioles
Prostaglandin F_{2a}	Constriction	Pulmonary, renal, and splanchnic veins
Prostacyclin	Dilatation	Systemic arterioles and veins
Endothelial derived relaxant factor	Local dilatation	Arterioles
Calcium, increased	Local constriction	Arterioles and veins
Potassium, increased	Local dilatation	Arterioles and veins
Magnesium, increased	Local dilatation (strong)	Arterioles and veins
Acidosis, severe	Local dilatation	Systemic arterioles and precapillary sphincters
	Constriction	Pulmonary arterioles
Alkalosis, severe	Dilatation	Arterioles
Hypoxia	Dilatation	Systemic arterioles and precapillary sphincters
	Constriction	Pulmonary arterioles
Hypercapnia	Dilatation	Systemic arterioles

circulation. Vasoconstriction is mediated by leukotrienes, thromboxane, and many prostaglandins.

Prostacyclin has generally been touted as a favorable prostaglandin because of its vasodilatory effects. It is a potent pulmonary and systemic vasodilator and has been reported to decrease pulmonary artery pressure and to relieve experimentally induced respiratory distress in dogs.[16] Prostacyclin seems to work in direct opposition to thromboxane A_2 because it inhibits platelet aggregation and leukocyte adherence to damaged vascular endothelium.[17]

Changes in capillary permeability occur either by mediator stimulation or by direct capillary endothelial damage. Mediators that stimulate increased capillary permeability include complement, serotonin, histamine, bradykinin, and PAF. Direct cell damage is caused by the products of neutrophils and macrophages such as ODFR, proteases, TNF, and IL-1. Many of the phagocytic neutrophils normally adhere to capillary walls, a phenomenon known as margination. Margination is enhanced by the kallikrein/kinin systems, which increases the neutrophil attraction and adherence properties of the venular endothelial surface. Migration of additional neutrophils to the site of injury

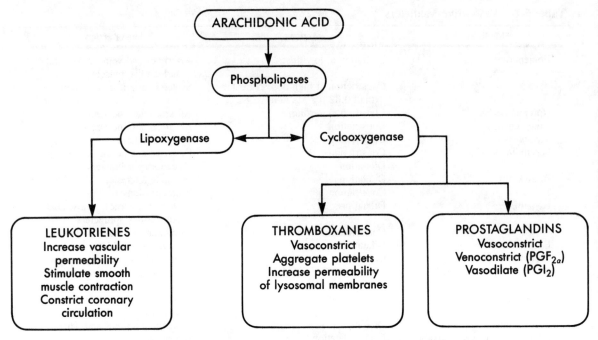

Fig. 5-2   Biologic activity of arachidonic acid metabolites.[4,14]

Table 5-2   Mediators Produced by Neutrophils and Macrophages

Cell type	Mediator	Action
Neutrophils	Platelet activating factor (PAF)	Increases capillary permeability
		Enhances neutrophil margination
		Induces platelet aggregation
Neutrophils and macrophages	Oxygen-derived free radicals (ODFR)	Phagocytosis
		Damages endothelium when antioxidant defenses depleted, thereby increasing permeability
	Proteases	Phagocytosis
		Destroys interstitial architectural proteins, thereby increasing permeability
	Arachidonic acid metabolites	See Fig. 5-2
Macrophages	Interleukin-1 (IL-1)	Attracts neutrophils
		Stimulates lymphocytes
		Elicits fever as an endogenous pyrogen
	Tumor necrosis factor (TNF)	Induces IL-1 release from endothelial cells and macrophages
		Produces hypotension

is dependent on local perfusion; therefore diminished perfusion present with hypovolemia resulting from hemorrhage or burns, venous stasis resulting from shock states, and blocked vasculature as a result of microvascular thrombi all impede cell movement. Neutrophil chemotaxis is compromised specifically in burn patients because complement component concentrations are reduced as a result of activation and consumption of complement in the burn wound.[18]

Blood flow is blocked by microthrombi formation, which is stimulated by kallikrein, PAF, and thromboxane. Many of these mediators are produced by more than one cell type or biochemical reaction. In addition, some mediators are able to reactivate the process by which they were originally formed, leading to increased mediator activity. See Chapter 3 for an in-depth discussion of the inflammatory/immune response (IIR) and inflammatory mediators.

Endothelial damage

Investigators postulate that the endothelial cell is the initial target cell in acute septic injury and acute lung injury as they occur in MSOF.[19,20] The capillary endothelial cells are susceptible to damage by many different mechanisms. Direct mechanical trauma and mechanical stress such as shear forces caused by changes in blood flow and/or pressure will activate the endothelium, causing the release of vasoactive mediators.[21]

Coagulation. Surface coagulation occurs when the smooth lining of the endothelium is disrupted, thereby setting the intrinsic clotting system into motion. Exposure of the subendothelial collagen is a powerful initiator of the clotting process. Microorganisms, endotoxin, lipid moieties, and other bacterial products and toxins stimulate host cells to release endogenous proteins or cytokines that damage the endothelium. Human endothelial cells are reported to generate procoagulants in response to endotoxin.[19]

Immune complexes and cellular interaction. Immune complex formation enhanced by the complement cascade is believed to trigger production of vasoactive mediators by endothelial cells. Complement fragment C5a interacts with neutrophils and the endothelial membrane, resulting in activation and aggregation of these leukocytes.[19] Leukocyte aggregates, platelet aggregates, and microthrombi cause mechanical obstructions of the vasculature. Neutrophils also cause damage to the vascular endothelium through the generation of oxygen radicals.[19,22]

Macrophages generate IL-1 and TNF, which damage the capillary endothelium. Each of these mediators can independently injure the vascular endothelium; however, studies have suggested that these cytokines may act synergistically to disrupt pulmonary vascular endothelium.[19] IL-1 stimulates neutrophils to increase thromboxane release and endothelial cells to produce prostaglandins and PAF.[19] TNF may evoke the synthesis and release of inflammatory mediators such as leukotrienes and PAF.[13]

Permeability changes. The capillary membrane is not only injured by these mediators but its permeability characteristics are also altered. PAF, serotonin, histamine, complement, and bradykinin directly increase vascular permeability, but other mediators produce this result by damaging the endothelium. Increased capillary permeability leads to third spacing and edema formation.

Vasomotor control. The endothelial cell has been shown to mediate the vasodilatory action of several substances, including acetylcholine, adenosine, serotonin, and catecholamines.[20] Direct vasomotor control by endothelial cells is postulated to occur by stimulus-induced contraction and regulation and/or interendothelial signal transmission along the capillary lining.[21] In other words, endothelial cells must be intact for vasoactive mediators to be effective. Endothelium-derived relaxation factor (EDRF) is the name given to the humoral agent that mediates the action of vasoactive substances. Based on the ability of nitrovasodilators to mimic EDRF through their stimulation of nitric oxide release, it has recently been postulated that EDRF and nitric oxide are the same substance.[23]

Neuroendocrine activation

The neuroendocrine response to trauma, sepsis, or shock includes the release of catecholamines, glucagon, glucocorticoids, aldosterone, renin, and angiotensin. Endogenous catecholamines are released from the adrenal medulla and peripheral adrenergic nerve endings following trauma, sepsis, or ischemia. Epinephrine and norepinephrine generally induce vasoconstriction by stimulating alpha receptors and can produce redistribution of blood flow within a given vascular bed. Specific effects on regional blood flow will be discussed in the next section.

Catecholamines also stimulate beta receptors, which directly affect cardiac function and blood flow and induce lipolysis and glycogenolysis.[24] Glucagon secretion is increased in response to catecholamines. This hormone stimulates glycogenolysis, gluconeogenesis, lipolysis, and amino acid transport to the liver for conversion to glucose precursors. Glucocorticoids are released from the adrenal cortex and prepare the body for the stress caused by the insult of trauma or disease. This preparation includes antiinflammatory effects such as stabilizing capillary, cellular, and lysosomal membranes as well as the nutritional components of gluconeogenesis, lipolysis, and protein mobilization. Aldosterone is also released into the bloodstream by the adrenal cortex in response to ACTH secretion by the anterior pituitary gland. This mineralocorticoid targets the distal renal tubules, sweat glands, salivary glands, and intestines to increase sodium reabsorption, thereby conserving extracellular fluid volume.[24]

The renin-angiotensin system is a complex humoral system with major cardiovascular effects including systemic vasoconstriction, positive inotropy, and increased capillary permeability.[25] Angiotensin II exhibits more potent cardiac activity than either angiotensin I or III; however, this action is not as strong as that produced by the catecholamines. Vasoconstriction involves all vascular beds including the coronary circulation. Angiotensin can produce redistribution of blood flow specifically in the kidney, where flow is shifted from cortical to medullary regions.[25]

Regional blood flow

Regional circulation may be redistributed in sepsis, trauma, or shock in response to the many vascular mediators already discussed. Vasodilatation and increased vascular permeability are affected at the local capillary level by the complement cascade, the kallikrein/kinin systems, and histamine release. Vasodilatation in sepsis is measured as a decrease in systemic vascular resistance, which then leads to a decrease in preload as a result of blood pooling in the periphery. The humoral systems stimulate the nonspecific immune response, resulting in neutrophil chemotaxis, phagocytosis, and release of proteases and oxygen radicals. Neutrophil activity leads to a further increase in capillary permeability and the production of monocyte/macrophage chemotactic substances. Proteases and arachidonic acid metabolites are common products of both neutrophils and macrophages. These products alter capillary permeability and generally cause vasoconstriction. Vasoconstriction is seen as an increase in systemic vascular resistance and will occur in cardiogenic or hypovolemic shock. Systemic vascular resistance remains low in sepsis. Blood flow in either sepsis or hypovolemia is further disrupted by the formation of microthrombi and cell aggregates. Fig. 5-3 depicts the many processes that contribute to maldistribution of circulating volume. This description of events is general because regional blood flow within organs varies in sepsis.

Hyperemia. Skeletal muscle is relatively unaffected in sepsis. The vascular bed in striated muscle dilates with exercise, a process known as functional hyperemia. *Functional hyperemia* also occurs in other vascular beds such as the splanchnic and cerebral circulations when the tissue served becomes highly active.

Reactive hyperemia occurs when the blood supply to tissues is occluded for a time and then is restored.[3] Blood flow then increases to about five times normal for a few seconds to a few hours, depending on the amount of time the flow was occluded. This phenomenon lasts long enough to repay almost exactly the oxygen debt accrued during the period of blockage.[3] Continued vasodilatation in reactive hyperemia is proposed to occur according to the following mechanisms: (1) blood flow–dependent vasodilatation, (2) conduction of a vasodilatory stimulus along the vessel wall from the distal to more proximal circulations through endothelial cell mediation, and (3) direct effects of a substance on vascular smooth muscle.[21] Reactive hyperemia is impaired in sepsis, so ischemic tissues may not have their oxygen demands met even if volume and flow are restored.

Principal vasodilators considered to play a role in reactive hyperemia are intermediates of the kinin and prostaglandin systems: bradykinin and prostaglandin I_2.[26] These intermediates are activated during occlusion and cause dilatation of precapillary arterioles. Hartl et al studied reactive hyper-

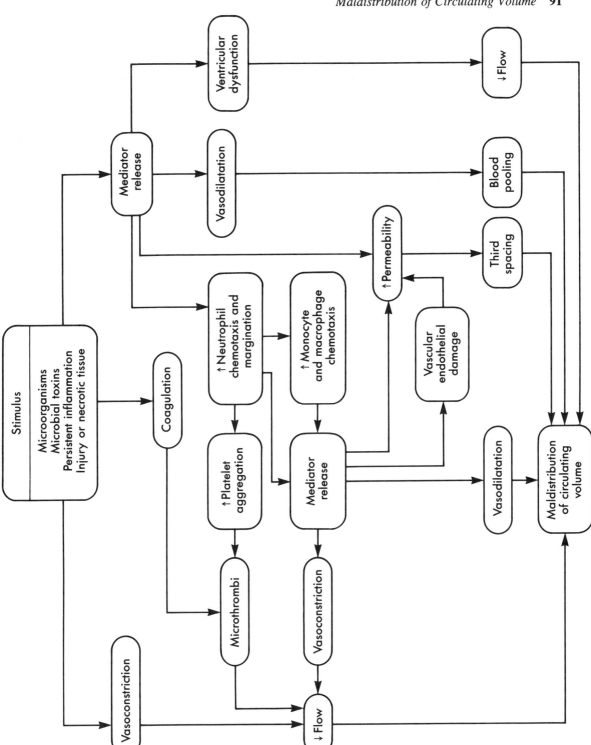

Fig. 5-3 Processes leading to maldistribution of circulating volume.

emia in 12 patients with septic conditions.[26] Nine of these patients developed MSOF with the loss of reactive hyperemia. The two patients with MSOF who survived were younger and demonstrated the return of reactive hyperemia with recovery.[26] The investigators concluded that: (1) the absence of reactive hyperemia in the septic state is not necessarily combined with impaired microvascular reactivity but may be related to generally poor clinical conditions such as severe MSOF; (2) the absence of reactive hyperemia precedes therapy-resistant hypotension, hypoxemia, and DIC, suggesting that the absence of reactive hyperemia is not caused by these conditions; and (3) provocation of reactive hyperemia may be a useful method to detect microvascular derangements in high-risk patients.[26] In other words, the loss of reactive hyperemia is an ominous sign in MSOF; however, the absence of reactive hyperemia is not diagnostic since other factors such as age will affect outcome.

Peripheral vascular paralysis. Normal peripheral vascular autoregulatory mechanisms are overridden in a condition referred to as "peripheral vascular paralysis."[7] This condition is present in the hyperdynamic stage of sepsis, which is characterized by an increased cardiac output, decreased systemic vascular resistance, altered metabolism with lactic acidosis, impaired oxygen use, and an increased microvascular permeability. Cardiac output is proposed to increase despite myocardial depression and the drop in systemic vascular resistance because fluid resuscitation has expanded the intravascular volume or because blood flow has been redirected into vascular circuits with shorter time constants. Blood is traveling faster through the vascular tree because systemic vascular resistance (SVR) is decreased and precapillary sphincters may be closed. Although this may contribute to an increased cardiac output, it may also contribute to the defect in intraorgan blood flow distribution.[7] With capacitance reduced by venoconstriction, intravascular volume is redistributed centrally; increased venous return to the right side of the heart results in increased cardiac output.

Myocardium. Flow-dependent vasodilatation is a normal response to brief periods of ischemia in the myocardium.[21] In sepsis, myocardial blood flow is redistributed from the subendocardial to the subepicardial layer.[25,27] This redistribution may be caused by myocardial edema, increased end diastolic pressure, or a release of vasoactive substances.[27] The left ventricular subendocardium, which receives most of its blood flow during diastole, is believed to be highly vulnerable to hypoperfusion and resulting ischemia because subendocardial blood flow becomes less than subepicardial flow when myocardial perfusion is compromised.[28] The intramyocardial vessels supplying the subendocardium are also subjected to the compressive effects produced by filling pressures and myocardial edema.

Adams et al reported on several animal studies in which endotoxin was infused and the left ventricular subendocardial-to-epicardial blood flow ratio remained normal or near normal despite a reduction in total coronary blood flow.[28] These findings were attributed to coronary autoregulation in which coronary blood flow was adequate to supply the energy requirements of the myocardium despite the shock state.[28] Human studies have been reported in which left ventricular coronary blood flow increased during septic shock.[29,30] These results were attributed to either excess coronary vasodilatation in relation to metabolic needs or the presence of a defect in myocardial oxygen extraction in the septic heart, which would then require an increase in coronary blood flow.[29] Excess coronary vasodilatation in relation to myocardial oxygen need indicates an abnormality in autoregulation; however, either excess coronary vasodilatation or a defect in myocardial oxygen extraction has the net result of an increase in left ventricular coronary blood flow. Global myocardial ischemia therefore does not appear to be the causative factor of myocardial depression in humans with sepsis as long as the mean arterial pressure remains equal to or greater than 60 mm Hg,[28,30] although patchy areas of ischemia and necrosis may be occurring.[29]

Right ventricular coronary blood flow also increased in animal studies; however, failing right ventricle autoregulation was suggested by a fall in the endocardial-to-epicardial blood flow ratio in the presence of mild pulmonary hypertension.[29] The right ventricle then becomes vulnerable to ischemia when ARDS-associated pulmonary hypertension occurs.

Coronary blood flow and myocardial ischemia are only parts of the question in examining myocardial dysfunction in shock. Another aspect to consider is that of contractility. Myocardial depression may be masked by the compensatory actions of epinephrine and norepinephrine on cardiac beta receptors. Beta-adrenergic blockade with propranolol uncovers this underlying myocardial depression.[28]

Myocardial depression is generally described in terms of left ventricular performance. Endotoxin's effect on left ventricular function has been well studied since endotoxin is one of the primary bacterial products present in patients with gram-negative bacterial sepsis. Endotoxemia in humans produces a hyperdynamic state with a high cardiac index and a low systemic vascular resistance index. In one study, left ventricular performance was depressed 5 hours after the administration of endotoxin and after volume loading as measured by decreased left ventricular ejection fraction and increased left end-diastolic and end-systolic volume indices.[31] Evaluation of left ventricular systolic function before and after volume loading in this same study confirmed the hypothesis that systolic left ventricular function is intrinsically abnormal in endotoxemia and that this is not simply related to preload or afterload.[31]

Right ventricular performance has been studied less; however, recent reports indicate that myocardial depression may be biventricular. Parker et al studied a group of septic patients and found that changes in the right ventricular ejection fraction and end-diastolic volume index generally followed the same direction as the comparable parameters of the left ventricle.[32] All patients were given intravenous fluids, and vasopressors were added if the mean arterial pressure remained below 60 mm Hg, thereby ruling out myocardial dysfunction resulting from hypoperfusion. The authors justify inclusion in the study of the patients receiving vasopressors because they found no differences in the hemodynamic data between patients receiving or not receiving vasopressor therapy.[32]

Ventricular dilatation occurs in sepsis and returns to normal as patients recover.[31,32] In sepsis, ventricular dilatation is seen as in increase in right and left end-diastolic volume indices. The stroke volume index remains normal, yet ejection fraction is decreased, probably because of humoral factors and increased end-diastolic volume. The compensatory mechanisms of the Starling effect help to maintain ventricular performance.[31]

Vasoactive substances also affect cardiac performance. PAF is known to cause coronary constriction; however, its role in sepsis and MSOF appears to be related to its negative inotropic effect.

Animal studies indicate that myocardial ischemia may increase the local production of PAF and render the heart more susceptible to its action, thereby perpetuating ischemic cellular injury.[10] Myocardial depressant factor (MDF) is another substance hypothesized to cause decreased cardiac contractility. Pancreatic ischemia is reported to stimulate the release of MDF into the circulation. The biologic actions of MDF are thought to include negative inotropy, splanchnic constriction, and depressed phagocytosis by the reticuloendothelial system.[25] Leukotrienes have been shown to produce a dose-dependent coronary vasoconstriction in animal models that is prevented by the administration of a leukotriene receptor antagonist.[14] Leukotriene C_4 appears to be more potent than leukotriene D_4 in this regard; however, both leukotrienes produce a negative inotropic effect that is not blocked by leukotriene receptor antagonists.[14] More studies are required to define the effect of endogenously produced mediators on cardiac blood flow and performance.

Pulmonary vasculature. The pulmonary vascular response to endotoxin is a two-phase process consisting of the initial vasoconstrictive phase followed by the phase of increased microvascular permeability. Vasoconstriction of the pulmonary arterioles is measured by pulmonary artery pressures and pulmonary vascular resistance. This constriction is mediated by many substances that are released during shock and sepsis; pulmonary hypertension is common in experimental endotoxemia.[32] Endotoxin stimulates arachidonic acid metabolism, which produces leukotrienes through the lipoxygenase pathway. Leukotrienes have been shown to affect contraction of the bronchial smooth muscle, enhance the action of histamine, and increase vascular permeability.[33]

In animal studies, leukotrienes increase both pulmonary vascular resistance and vascular permeability; however, the change in pulmonary vascular resistance is transient and may be blocked by leukotriene receptor antagonists or indomethacin.[14] The pulmonary venoconstrictor effect of arachidonic acid metabolism is therefore likely to be mediated by cyclooxygenase products such as thromboxane, since the constriction is reported to be inhibited by cyclooxygenase and thromboxane synthetase inhibitors.[34,35] Ibuprofen has recently been shown to inhibit pulmonary hypertension and the hyperdynamic response to endotoxin in sheep.[36]

Ibuprofen did not attenuate the microvascular leak, leading the authors to conclude that the ibuprofen effect may be due to a response other than decreased prostanoid production.[36]

Sensitivity to endotoxin varies among species, with the sheep model considered closest to the human response. A recent study of normal volunteers administered endotoxin reported no changes in pulmonary artery pressures (PAP) or pulmonary capillary wedge pressure (PCWP) when compared with controls.[31] PAP and PCWP increased in both groups with volume loading; however, no significant differences were noted.[31] Another recent study of patients in septic shock reported a mean PAP of 22 mm Hg.[32] This value returned to normal in survivors but remained high in nonsurvivors.[32] Pulmonary vascular resistance index did not change significantly in either survivors or nonsurvivors.[32] The differences reported in these studies may reflect measurements taken during different phases of sepsis.

Alveolar hypoxia causes reflex pulmonary hypertension because precapillary arteries constrict and blood flow is directed to other areas of the lung. Although leukotrienes have been implicated as mediators of this response, their exact role is unconfirmed. Studies with dogs demonstrate the expected increases in pulmonary vascular resistance and leukotriene concentrations in bronchoalveolar lavage fluid after induced alveolar hypoxia; however, administering a leukotriene inhibitor did not alleviate the pulmonary vasoconstriction even though leukotriene concentrations were controlled.[14] Reflex pulmonary hypertension resulting from alveolar hypoxia may be mediated by several substances released by perivascular mast cell degranulation such as thromboxane, serotonin, and histamine.[34]

Endotoxin-induced pulmonary endothelial damage is caused by neutrophil release of leukotrienes, but this damage may also occur through alternate pathways.[37] Alveolar macrophages may be stimulated by endotoxin to produce oxygen free radicals, proteolytic enzymes, or both.[37] Oxygen radical formation in the neutrophil occurs during a process known as "respiratory burst" that is enhanced in the presence of alveolar macrophages. The result is an overwhelmed antioxidant balance and damage to the pulmonary vascular endothelium.[19,22] Oxidant injury is also perpetrated by the xanthine-hy-poxanthine pathway, which will be discussed in the section on postischemic reperfusion injury.

Neutrophils sequestered in response to the initial injury are hypothesized to cause oxidant lung injury by two mechanisms: first, neutrophil-produced peroxide diffuses directly into pulmonary endothelial cells; and, second, a more potent oxidizing agent, the hydroxyl radical, is produced when neutrophil peroxide is produced in the presence of free iron.[38] Catalase, an endogenous lung tissue antioxidant, has been demonstrated to be greatly reduced after endotoxemia in sheep; therefore lung tissue may be susceptible to subsequent peroxide injury before catalase activity is restored.[38] Endotoxin stimulates lymphocytes to produce lymphokines, which have a chemotactant effect on neutrophils, thus increasing neutrophil activity and, consequently, endothelial damage in the septic lung.[11]

The cyclooxygenase pathway of arachidonic acid is also stimulated by endotoxin. Thromboxane A_2, a metabolite of this pathway, causes pulmonary vasoconstriction, mediates bronchoconstriction, increases membrane permeability, and aggregates platelets and neutrophils.[4,11] Increased levels of thromboxane A_2 are reported to be associated with the pulmonary hypertension, hypoxia, and increased airway resistance that occur in endotoxemia.[4] Differences in response to thromboxane exist among species, but a prospective study of 106 septic surgical patients revealed that the transpulmonary thromboxane B_2 gradient correlated with the degree of pulmonary hypertension.[4] Thromboxane B_2 is the stable, measurable end-metabolite of the short-lived, physiologically active mediator thromboxane A_2.

Prostacyclin (PGI_2), another active metabolite from the cyclooxygenase pathway of arachidonic acid, inhibits thromboxane and is a potent pulmonary vasodilator.[11] This mediator has been used experimentally to treat the pulmonary hypertension associated with endotoxemia.[17] It is likely that, under normal circumstances, a balance among the endogenous constrictor and dilator prostaglandins may be necessary to maintain normal pulmonary and systemic vascular tone.

Increased pulmonary vascular permeability is the second phase occurring in traumatic and septic shock. As mentioned, this change is thought to be mediated by several substances including oxidants, leukotrienes, thromboxane, histamine, serotonin, and bradykinin. Conflicting studies have been reported regarding the role of leukotrienes in altering vascular permeability.[34] Further investigation is indicated to determine whether leukotrienes increase vascular permeability directly or increase transvascular fluid filtration by increasing the microvascular hydrostatic pressure.[34] Thromboxane A_2 inhibition has recently been shown to decrease lymph protein clearance in sheep that had received an infusion of endotoxin.[35] This study suggests that phase II increases in microvascular permeability may be attenuated by the specific inhibition of thromboxane A_2, whereas cyclooxygenase inhibition was unsuccessful.[35]

In summary, changes occurring in the pulmonary vasculature include vasoconstriction, increased hydrostatic pressure, increased capillary permeability, increased fluid movement, and microthrombi formation. These changes potentiate ventilation to perfusion (V/Q) mismatching, intrapulmonary shunting, and poor oxygenation status.

Splanchnic circulation. The splanchnic circulation serves the gastrointestinal tract, the spleen, the pancreas, and the liver. Blood flow to the splanchnic circulation is greatly reduced during trauma, shock, or sepsis. Leukotrienes have been shown to be potent mesenteric vasoconstrictors.[14,29] The bowel is reported to lose reactive hyperemia and thus the ability to augment blood flow after an ischemic event.[29] This finding supports the work of Hartl et al, who reported a loss of reactive hyperemia in septic patients before the development of MSOF.[26]

Decreased blood flow to the gastrointestinal tract results in an ileus; however, prolonged ischemia may result in mucosal erosions because of mucosal barrier breakdown, changes in intramural pH, and diminished epithelial regeneration.[39] These lesions are found primarily in the stomach, jejunum, and ileum and are presumed to occur as a result of high alpha-receptor activity in the splanchnic vascular bed, which leads to a selective decrease in circulation to the mucosal layer.[40] Blunt and penetrating abdominal trauma can cause intestinal disruption and fecal contamination of the peritoneal cavity. Translocation of enteric bacteria and endotoxin from the bowel lumen to the portal circulation is reported to occur when bowel integrity is compromised by decreased blood flow.[7,41] The liver is then challenged to clear these bacteria and their toxins before they reach the central circulation.

Hepatic ischemia is believed to occur in sepsis despite the normotensive, hyperdynamic state. Animal studies report that a fall in hepatic blood flow was associated with a fall in energy charge and an elevation of the tissue lactate-to-pyruvate ratio.[29] Despite decreased blood flow, metabolic demands on the liver are increased in sepsis and shock as vasoactive mediators stimulate gluconeogenesis and protein synthesis, especially acute phase proteins. Decreased hepatic perfusion decreases the performance of vital functions of the liver, including phagocytosis by Kupffer cells, detoxification of drugs and hormones, and removal of activated clotting factors.[39]

Intraorgan hepatic blood flow is congested and associated with dilatation of sinusoids, particularly in the centrilobular region.[40] As blood moves from the lobule's periphery to the central lobular region, the hepatocytes are continuously extracting oxygen; therefore less oxygen may reach the centrilobular region and predispose the region to ischemic damage.[40] Hepatocyte lipid accumulation is another change seen in the ischemic liver.[40] This intracellular lipid accumulation, or fatty change, indicates an abnormality in the liver's ability to process lipid. Fatty change may occur in other organs, but it is most commonly seen in the liver because the liver is the primary fat-metabolizing organ.

Hepatic perfusion deficits may stem from several mechanisms. Microcirculatory aggregates of platelets, leukocytes, and fibrin have been identified in the liver.[6,42] Thromboxane A_2 has been implicated in reducing hepatic blood flow in sepsis; however, the level at which this mediator produces its effect (prehepatic, hepatic and/or mesenteric vascular, or intrahepatic) has not been determined.[43]

Following reperfusion of the splanchnic bed, many toxic mediators released by the liver and other GI organs during the ischemic period enter the circulation. After exposure to bacteria and endotoxin, hepatic macrophages release interleukin-1, which causes the liver to produce C-reactive protein.[39] This protein is considered to be proteolytic, but its role in MSOF is unclear. Two mediators released by the ischemic intestine, serotonin and thromboplastin, activate the clotting cascade and promote the development of disseminated intravascular coagulopathy. The ischemic pancreas releases pancreatic enzymes and myocardial depressant factor into the circulation during shock. Myocardial depressant factor is reported to further increase splanchnic vasoconstriction and depress myocardial contractility.[25]

Renal vasculature. Renal blood flow is normally greater than the metabolic need of the kidney in order to maintain glomerular filtration. In shock, the hypoperfused kidneys may lose the capacity for autoregulation if the mean arterial pressure falls below 70 mm Hg.[44] Blood flow is redistributed from the outer to the inner cortex as a result of sympathetic stimulation and angiotensin production.[45] The result of this redistribution is tubular ischemia because the glomeruli and most of the tubular components are located in the outer cortex.[44] In hyperdynamic sepsis, renal blood flow is reported to increase and yet still not meet the increased renal metabolic needs in sepsis.[29] Vasoconstricting prostaglandins are thought to be responsible for the increased renin-angiotensin activity; therefore in this hypothesis an increase in prostacyclin or a reduction in thromboxane would increase glomerular filtration. This anticipated increase in glomerular filtration rate was reported in a study in which a thromboxane synthetase inhibitor was infused into septic sheep.[46]

Cerebral circulation. The brain is one of the organs preferentially perfused in shock. Cerebral blood flow increases if SaO_2 falls below 90% or if PaO_2 falls below 60 mm Hg. Autoregulatory mechanisms maintain a constant cerebral blood flow over a mean arterial pressure range of 50 to 130 mm Hg; however, global ischemia and partial ischemia will occur with cardiac arrest and shock, respectively. The brain relies on a continual supply of oxygen; consequently, hypoperfusion permits a rapid depletion of the high-energy substrates ATP and phosphocreatine. The ATP-dependent sodium-potassium pump fails, allowing potassium to leak out of the cell. Calcium enters the cell at a critical level of extracellular potassium and activates phospholipase.[47]

Phospholipase activates arachidonic acid metabolism, which will produce thromboxane A_2, leukotrienes, and oxygen-derived free radicals in the case of partial ischemia because oxygen is available to support the reaction. Thromboxane and leukotrienes cause cerebral vasoconstriction, and oxygen-derived free radicals cause further damage to the cell membrane and vascular endothelium.

Postischemic reperfusion injury

Xanthine oxidation. Postischemic reperfusion injury refers to alterations in cellular metabolism that occur during ischemic periods and the consequent inability to metabolize the toxic metabolites after reperfusion. The metabolites produced include oxygen-derived free radicals (ODFR) in which oxygen has been reduced by one, two, or three electrons. Although neutrophils and macrophages form oxygen radicals through the NADPH oxidase system during phagocytosis, another pathway involving the energy form adenosine triphosphate (ATP) generates oxygen radicals during reperfusion injury. During ischemia, ATP is metabolized to hypoxanthine, and xanthine dehydrogenase is converted to xanthine oxidase (Fig. 5-4). Xanthine oxidase catalyzes the oxidation of hypoxanthine to xanthine and uric acid when reperfusion of the tissues supplies the oxygen to support the reaction.[48] Oxygen radicals are formed as by-products of xanthine oxidation.[48]

Current research of oxidant-induced cell injury focuses on the early phase of trauma, since generalized inflammation and tissue changes are present very early after an injury has occurred.[49] Oxidant release in burn tissue is hypothesized to trigger systemic complement activation, which results in distant organ inflammation and further oxidant release.[49] Free iron is reported to react with the oxygen radicals generated by the xanthine oxidase pathway to produce a more potent oxidant, the hydroxyl ion.[50]

Deferoxamine, an approved iron chelator, has recently been shown to provide protection from oxidant injury in a sheep model of a burn injury.[50] This conclusion was reached because animals infused with deferoxamine complexed with hetastarch after a burn injury demonstrated improved cardiac function, decreased red cell hemolysis, and no evidence of lung or liver tissue lipid peroxidation as compared with animals receiving standard fluid management after a burn injury.[50] The study animals' resuscitation requirements decreased significantly, indicating less non-burn tissue fluid loss and increased oxygen consumption to meet the increased oxygen demands after the injury.[50] Along with cyclooxygenase inhibition, ibuprofen protects lung tissue from septic injury by chelating iron.[51] Ibuprofen may then protect tissues from oxygen radicals in a dual fashion by preventing initial oxidant production early after an injury and later

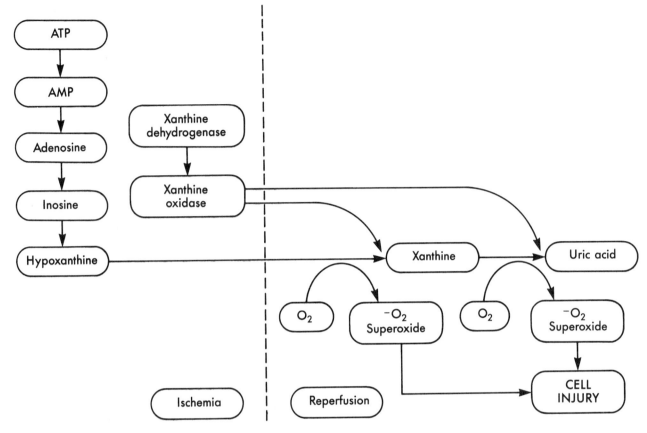

Fig. 5-4   Free radical production by xanthine oxidase pathway. *AMP,* Adenosine monophosphate; *ATP,* adenosine triphosphate. (From Black L, Coombs VJ, Townsend SN. Reperfusion and reperfusion injury in acute myocardial infarction. Heart Lung 1990; 19:279.)

oxidant generation through the arachidonic acid pathway.

Effects. Under normal conditions, intracellular antioxidant defenses protect tissues; however, these defenses are overwhelmed after ischemia with reperfusion, and tissue damage results. The effects of oxygen radical generation have been categorized into primary and secondary effects. Primary effects directly damage the cell and its function by peroxidation of the lipid moiety of the cell membrane. Hydroxyl radicals induce changes in proteins and nucleic acids causing enzyme inactivation and DNA strand breaks. Secondary effects are those that activate proteases and phospholipases through a disturbance in cellular calcium homeostasis. Phospholipases destroy the cellular infrastructure

and activate xanthine oxidase and NADPH oxidase, thereby perpetuating oxygen radical production.[48] Phospholipases also release free fatty acids, which cause an intracellular acidosis and increased arachidonic acid metabolism.

Myocardium. Postischemic reperfusion injury occurs primarily in the heart, the liver, the gut mucosa, and the kidneys. Evidence of reperfusion injury in the heart was reported by Bulkley and Hutchins at autopsies of patients who had died after coronary artery bypass graft surgery.[52] Two types of necrosis were described: a contraction band necrosis in areas that had been revascularized and a coagulation necrosis distal to obstructed vessels that were not bypassed.[52] Other processes in addition to ODFR production have been proposed to explain cardiac reperfusion injury. These processes include marked calcium entry into the cell at the moment of reperfusion, cell swelling resulting from the influx of sodium and water, and white cell plugging of capillaries and arterioles.[53] Oxygen radicals have also been implicated in depression of myocardial contractility after severe burns.[54]

Liver. Hepatic reperfusion after an ischemic period may produce not only liver injury but also widespread tissue injury. The ischemic liver releases many cytoplasmic enzymes upon reperfusion. It has been shown that xanthine dehydrogenase and xanthine oxidase are included in this hepatocellular enzyme release and stimulate the production of free oxygen metabolites.[55] The oxygen radicals produced as a result of circulating xanthine oxidase could directly injure the vascular endothelium, activate oxidant-producing inflammatory cells that could travel to and injure tissues distal to the site of origin, and produce oxygen radicals in the plasma, which has limited antioxidant defense mechanisms.[55] Allopurinol, a xanthine oxidase inhibitor, may be beneficial in the case of systemic shock because of its extracellular antioxidant effects.[55]

Another mediator reportedly released from ischemic hepatic macrophages is tumor necrosis factor.[42] Tumor necrosis factor has been shown in the rat to be associated with both hepatic and pulmonary injury after hepatic lobular ischemia and reperfusion.[42] Pretreatment with anti-TNF monoclonal antibodies in the animals studied reduced SGPT levels and completely inhibited pulmonary edema.[42] This study suggests that TNF increases the vascular endothelium's susceptibility to neutrophil-derived mediators such as ODFR; therefore TNF may potentiate further pulmonary damage.[42]

Brain. The ischemia-reperfusion sequence in the brain is followed by a prolonged postischemic hypoperfusion period associated with a profound increase in cerebral vascular resistance.[47] This cerebral vasoconstriction is attributed to cerebral edema, increased intracellular calcium, and increased levels of thromboxane A_2 in tissue as well as in the cerebral vasculature. Evidence exists to support the potential therapeutic effects of calcium channel blockers in cerebral ischemia. Postulated beneficial mechanisms include nonspecific cerebral vasodilatation, blockade of calcium activation of phospholipase, and antagonism of calcium-induced vasoconstriction.[47]

CLINICAL PRESENTATION AND ASSESSMENT
Stages of MSOF

Simply defined, MSOF is the failure of two or more organ systems. The definition of organ failure as it applies to a specific organ is more difficult to state because of the lack of consensus among reports. MSOF has been described as a syndrome with sequential progression; therefore therapy in this syndrome is best begun before organ failure declares itself. The stages of MSOF as described by DeCamp and Demling are: stage 1, clinical presentation of early sepsis; stage 2, multiple organ dysfunction; stage 3, late organ failure or established MSOF; and stage 4, the preterminal stage.[56]

Early sepsis stage and multiple organ dysfunction. The first stage of MSOF resembles early sepsis; however, a differentiation needs to be made between septicemia, septic shock, and sepsis syndrome. Septicemia is diagnosed clinically when microorganisms are identified in the bloodstream. Septicemia has been induced experimentally with infusion of either microorganisms or their endotoxins into the bloodstream. Septic shock occurs with severe infection, causing altered central hemodynamics and oxygen use. Sepsis syndrome describes nonbacteremic sepsis (absence of positive blood cultures) with symptoms such as hypotension, metabolic abnormalities, hyperthermia or hypothermia, leukocytosis or leukopenia, mental confusion, hyperventilation with hypocapnia, pulmonary edema, and a falling platelet count with or without evidence of disseminated intravascular coagulation.[7] These patients present a classic septic shock picture, but no infectious process is found. Once a general inflammatory response is begun, it may become self-perpetuating by processes already described. The patient then progresses from sepsis syndrome to MSOF.[57]

Septic shock has been classically divided into the two phases of hyperdynamic and hypodynamic shock (Table 5-3); although recent research indicates that only 10% of those who do not survive septic shock experience a true hypodynamic state.[58] The falling cardiac output (CO) commonly attributed to a "hypodynamic" phase of myocardial failure is more often related to volume status, and with adequate fluid resuscitation, most septic patients remain in the hyperdynamic phase.[58] The hyperdynamic phase is characterized by a decreased systemic vascular resistance (SVR) and increased CO.

Table 5-3 Phases of Sepsis[57, 59, 60]

	Septicemia	Hyperdynamic	Hypodynamic/preterminal
Cardiovascular	Sinus tachycardia Bounding pulse CO/CI increased Pulse pressure widens	Sinus tachycardia Warm, dry, flushed skin CO/CI normal or increased BP <90 mm Hg or 50 mm Hg below baseline PAP decreased PCWP decreased SI decreased SVR decreased PVR increased Mixed venous O_2 saturation increased	Tachycardia Dysrhythmias Weak, thready pulses Cold, pale, clammy skin CO/CI decreased Profound hypotension PAP increased PCWP increased SI decreased SVR usually increased but may be decreased PVR increased Mixed venous O_2 saturation decreased
Pulmonary	Tachypnea Hyperventilation Respiratory alkalosis	Tachypnea Respiratory depth decreased Hypoxemia Respiratory and metabolic acidosis Breath sounds diminished with crackles	Shortness of breath, if not intubated Respiratory depth decreased Refractory hypoxemia Respiratory and metabolic acidosis Breath sounds diminished with crackles and wheezes
Renal	May be within normal limits	Urine output <0.5 mL/kg/hr Occasionally, inappropriate polyuria Osmolality increased	Oliguria Anuria BUN and creatinine increased
Metabolic	Temperature elevated Hyperglycemia	Temperature elevated Hyperglycemia	Temperature subnormal Hyperglycemia or hypoglycemia Serum amylase, lipase, and LFTs elevated
Hematologic	Leukopenia followed by rebound leukocytosis with a shift to the left	WBC increased Clotting factors decreased	WBC increased or decreased Clotting factors decreased Thrombocytopenia RBC decreased
CNS	Apprehension Mental cloudiness Delayed responses	Confusion Disorientation	Obtundation

Abbreviations: *LFT*, liver function test; *CNS*, central nervous system.

Vasodilatation occurs in both the venous and the arterial vascular beds, causing both a decrease in SVR and preload. Cardiac output is maintained or increased as the heart rate increases to compensate for the hypotension. Other factors contributing to the maintenance of CO despite a fall in SVR and preload are reexpansion of the relative blood volume by fluid resuscitation and diversion of blood flow into vascular circuits with shorter time constants.[7] This maldistribution of blood flow is out of proportion to the metabolic needs of some tissues and clearly not enough to meet the needs of bypassed tissues. The arteriovenous oxygen difference begins to narrow because some tissues receive little oxygen and others may have such a rapid transit time that adequate oxygen unloading is impaired.[57]

The hypodynamic phase of septic shock, as classically described, includes a low CO and compensatory rise in SVR. If the patient is unable to compensate, both CO and SVR will be low. This terminology (hyperdynamic vs. hypodynamic) is now used to describe CO values only and cannot be based on blood pressure and peripheral responses, such as skin temperature or organ perfusion. The CO may be high, and thus hyperdynamic, even in the presence of falling urine output and other signs of hypoperfusion (decreased level of consciousness, GI bleeding, or increased liver function tests). Thus "hyperdynamic" does not apply to *adequacy* of CO or circulation but only to the cardiac output's absolute value relative to normal. As stated, research indicates that only 10% of those who do not survive septic shock experience the true, low CO, hypodynamic (myocardial failure) phase. Forty percent succumb to unresponsive hypotension secondary to refractory systemic vasodilatation, with the other 50% mortality attributed to MSOF.[58]

A classic picture of progressive and refractory shock is presented when hypodynamic septic shock does occur. Heart rate continues to increase, but myocardial contractility is further depressed by circulating mediators. Preload is greatly reduced because of maldistribution of blood flow and third spacing related to increased vascular permeability.

Organ failure stage. Universal criteria for diagnosing individual organ failure are not established. Although many definitions for organ failure exist, it is possible to identify some consistency in the criteria used in the definitions. In cardiovascular failure, indicators generally include bradycardia, cardiac index less than 2 L/min/m^2, mean arterial pressure less than 50 or 60 mm Hg, and occurrence of a lethal ventricular dysrhythmia such as ventricular tachycardia, ventricular fibrillation, or asystole.[61,62] Other indicators associated with cardiovascular failure are decreased right and left ventricular ejection fraction, an increase in left ventricular end-diastolic and end-systolic volume, and a decrease in ventricular stroke work.[62]

Respiratory failure occurs as a result of increased vascular permeability and direct endothelial damage. The lungs are the first organ to receive the toxic mediators released into the bloodstream by the ischemic liver. Mediator-induced damage results in noncardiogenic pulmonary edema, which is often followed by ARDS and nosocomial pneumonia. The clinical definition of respiratory failure used by Knaus and Wagner states that the patient would exhibit one or more of the following: respiratory rate ≤ 5/min or ≥ 49/min, Paco$_2$ ≥ 50 mm Hg, alveolar-arterial oxygen tension difference ≥ 350 mm Hg with Fio$_2$ = 1.0, or ventilator or continuous positive airway pressure (CPAP) dependence for more than 48 hours.[61]

Failure of the liver is determined by an elevated bilirubin, the presence of ascites, and evidence of encephalopathy.[57] In the acute situation, dying hepatocytes release the enzymes SGOT, SGPT, and LDH.[39] Prothrombin time will begin to increase and serum albumin levels will fall below 2.0 g/dL.[62] The ability of the liver to tolerate an ischemic insult, whether a result of hypovolemic shock or maldistribution of blood flow induced by the septic shock/sepsis syndrome, will depend on the hepatic reserve. This reserve is reduced with preexisting disease such as hepatitis or cirrhosis. Iatrogenic injuries can also occur with the use of hepatotoxic drugs such as acetaminophen, diazepam, and inhalation anesthetics.[39,57]

The clinical signs of renal failure are generally agreed to be urine output ≤ 0.5 mL/kg/hr, serum BUN ≥ 100 mg/dL, and serum creatinine ≥ 3.5 mg/dL.[61] As fluid resuscitation techniques have improved, the major cause for acute renal failure has moved from prerenal factors to renal factors such as nephrotoxic drugs.

Central nervous system dysfunction is manifested by changes in the level of consciousness. The patient may be confused, agitated, or respond slowly to verbal stimuli. Failure may be quantified by a Glasgow coma scale; score ≤ 6, in the absence of sedation, indicates neurologic failure.[61] Hematologic failure is more difficult to quantitate. A white blood cell count ≤ 1000/mm^3, a platelet count $\leq 50,000$/mm^3, and a fibrinogen level below 100 mg/dL all have been identified as indicators of hematologic failure.

THERAPEUTIC MANAGEMENT

Therapeutic management of maldistribution of circulating volume concentrates on restoring effective circulating blood flow and oxygen transport to all tissues. In hypovolemic shock and the early stages of sepsis and inflammation, decreased preload must be treated along with its precipitating cause. Volume expansion and fluid challenges are used to correct decreased preload with the addition of inotropic support if fluid therapy alone does not improve the patient's status. Increased capillary permeability continues in the latter stages of sepsis, allowing intravenous fluids to cross into the interstitial space, which produces edema and compromises flow by compressing the microvasculature. Further manipulation of vascular tone by vasoactive agents is required. Many hemodynamic parameters are used to monitor cardiovascular status; however, optimal tissue perfusion is best monitored by oxygen supply-demand measurements such as oxygen consumption.[57]

Fluid resuscitation

Crystalloids. Preload is increased by intravascular volume loading with intravenous fluids classified as crystalloids and colloids. Crystalloids are commonly the first resuscitation fluids administered after intravenous access is established in trauma.[63] Crystalloids, such as normal saline and lactated Ringer's solution, contain electrolytes but no plasma proteins and, consequently, will diffuse into the interstitial space, causing edema. Diffusion of crystalloids into the interstitial space necessitates that more fluid be administered than the amount lost. The American College of Surgeons Committee on Trauma advocates that crystalloid solutions be infused to replace three times the estimated blood loss because only one part will remain in the intravascular space while two parts will diffuse into the interstitital space.[64] Other authors recommend the prompt administration of 2 to 3 L of crystalloid during evaluation of the clinical situation.[57,65,66] Continued resuscitation and definitive diagnosis can then be guided by the patient's response to the fluid challenge. If more than 25% of blood volume is lost, blood products must also be transfused in order to maintain intravascular volume; red blood cells are transfused to maintain oxygen-carrying capacity.

Burn shock formulas in current use recommend crystalloid administration in the form of lactated Ringer's solution. Over the first 24 hours, the volume requirements are calculated as 2 to 4 mL/kg per percentage of total burn body surface area. One-half the calculated amount is given in the first 8 hours after burn injury, since this is the period when the greatest fluid, electrolyte, and protein shifts occur. Fluids are not bolused unless the patient develops grossly inadequate perfusion, because a bolus will transiently increase capillary hydrostatic pressure and increase the rate of loss into the burn wound.[67] If the patient develops grossly inadequate perfusion, a bolus of colloid solution should be given.[68] Current studies demonstrate advantages of colloid addition to early resuscitation regimens of a burn injury.[69,70] The advantage relates specifically to the nonburn tissue that regains normal permeability characteristics soon after injury. Hypoproteinemia accentuates edema formation in these tissues, thereby increasing morbidity.[69]

Fluid resuscitation with crystalloids carries with it the potential to cause both pulmonary and peripheral edema. Colloid oncotic pressure reduction by dilution of plasma proteins with crystalloid solutions is the postulated mechanism for pulmonary edema formation.[65] When volume administration is monitored to prevent volume overload, there is no difference in lung function in fluid resuscitation of shock using crystalloids or colloids.[65] Rainey and English identify the major pitfall to avoid in crystalloid resuscitation as inadequate fluid administration, since edema is expected with these fluids and is not considered a sign of intravascular volume overload.[65] Crystalloid resuscitation has the beneficial effect of reducing blood viscosity and thereby improving blood flow through the microvasculature. In addition, electrolyte solutions are beneficial because they are nonallergenic, inexpensive, and readily available.

Hypertonic saline. Hypertonic saline is another electrolyte solution used in fluid resuscitation. This solution produces a large osmotic force that pulls fluid from the intracellular space to the extracellular space in order to achieve an iso-osmolar state. Total fluid requirements are reduced with the use of hypertonic saline resuscitation. Complications of hypertonic saline resuscitation are related to those of the hyperosmolar state. Current recommendations are that serum sodium levels should not be allowed to exceed 160 mEq/L during the use of hypertonic saline.[71] Free water cannot be given during hypertonic saline resuscitation because this dilutes the solution to a more isotonic concentration necessitating an increase in the total amount of fluid infused.

Colloids. Colloids are generally considered to be plasma proteins; however, synthetic substitutes are also included in this category. Plasma proteins are available in the form of albumin, plasma protein fraction, fresh frozen plasma, and whole blood. Fresh frozen plasma and whole blood carry the risk of disease transmission, whereas this risk is eliminated in heat-treated products such as albumin and plasma protein fraction. Heating also inactivates the clotting factors in albumin and plasma protein fraction. Plasma protein fraction, also known as plasmanate, differs from albumin because it contains some globulins as well as albumin. Hypotension associated with plasmanate administration is attributed to kinins or prekallikrein activator present among the globulin proteins.[65] Synthetic or nonprotein colloids available are dextran and hetastarch. Colloids are well known for their volume-expanding ability.

Albumin. Albumin is a small protein that generates about 80% of the plasma oncotic pressure.[65] Endogenous albumin is present in both the intravascular and interstitial spaces. Interstitial albumin may be either tissue-bound or nonbound. Free interstitial albumin returns to the intravascular compartment through lymphatic drainage, which increases during intravascular volume depletion.[65] Albumin is produced in the liver, but synthesis is depressed during injury or stress since hepatocytes increase production of acute phase reactants. In such situations, interstitial protein stores translocate into the intravascular space to correct up to a 50% depletion of intravascular albumin.[65]

Clinically, albumin is available as 5% and 25% solutions. Comparing volumes containing 25 grams of albumin, a 500 mL solution of 5% albumin is isooncotic and increases the intravascular space by 450 to 500 mL providing that microvascular permeability is normal. The 25% solution is 100 mL and also increases the intravascular volume by about 450 mL; however, the additional 350 mL must translocate from the interstitial space.[65] In hypovolemic shock or early sepsis, this translocation of fluid does not occur rapidly enough, so the 5% solution is the fluid of choice.

Dextran. Dextran and hetastarch are nonprotein colloids that generate oncotic force. Dextran is a high–molecular weight polysaccharide produced from glucose and is commercially available as dextran 40 or dextran 70 in which the molecular weights are 40,000 and 70,000, respectively. The amount of time dextran molecules remain in the intravascular space is determined by their size. Although dextran solutions are labeled according to mean molecular weight, both solutions contain a range of molecular weights. Smaller particles are rapidly excreted by the kidney, causing an osmotic diuresis, but larger particles remain in the circulation longer than 24 hours.

Dextran improves microcirculatory blood flow by coating endothelial and cellular surfaces.[65] This reduces sludging and cell aggregation. The platelet functions of adherence and degranulation are inhibited by dextran, thus decreasing thrombus formation. By the same mechanism, aggressive dextran infusion can cause a clotting deficiency. Dextran has antigenic cross-reactivity with bacterial polysaccharide antigens and is reported to cause anaphylaxis.[65] A small portion of the population has circulating dextran antibodies. Allergic reactions may be prevented with the prior infusion of a small dextran molecule known as PROMIT, which will bind with circulating dextran antibodies.

Hetastarch is another synthetic colloid with volume-expanding capability comparable to 5% albumin.[72] This solution has about the same incidence of anaphylaxis as albumin and has the potential to cause bleeding complications if administered in amounts greater than 2 L per day.[72] As with dextran, hetastarch causes an osmotic diuresis and does not replace natural proteins. Hetastarch continues to expand the plasma volume for 24 to 36 hours after administration.[72]

Crystalloid vs. colloid. The primary goal in fluid resuscitation is to increase the circulating volume without producing pulmonary edema. Given normal capillary permeability, colloids expand the plasma volume more effectively than crystalloids. Whether crystalloid or colloid solutions are more effective in avoiding pulmonary edema has been debated with beneficial and adverse effects demonstrated for either solution. Current knowledge indicates that expansion of plasma volume to above the preshock level improves survival significantly.[73] In sepsis, it is recommended that cardiac output and oxygen transport be increased to twice

Table 5-4 Vascular Effects of Adrenergic Receptor Stimulation

Receptor	Location	Effect
Alpha₁	Postsynaptic vascular smooth muscle receptors	Vasoconstriction in peripheral and pulmonary circulations
Alpha₂	Presynaptic receptor on sympathetic nerve ending	Inhibition of norepinephrine release
Beta₁	Postsynaptic myocardial receptors	Increased heart rate and contractility Increased coronary vasodilatation
	Renal juxtaglomerular cells	Release of renin
Beta₂	Postsynaptic vascular and bronchial smooth muscle receptors	Vasodilatation in peripheral circulation Bronchodilatation
Dopaminergic	Postsynaptic renal and mesenteric vascular smooth muscle receptors	Vasodilatation of renal and mesenteric circulations

the normal levels in order to maintain oxygen consumption at about one-and-one-half times normal, which is an initial estimate of the need of the patient with sepsis.[57] Overall, the outcome of shock resuscitation is related to interacting factors such as type and severity of shock, selection and volume of infusion solution given, duration of infusion, and volume of infusion distribution over time.[73]

Neither crystalloid nor colloid solutions, excluding whole blood, replace the oxygen-carrying capacity of red blood cells. Fresh frozen plasma will replace clotting factors and is indicated in correcting specific coagulation deficiencies; however, plasma will not improve oxygen delivery. Packed red blood cells rather than whole blood are used to improve oxygen delivery since they are specific therapy. The concept of optimal hematocrit relates to the ability of the circulation to provide optimal tissue oxygenation. Optimal tissue oxygenation must be balanced with promotion of flow through the microcirculation. The first goal is accomplished with an increased hematocrit and the latter by keeping the blood less viscous (i.e., with a lower hematocrit). Consequently, a range of values has been reported as optimal for hematocrit.[29,57,74] It is not yet established if one value is indeed optimal for all organs. The septic bowel is reported to have an increased hematocrit requirement of about 48%.[29] Other authors define optimal hematocrit in sepsis to be 30% to 42%.[57,74]

Pharmacologic therapy

Pharmacologic therapy intended to correct the maldistribution of circulating volume in MSOF involves drugs that manipulate preload, afterload,

and contractility. Initially, decreased preload is managed by fluid resuscitation techniques as previously described. If fluid therapy does not result in clear improvement, inotropic support is added to increase myocardial contractility and reverse excessive vasodilatation. The majority of drugs used to support cardiovascular status in shock and MSOF act on adrenergic receptors. Table 5-4 summarizes the different types of receptors and the vascular effects of their stimulation. Table 5-5 categorizes the vasoactive drugs discussed in this section.

Dopamine. Dopamine is generally the first vasoactive drug infused to improve myocardial contractility and, consequently, tissue perfusion in the shock state. The effects of dopamine are dose dependent. Dopaminergic receptors are stimulated at doses of 2 to 3 μg/kg/min. The improved blood flow to the renal and mesenteric vascular beds increases urine output and restores liver function.[39] The chronotropic and inotropic effects of increased heart rate and contractility predominate in the moderate dose range of 5 to 10 μg/kg/min. When the dose is in the high range of 10 to 15 μg/kg/min, alpha vasoconstriction is in effect with minimal beta₁ activity and an overwhelming of dopaminergic effects. A point to remember with all vasoactive medications is that different patients respond individually to specific doses.

Dobutamine. Dobutamine has its major effect on contractility rather than on heart rate or blood vessels because it primarily stimulates beta₁ receptors. At higher infusion rates of 5 to 15 μg/kg/min, mild beta₂ and some alpha activity causes slight vasodilatation and improved coronary blood

Table 5-5 Categories of Vasoactive Drugs

Drug	Chronotropic	Inotropic	Dopaminergic	Vasopressor	Vasodilator
Dopamine	Moderate dose	Moderate dose	Low dose	High dose	Low dose
Dobutamine	High dose	Moderate dose	—	—	High dose
Epinephrine	All doses	Low dose	—	High dose	Low dose
Isoproterenol	All doses	All doses	—	—	All doses (cardiac, skeletal, and pulmonary circulations)
Norepinephrine	Low dose, may cause reflex bradycardia	Low dose	—	Moderate to high dose	—
Amrinone	—	All doses	—	—	All doses
Phenylephrine	May cause reflex bradycardia	—	—	All doses	—
Nitroprusside	May cause reflex tachycardia	—	—	—	All doses

flow.[75] Fluid requirements are reported to be increased when dobutamine is infused at a dose of 6 μg/kg/min; however, oxygen transport and oxygen consumption improved significantly.[76] When dobutamine and dopamine were compared at the same dose, dobutamine reduced PCWP, but dopamine maintained wedge pressure.[77] Dobutamine reduction of PCWP occurred at a dose of 7.5 μg/kg/min, at which point, oxygen delivery and oxygen transport variables also improved significantly over baseline.[77]

Combination therapy is frequently used to achieve an optimal cardiovascular effect. This approach avoids the administration of high doses that are known to cause undesirable effects. Since dobutamine is shown to be beneficial in improving oxygen delivery and oxygen consumption, it is combined with low-dose dopamine to perfuse the mesentery. Optimal tissue perfusion goals may then be attainable.

Digoxin. Digoxin is indicated to improve myocardial contractility. The effect of this drug is not immediate; however, it is an important addition because digoxin's action is not dependent on adrenergic receptors. Adrenergic receptor sensitivity is reported to be depressed during endotoxin shock.[78] Consequently, larger doses of vasoactive agents may be required in order to achieve the same effect. This depressed sensitivity would not affect the inotropic action of digoxin.

Epinephrine. Epinephrine in low doses stimulates beta$_1$ and beta$_2$ adrenergic receptors, causing increased heart rate and force of contraction, which produces an increased cardiac output. Other effects of epinephrine at this dose are dilatation of the bronchi and of the blood vessels of cardiac and skeletal muscle. In doses greater than 0.02 μg/kg/min, epinephrine causes more alpha constriction, thereby increasing afterload and blood pressure. Epinephrine is known to stimulate beta$_1$ receptors more than beta$_2$ receptors; therefore, it will increase cardiac work more than it increases coronary blood flow.[75] Myocardial ischemia may result secondary to this imbalance of oxygen supply and demand.

Isoproterenol. Isoproterenol is classified as a pure beta drug because it only stimulates beta receptors. Based on the actions produced by beta stimulation, isoproterenol will improve contractility, increase heart rate, and produce vasodilatation in the cardiac, skeletal, and pulmonary circulations. This vasodilatation can be detrimental to the splanchnic bed and other organs that are not preferentially dilated. Because isoproterenol both increases fluid requirements by its vasodilatory effects and increases myocardial oxygen consumption, it is not generally recommended for use in shock.

Norepinephrine. Norepinephrine stimulates alpha$_1$ and beta$_1$ receptors. Again, low-dose and high-dose effects occur such that beta stimulation is seen at low doses and mixed alpha and beta effects occur at high doses. Norepinephrine increases cardiac work, and its potent vasoconstrictor effects can compromise blood flow to the kidney and other tissues and cause the movement of intravascular fluid into the interstitial space.[75] These considerations have limited the use of this drug in the shock state.

Amrinone. Amrinone is another inotrope with limited use in shock. Amrinone increases contractility by inhibition of phosphodiesterase. This drug also decreases both preload and afterload because it directly relaxes both venous and arteriolar smooth muscle.[75] Reductions in preload and afterload are desirable in congestive heart failure but will exacerbate hypotension in shock. In the hypodynamic phase of septic shock, amrinone may be helpful because it decreases afterload and increases contractility. Because amrinone does not depend on adrenergic receptor activity, which is depressed in sepsis, it may be more effective than adrenergic drugs such as dobutamine, dopamine, and epinephrine.

Phenylephrine. Vasoconstrictor therapy may be indicated to increase vascular tone and systemic vascular resistance in distributive shock. Many of the inotropic agents previously discussed have vasoconstrictor properties when dosage is increased. Phenylephrine is a pure alpha-adrenergic drug that constricts blood vessels in the skin, kidneys, lungs, and gastrointestinal tract. This drug increases coronary blood flow, but its use is limited to situations where cardiac output is adequate and vasoconstriction is necessary for blood pressure support.[75] Cardiac output must be monitored closely with the administration of vasoconstrictor agents in order to avoid increases in afterload that can compromise cardiac output. In one study of endotoxin shock, phenylephrine, norepinephrine, and dopamine were shown to have no effect on organ blood flow.[78] These agents neither decreased blood flow to any organ nor increased blood flow to any organ with reduced flow.[78]

Nitroprusside. Vasodilators are used to decrease severe elevations of systemic vascular resistance that may occur in the hypodynamic phase of septic shock. The rationale for use of nitrates or nitroprusside is to increase cardiac output by afterload reduction. Nitroprusside is known as a balanced vasodilator because it reduces both pulmonary venous and systemic venous pressure.[79] Reduction of pulmonary venous pressure may override hypoxic pulmonary vasoconstriction, thereby increasing the shunt fraction. Nitroprusside causes direct relaxation of arterial and venous smooth muscle and is not dependent on adrenergic receptors to produce its effect.[79]

Monitoring

In hypovolemic shock and early sepsis, monitoring is directed toward the assessment of preload, tissue perfusion, and tissue oxygenation. Defining optimal preload necessitates collecting data best obtained from a pulmonary artery catheter. Increases in filling pressures are required to generate a cardiac output about twice normal in order to provide adequate tissue oxygenation.[57] The Starling curve needs to be defined in sepsis so the optimal filling pressure for the individual patient may be provided. PCWP also must be increased in the interest of optimizing left ventricular function. The recommended value for PCWP is 12 to 18 mm Hg.[74] Adequacy of perfusion may be signaled by a reversal of lactic acidosis, although some clinicians believe lactate levels and acidosis are affected by too many other factors and may not be true indicators of tissue oxygenation. Mean arterial blood pressure should exceed 80 mm Hg to maintain organ perfusion. Oxygenation is best monitored by evaluating oxygen delivery and oxygen consumption.

Prevention

The approach to prevention of postoperative organ failure has been stated by Waxman;[80] however, many of the points are applicable in the treatment of MSOF from any cause.[80] The recommendations include aggressive preoperative fluid resuscitation; monitoring of oxygen delivery and oxygen consumption; minimization of intraoperative oxygen deficits; assessment of cardiopulmonary reserve; support of physiologic compensatory mechanisms such as increases in cardiac output, oxygen delivery, and oxygen consumption; prevention of sepsis; aggressive nutritional therapy; and support of individual organ systems.[80]

When this approach is generalized to trauma or sepsis, the major points include close monitoring of oxygen transport variables, especially in patients with decreased cardiopulmonary reserves as well as diminished reserves in other organ systems; aggressive support of oxygen delivery and oxygen consumption with timely and appropriate fluid resuscitation and support of individual organ systems; aggressive nutritional support; and prevention or resolution of sepsis. The prevention or resolution of sepsis requires that the source be controlled either by surgical intervention, if the source can be found, or by administration of antimicrobials if the septic source cannot be removed immediately, as might be the case in burns or peritonitis.

INVESTIGATIONAL THERAPIES

Unconventional pharmacologic therapy in shock includes the administration of glucagon, naloxone, and calcium antagonists.

Glucagon. Glucagon exerts an inotropic effect on the heart and is indicated in low output states induced by beta blockade. The mechanism of glucagon's inotropic effect is not confirmed but it is thought to occur by activation of adenyl cyclase, thereby increasing cyclic adenosine monophosphate (AMP).[81] Cyclic AMP then induces cell contraction. Catecholamines are dependent upon the beta receptor in order to effect an increase in cyclic AMP.

Naloxone. Naloxone's role in septic shock is still under investigation; however, it is used only as adjunctive therapy in reversing the hypotension of septic shock. This narcotic antagonist is thought to be beneficial in shock because it antagonizes the cardiovascular actions of endogenous opiates. Factors reported to affect the success of naloxone therapy in septic shock include the length of time hypotension was present before naloxone administration and the amount of antagonist given.[82] The presence and concentration of other circulating mediators that contribute to cardiovascular instability may also contribute to the success or failure of naloxone therapy. A current study reported hemodynamic improvement with naloxone but found no overall effect on mortality.[83]

Calcium antagonists. Calcium homeostasis is disrupted in shock, resulting in increased intracellular calcium levels. Intracellular calcium accumulation activates several intracellular processes that can lead to cell destruction, organ dysfunction, and death.[84] Calcium antagonists have been used successfully in the treatment of myocardial ischemia. Now researchers are demonstrating improved cardiovascular function and survival associated with the administration of calcium channel antagonists in endotoxin shock.[84]

Future. Future therapy to correct the maldistribution of circulating volume will focus on methods to maximize blood flow through the microcirculation. This may include infusing prostacyclin to dilate vascular beds or administering arachidonic acid metabolite inhibitors and antagonists. ODFR scavengers will reduce the damage done to the endothelium by toxic oxygen species. Antiinflammatory therapy may include antiendotoxin antibodies and neutralization of tumor necrosis factor. Many of these theoretical therapies will prove to be unworkable; however, new discoveries will occur to change our thinking about the etiology, treatment, and prognosis of MSOF.

CONCLUSION

Maldistribution of circulating volume leading to MSOF is a complex event involving treatment regimens, clinical conditions such as hemorrhage, and the release of vasoactive mediators. These mediators, derived from humoral, cellular, and biochemical pathways, affect the microvascular, organ, and regional circulations. Humoral mediators released at the site of injury or inflammation cause vasodilatation, permeability changes, and coagulation. Local mediators also enhance neutrophil chemotaxis and margination. The activated neutrophil releases macrophage chemotactic substances and vasoactive mediators such as PAF, ODFR, and proteases, which cause further tissue damage and maldistribution of circulating volume. Macrophages produce cytokines such as IL-1 and TNF as well as ODFR and proteases. Neutrophil- and macrophage-generated mediators affect the heart, lungs, liver, kidneys, and brain. Reperfusion of these organs after shock may not result in a return to normal functioning but may instead initiate postischemic reperfusion injury. Current therapy of maldistribution of circulating volume concentrates on treatment of symptoms by restoring effective circulating blood flow and oxygen transport to all tissues. This is accomplished by fluid resuscitation and pharmacologic manipulation of the vasculature. Investigational therapies focus on preventing mediator-induced cellular damage and maldistribution of circulating volume, which leads to organ dysfunction and MSOF.

REFERENCES

1. Cerra FB. Hypermetabolism-organ failure syndrome: A metabolic response to injury. Crit Care Clin 1989;5:289-302.
2. Webb WR, Brunswick RA. Microcirculation in shock—clinical review. In: Cowley RA and Trump BF, eds. Pathophysiology of Shock, Anoxia, and Ischemia. Baltimore: Williams and Wilkins, 1982:181-185.
3. Guyton AC. Local control of blood flow by the tissues and humoral regulation. In: Guyton AC, ed. Textbook of Medical Physiology, 8th ed. Philadelphia: W.B. Saunders Co., 1991:185-193.
4. Petrak RA, Balk RA, Bone RC. Prostaglandins, cyclooxygenase inhibitors, and thromboxane synthetase inhibitors in the pathogenesis of multiple systems organ failure. Crit Care Clin 1989;5:303-314.
5. Ruffolo RR. Cardiovascular adrenoreceptors: Physiology and critical care implications. In: Chernow B, ed. Pharmacologic Approach to the Critically Ill, 2nd ed. Baltimore: Williams and Wilkins, 1988:166-183.
6. Fry DE. Multiple system organ failure. Surg Clin North Am 1988;68:107-122.
7. Pinsky MR, Matuschak GM. MSOF: Failure of host defense homeostasis. Crit Care Clin 1989;5:199-220.
8. Bell TN. Disseminated intravascular coagulation and shock. Crit Care Nurs Clin North Am 1990;2:255-268.
9. LaLonde C, Demling RH, Pecquet Goad ME. Tissue inflammation without bacteria produces increased oxygen consumption and distant organ lipid peroxidation. Surgery 1988;104:49-56.
10. Lefer AM. Induction of tissue injury and altered cardiovascular performance by platelet-activating factor: Relevance to multiple systems organ failure. Crit Care Clin 1989;5:331-352.
11. Stroud M, Swindell B, Bernard GR. Cellular and humoral mediators of sepsis syndrome. Crit Care Nurs Clin North Am 1990;2:151-160.
12. Tribett D. Immune system function: Implications for critical care nursing practice. Crit Care Nurs Clin North Am 1989;1:725-740.
13. Beutler B. Cachectin in tissue injury, shock, and related states. Crit Care Clin 1989;5:353-367.
14. Sprague RS et al. Proposed role for leukotrienes in the pathophysiology of multiple systems organ failure. Crit Care Clin 1989;5:315-329.
15. Lefer AM. Eicosanoids as mediators of ischemia and shock. Fed Proc 1985;4:275-280.
16. Kadowitz PP et al. Pulmonary and systemic vasodilator effects of the new prostaglandin, PGI_2. J Appl Physiol 1978;45:408-413.
17. Bihari D et al. The effects of vasodilation with prostacyclin on oxygen delivery and uptake in critically ill patients. N Engl J Med 1987;317:397-403.
18. Robins EV. Immunosuppression of the burned patient. Crit Care Clin North Am 1989;1:767-774.
19. Jacobs RF, Tabor DR. Immune cellular interactions during sepsis and septic injury. Crit Care Clin 1989;5:9-26.
20. Schumacker PT, Samsel RW. Oxygen delivery and uptake by peripheral tissues: Physiology and pathophysiology. Crit Care Clin 1989;5:255-269.
21. Duling BR et al. Vasomotor control: Functional hyperemia and beyond. Fed Proc 1987;46:251-263.
22. Vaughan PP, Brooks Jr C. Adult respiratory distress syndrome: A complication of shock. Crit Care Nurs Clin North Am 1990;2:235-253.
23. Palmer RMJ, Ferrige AG, Moncade S. Nitric oxide release accounts for the biological activity of endothelium-derived relaxation factor. Nature 1987;327:524-526.
24. Gotch PM. The endocrine system. In: Alspach JG, Williams SM, eds. Core Curriculum for Critical Care Nursing. Philadelphia: WB Saunders Co, 1985:451-494.
25. Lefer AM. Vascular mediators in ischemia and shock. In: Cowley RA, Trump BF, eds. Pathophysiology of Shock, Anoxia, and Ischemia. Baltimore: Williams and Wilkins, 1982:165-181.
26. Hartl WH et al. Reactive hyperemia in patients with septic conditions. Surgery 1988;103:440-444.
27. Alexander F, Hechtman HB. Pulmonary and cardiovascular responses. In: Clowes Jr GHA, ed. Trauma, Sepsis, and Shock: The Physiological Basis of Therapy. New York: Marcel Dekker, Inc, 1988:161-185.
28. Adams HR, Parker JL, Laughlin MH. Intrinsic myocardial dysfunction during endotoxemia: Dependent or independent of myocardial ischemia? Circ Shock 1990;30:63-76.
29. Bersten A, Sibbald WJ. Circulatory disturbances in multiple systems organ failure. Crit Care Clin 1989;5:233-254.
30. Cunnion RE et al. The coronary circulation in human septic shock. Circulation 1986;73:637-644.
31. Suffredini AF et al. The cardiovascular response of normal humans to the administration of endotoxin. N Engl J Med 1989;321:280-287.
32. Parker MM et al. Right ventricular dysfunction and dilatation, similar to left ventricular changes, characterize the cardiac depression of septic shock in humans. Chest 1990;97:126-131.
33. Myers JL. Anaphylactic shock. In: Perry AG, Potter PA, eds. Shock: Comprehensive Nursing Management. St. Louis: Mosby–Year Book, 1983:194-212.
34. Garcia JGN et al. Leukotrienes and the pulmonary microcirculation. Am Rev Resp Dis 1987;136:161-169.
35. Henry CL et al. Attenuation of the pulmonary vascular response to endotoxin by a thromboxane synthesis inhibitor (UK-38485) in unanesthetized sheep. J Surg Res 1991;50:77-81.
36. Demling RH, LaLonde C, Pequet Goad ME. Effect of ibuprofen on the pulmonary and systemic response to repeated doses of endotoxin. Surgery 1989;105:421-429.
37. Brigham KL, Meyrick BO. Endotoxin and lung injury. Am Rev Respir Dis 1986;133:913-927.
38. Daryani R et al. Changes in catalase activity in lung and liver after endotoxemia in sheep. Circ Shock 1990;32:273-280.
39. Collins AS. Gastrointestinal complications in shock. Crit Care Nurs Clin North Am 1990;2:269-277.
40. Teplitz C. The pathology and ultrastructure of cellular injury and inflammation in the progression and outcome of trauma, sepsis, and shock. In: Clowes, Jr GHA, ed. Trauma, Sepsis, and Shock: The Physiological Basis of Therapy. New York: Marcel Dekker, 1988:71-120.
41. Border JR, Hassett JM. Multiple systems organ failure: History, pathophysiology, prevention, and support. In: Clowes Jr GHA, ed. Trauma, Sepsis, and Shock: The Physiological Basis of Therapy. New York: Marcel Dekker, 1988:335-356.
42. Colletti LM et al. Role of tumor necrosis factor-α in the

pathophysiologic alterations after hepatic ischemia/reperfusion injury in the rat. J Clin Invest 1990;85:1936-1943.
43. Schirmer WJ et al. Imidazole and indomethacin improve hepatic perfusion in sepsis. Circ Shock 1987;21:253-259.
44. Lancaster LE. Renal response to shock. Crit Care Nurse Clin North Am 1990;2:221-233.
45. Burke TJ et al. Renal response to shock. Ann Emerg Med 1986;15:1397-1400.
46. Cumming AD et al. The protective effect of thromboxane synthetase inhibition on renal function in systemic sepsis. Am J Kidney Dis 1989;18:114-119.
47. Prough DS, DeWitt DS. Cerebral protection. In: Chernow B, ed. The Pharmacologic Approach to the Critically Ill, 2nd ed. Baltimore: Williams and Wilkins, 1988:198-218.
48. Ernster L. Biochemistry of reoxygenation injury. Crit Care Med 1988;16:947-953.
49. Demling RH, LaLonde C. Early postburn lipid peroxidation: Effect of ibuprofen and allopurinol. Surgery 1990;107:85-93.
50. Demling RH et al. Fluid resuscitation with deferoxamine prevents systemic burn induced oxidant injury. J Trauma 1991;31:538-543.
51. Kennedy TP et al. Ibuprofen prevents oxidant lung injury and in vitro lipid peroxidation by chelating iron. J Clin Invest 1990;86:1565-1573.
52. Bulkley BH, Hutchins GM. Myocardial consequences of coronary artery bypass graft surgery: The paradox of necrosis in areas of revascularization. Circulation 1977;56:906-913.
53. Black L, Coombs VJ, Townsend SN. Reperfusion and reperfusion injury in acute myocardial infarction. Heart Lung 1990;19:274-286.
54. Horton JW, White J, Baxter CR. The role of oxygen-derived free radicals in burn-induced myocardial contractile depression. J Burn Care Rehabil 1988;9:589-598.
55. Yokoyama Y et al. Circulating xanthine oxidase: Potential mediator of ischemic injury. Am J Physiol 1990;258:G564-570.
56. DeCamp MM, Demling RH. Posttraumatic multisystem organ failure. JAMA 1988;260:530-534.
57. Demling RH, Wilson RF. Sepsis and organ failure. In: Demling RH, Wilson RF, Decision Making in Surgical Critical Care. Philadelphia: BC Decker, 1988:172-210.
58. Parrillo JE et al. Septic shock in humans: Advances in the understanding of pathogenesis, cardiovascular dysfunction, and therapy. Ann Intern Med 1990;113:227-242.
59. Summers G. The clinical and hemodynamic presentation of the shock patient. Crit Care Nurs Clin North Am 1990;2:161-166.
60. Rice V. The clinical continuum of septic shock. Crit Care Nurse 1984;4:86-109.
61. Knaus WA, Wagner DP. Multiple systems organ failure: Epidemiology and prognosis. Crit Care Clin 1989;5:221-232.
62. Dorinsky PM, Gadek JE. Multiiple organ failure. Clin Chest Med 1990;11:581-591.
63. Beckwith N, Carriere SR. Fluid resuscitation in trauma: An update. J Emerg Nurs 1985;11:293-299.
64. Maier RV. Evaluation and resuscitation. In: Moore EE, ed. Early Care of the Injured Patient, 4th ed. Toronto: BC Decker, 1990:56-73.
65. Rainey TG, English JF. Pharmacology of colloids and crystalloids. In: Chernow B, ed. The Pharmacologic Approach to the Critically Ill, 2nd ed. Baltimore: Williams and Wilkins, 1988:219-240.
66. Trunkey DD, Sheldon GF, Collins JA. The treatment of shock. In: Zuidema GD, Rutherford RB, and Ballinger WF, eds. The Management of Trauma, 4th ed. Philadelphia: WB Saunders, 1985:105-125.
67. Robins EV. Burn shock. Crit Care Nurse Clin North Am 1990;2:299-307.
68. Demling RH, LaLonde C. Restoration and maintenance of hemodynamic stability. In: Demling RH, LaLonde C. eds, Burn Trauma. New York: Theime Medical Publishers, Inc, 1989:24-41.
69. Demling RH et al. Effect of nonprotein colloid on postburn edema formation in soft tissues and lung. Surgery 1984;95:593-602.
70. Carvajal HF, Parks DH. Optimal composition of burn resuscitation fluids. Crit Care Med 1988;16:695-700.
71. Demling RH. Fluid resuscitation. In: Boswick JA Jr, ed. The Art and Science of Burn Care. Rockville, MD: Aspen, 1987:189-202.
72. Rackow EC et al. Fluid resuscitation in circulatory shock: A comparison of the cardiorespiratory effects of albumin, hetastarch, and saline solutions in patients with hypovolemic and septic shock. Crit Care Med 1983;11:839-850.
73. Dawidson IJA et al. Lactated Ringer's solution versus 3% albumin for resuscitation of a lethal intestinal ischemic shock in rats. Crit Care Med 1990;18:60-66.
74. Iverson RL. Septic shock: A clinical perspective. Crit Care Clin 1988;4:215-228.
75. Burns KM. Vasoactive drug therapy in shock. Crit Care Nurse Clin North Am 1990;2:167-178.
76. Vincent JL, DeBacker D. Initial management of circulatory shock as prevention of MSOF. Crit Care Clin 1989;5:369-378.
77. Shoemaker WC et al. Comparison of hemodynamic and oxygen transport effects of dopamine and dobutamine in critically ill surgical patients. Chest 1989;96:120-126.
78. Breslow MJ et al. Effect of vasopressors on organ blood flow during endotoxin shock in pigs. Am J Physiol 1987;252:H291-298.
79. Parrillo JE. Vasodilator therapy. In: Chernow B, ed. The Pharmacologic Approach to the Critically Ill, 2nd ed. Baltimore: Williams and Wilkins, 1988:346-364.
80. Waxman K. Postoperative multiple organ failure. Crit Care Clin 1987;3:429-440.
81. Daley KA, Ruksnaitis N. Glucagon: A first-line drug for cardiotoxicity caused by beta blockade. J Emerg Nurs 1986;12:387-392.
82. Schumann LL, Remington MA. The use of naloxone in treating endotoxic shock. Crit Care Nurs 1990;10:63-71.
83. Hackshaw KV, Parker GA, Roberts JW. Naloxone in septic shock. Crit Care Med 1990;18:47-51.
84. Malcolm DS et al. Calcium and calcium antagonists in shock and ischemia. In: Chernow B, ed. The Pharmacologic Approach to the Critically Ill, 2nd ed. Baltimore: Williams and Wilkins, 1988:889-900.

6 Imbalance of Oxygen Supply and Demand

Barbara Clark Mims

An imbalance between oxygen delivery to peripheral tissues and tissue oxygen demand is a critical factor in the pathogenesis of MSOF in sepsis and critical illness.[1-4] Normal cellular function and long-term viability of the human organism require continuous transport of oxygen and substrate to the mitochondria.[2,5] Here oxidative phosphorylation occurs through the Krebs tricarboxylic acid cycle, generating the high-energy phosphate bonds of adenosine triphosphate (ATP). ATP provides the energy required to maintain cellular integrity and to support such physiologic processes as protein synthesis, muscular contraction, and active transport.[5] In cases of oxygen deprivation, ATP may be generated through increased glycolysis, a process that produces much less energy per mole of substrate than does oxidative phosphorylation. In addition, increased glycolysis leads to metabolic acidosis since glycolytic pathways produce pyruvate and subsequently lactate in anaerobic conditions. Excessive hydrogen ions are also released as ATP is broken down and not regenerated because of limited oxygen supply. An alternative to glycolysis involves the creatine kinase reaction, in which phosphocreatine (a high-energy phosphate compound) provides a high-energy phosphate bond to convert adenosine diphosphate (ADP) to ATP. This reaction occurs in the skeletal muscles, heart, and brain and is limited by the phosphocreatine stores.[5]

If energy supplied to meet the tissue demands is insufficient, cellular injury will occur because electrochemical gradients are lost and active transport across cell membranes falls.[3] Cellular injury leads to impaired tissue function and the triggering of an inflammatory process. As inflammatory mediators are released, the delivery of oxygen and substrate is further reduced, leading to a massive disruption of organ system function. The etiology of MSOF is complex and multifaceted, and hypoxic tissue

injury plays an important role. It is theorized that this hypoxic tissue injury may be initiated by injury to the endothelial cell.[3]

PHYSIOLOGY OF OXYGEN EXTRACTION
Compensatory mechanisms

In healthy tissues, when oxygen transport is normal or increased, oxygen consumption is independent of oxygen transport (Fig. 6-1).[3-5] In other words, if tissue demands are being met, delivering more O_2 will not change the amount being consumed. The tissues extract the needed amount, while the remainder is returned unused to the right side of the heart.

As oxygen availability to the tissues decreases, oxygen consumption is initially maintained by an increase in the oxygen extraction ratio.[3,6] However, when oxygen delivery falls below a critically low level, tissue extraction cannot increase in proportion to the reduced oxygen transport; therefore oxygen consumption falls. In tissues where phosphocreatine is present, ATP is generated by the creatine kinase reaction until the stores are depleted.[5] Only then does significant glycolysis occur, which suggests that lactic acidosis might be a relatively late consequence of an inadequate oxygen transport.

Pathologic supply dependency

The relationship between oxygen transport and oxygen consumption may be affected by many clinical conditions, including sepsis,[2,5] ARDS,[2,6-8] and MSOF.[3,9,10] In these conditions, oxygen uptake by the tissues changes significantly with changes in oxygen transport, even at normal or increased levels of oxygen delivery (Fig. 6-2).[10,11] This has been termed pathologic supply dependency.[5,9] The amount consumed depends on the amount delivered. Compensatory mechanisms are either inad-

109

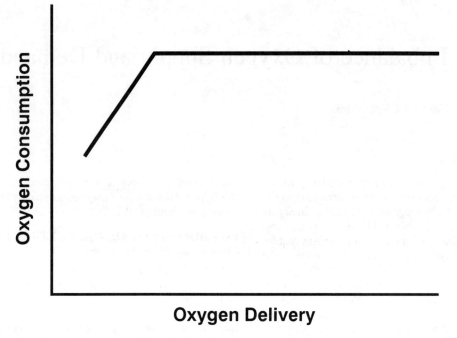

Fig. 6-1 Supply-independent oxygen consumption. Theoretic relationship between oxygen delivery and oxygen consumption in healthy tissues.

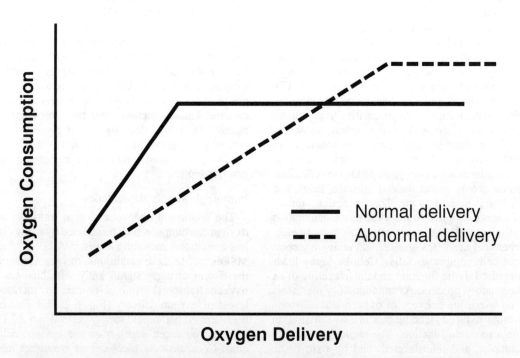

Fig. 6-2 Supply-dependent oxygen consumption. Theoretic relationship between oxygen delivery and oxygen consumption in pathologic oxygen supply dependency.

equate or dysfunctional. Mohsenifar et al[12] reported that patients with ARDS demonstrated oxygen supply dependency when oxygen delivery fell below 21 mL/kg/min. By contrast, in patients undergoing coronary artery bypass surgery, oxygen consumption has been shown to be independent of oxygen transport until delivery falls below 8 mL/kg/min.[13] Although these data are useful for illustrating the concept of pathologic supply dependency, note that the units mL/min/m^2 are used more frequently in clinical practice than the units mL/kg/min.

Maldistribution of flow. Pathologic supply dependency may be partially a result of a maldistribution of blood flow at the regional or microcirculatory level.[6] Normally when oxygen transport falls, two mechanisms act to prevent tissue hypoxia. First, regional redistribution of blood flow to the organs with the highest metabolic requirements occurs from a balance between extrinsic nervous system control and local tissue regulation of arteriolar tone. The second mechanism involves the regulation of perfused capillary density by intrinsic vascular control within tissues. A large fraction of available capillaries is normally not perfused. In normal tissues, as tissue PO_2 falls, the density of perfused capillaries increases by regulatory mechanisms that relax precapillary sphincter tone. If this ability to regulate flow distribution is lost, some capillaries may be overperfused while others are underperfused. Even in normal tissues, the transit time of blood flow through capillaries varies widely. If this variation in transit times increases as a result of disease, the transit time through some capillaries may lengthen to the point that capillary PO_2 falls below a critical level needed to maintain molecular diffusion.

Rapid transit times (hyperdynamic state) may also contribute to defects in diffusion because the hemoglobin may not have enough time to unload its oxygen.[5] As a result, local oxygen consumption falls. Tenney[14] has demonstrated that when oxygen delivery is low, increasing capillary density is more effective than increasing blood flow in restoring mean tissue PO_2. If the recruitable capillary surface is limited by microembolization or loss of precapillary sphincter regulatory capacity, tissue anoxia can occur. Clinical conditions such as ARDS, sepsis, shock, and trauma stimulate intravascular coagulation and precipitate microembolization, thus

contributing to a reduced oxygen extraction capacity.[6]

Arteriovenous shunting. The second mechanism hypothesized to contribute to the pathologic supply dependency is arteriovenous shunting of blood,[6] involving arteriovenous channels in the microcirculation. Blood might be routed past exchanging capillaries by way of these channels, decreasing oxygen delivery and consumption at the cellular level. Arteriovenous shunting continues to be controversial, because no true anatomic shunts have been unequivocally demonstrated in healthy animals or humans or animals or humans with sepsis.[5]

Summary

Clearly, abnormal oxygen transport at the microcirculatory level plays a role in the oxygen supply/demand imbalance seen in sepsis and MSOF. The etiology, pathogenesis, and extent of that role remain to be elucidated. In addition, cardiac failure, lung failure, decreased blood oxygen-carrying capacity, or vascular disease that limits perfusion to certain anatomic regions may also contribute. Recent evidence indicates that in certain clinical conditions, tissue anoxia may also occur as a result of an inability of the tissues to extract oxygen in sufficient quantities to meet tissue oxygen requirements.[2,6]

OXYGEN TRANSPORT AND UTILIZATION IN SEPSIS AND INFLAMMATION
Pathophysiology

In the early stages of sepsis, patients manifest an increased cardiac output (CO) and increased oxygen transport with a concomitant decrease in systemic vascular resistance (SVR) and oxygen extraction ratio.[2,5] If the syndrome continues, the cardiac output falls and oxygen transport decreases significantly.[5] Although CO is elevated in the hyperdynamic state, myocardial depression is actually present secondary to direct action of mediators such as myocardial depressant factor and tumor necrosis factor. Although this myocardial depression contributes to the low cardiac output seen in the terminal stages of septic shock and MSOF, the most likely source of a falling CO in the hyperdynamic state is volume depletion.[15]

As previously described, there is a pathologic oxygen supply dependency in sepsis.[3,16] As a result, oxygen delivery and oxygen consumption track each other over a very wide range of oxygen delivery values.[5,10] Lactic acidosis is common, which suggests that oxygen demands remain unmet even though oxygen delivery is increased.

Three possible theories have been offered to explain oxygen extraction and utilization abnormalities in sepsis. These include: (1) an abnormality of the cells' bioenergetic mechanisms, rendering them incapable of using oxygen; (2) shunting of blood around metabolizing tissues or redirection of blood flow through nonnutritive vascular beds; (3) impaired oxygen diffusion from systemic capillaries resulting from hyperdynamic circulation.[5]

Cellular defect. Considerable controversy surrounds the issue of whether or not sepsis affects the ability of the cells to use oxygen. Some studies have demonstrated an impairment of oxidative metabolism in sepsis, but others have shown that the oxidative capacity of the mitochondria is normal.[5]

Maldistribution of flow. The maldistribution of blood flow in sepsis may be in part a result of microvascular occlusion. This occurs secondary to activation of inflammatory mediators, which results in endothelial damage, granulocyte and platelet agglutination, and capillary occlusion.[17] Capillary occlusion causes a reduction in the cross-sectional area of the capillary, which increases the diffusion distance to the tissues and interferes with capillary recruitment.[5] This is critical because capillary recruitment is an essential mechanism by which the organism increases oxygen extraction in times of oxygen need.

Loss of local autoregulation. A second mechanism contributing to the maldistribution of flow is the loss of autoregulatory ability.[18] When this occurs, blood flow is no longer diverted to the tissues with the highest metabolic need for oxygen. Loss of autoregulation may occur when vasoactive substances such as prostaglandins are released into the circulation and interfere with local control of vascular tone.[5] Other factors that occur in sepsis and damage the endothelium and underlying smooth muscle include hypoxia, inflammation, complement activation, O_2 radical production, and lipid peroxidation. These factors can interfere with the matching of O_2 delivery to tissue oxygen needs by interfering with vascular smooth muscle tone and possible interactions between the endothelium and the smooth muscle. The fall in SVR indicates that the autoregulatory ability is lost.[5] Clinical studies have shown that the fall in SVR correlates with a reduction in the ability of the tissues to extract oxygen.[19]

Impaired oxygen diffusion. The third factor that may contribute to abnormal oxygen consumption in sepsis is an impairment of oxygen diffusion into the tissues. This may occur when tissue inflammation and edema widen the diffusion distance from the capillaries to the cells. This may be compounded by increases in capillary flow secondary to the hyperdynamic state.[5] The shorter capillary transit time may not allow enough time for the oxygen to unload from the hemoglobin.[20,21]

Although the exact mechanism responsible for the abnormal oxygen utilization in sepsis is unclear, it is significant that oxygen consumption increases as oxygen delivery increases. This implies that the abnormality is more likely with the delivery of oxygen to the tissues than with the ability of the cells to use oxygen.[5,22,23]

Sequelae

The identification of a pathologic supply dependency is an ominous sign in the critically ill.[5] One study identified a 70% mortality rate in ICU patients with supply dependency, as compared to 30% in patients without supply dependency.[24] Another study found a greater increase in oxygen consumption subsequent to an increase in oxygen transport in patients who died than in those who survived. This suggests that when supply dependency exists, it indicates a significant defect in tissue oxygenation, which may lead to MSOF.[10]

Clinical studies have demonstrated that all tissues do not demonstrate the same degree of supply dependency in response to endotoxin.[3,16,25] The oxygen demand of skeletal muscle appears to be increased in sepsis, but its ability to extract oxygen remains largely intact.[3] The oxygen demand of the splanchnic tissues increases in sepsis, and these tissues demonstrate a significant impairment in their ability to extract and use O_2. Since the gastrointestinal mucosa normally borders on hypoxia, the increased demand for oxygen coupled with the impairment in oxygen extraction and utilization leads to rapid development of intestinal mucosal injury during shock and sepsis. This sets the stage for the release of toxic substances from the gut into the systemic circulation and for translocation of bacteria from the gut lumen into the portal circulation or lymphatics.[1]

Pathogenesis: endothelial damage

The oxygen extraction defects described above may be mediated in part by endothelial cell damage.[3] Normally, the endothelium releases a substance called endothelium–derived relaxation factor (EDRF).[26,27] EDRF mediates the vasodilatory properties of a number of substances, including acetylcholine, adenosine, serotonin, and catecholamines.[3,28] Complement activation leads to aggregation of neutrophils in peripheral tissues in MSOF. The neutrophils then release toxic oxygen-derived free radicals, which damage the peripheral endothelial cells. When damaged, the endothelial cells may not be able to release EDRF in response to local metabolic feedback, which impairs the ability of the microvasculature to regulate the distribution of blood flow among capillaries. Transit times between capillaries would then vary, and some would be overperfused while others would be underperfused in relation to tissue oxygen requirements. If oxygen transport was then reduced, poorly perfused tissues would become supply dependent even if total oxygen transport was still normal.[3]

The presence of even small amounts of endotoxin may activate neutrophils, which then release toxic oxygen radicals and lysozymes.[2,29,30] These substances cause endothelial damage and activate the arachidonic acid cascade, resulting in altered control of the microcirculation, microembolization, and plugging of capillaries with leukocytes. These actions increase the diffusion distance between erythrocytes and mitochondria, thus decreasing oxygen transport at the cellular level.[2]

Oxygen consumption during sepsis has been variously reported to be normal, decreased, or increased.* Tissue oxygen requirements are thought to be elevated during sepsis.[34,35] However, oxygen consumption may not increase in response to the increased tissue oxygen requirements because of failure of the peripheral tissues to increase the extraction ratio.[16,33]

CLINICAL ASSESSMENT OF OXYGEN SUPPLY/DEMAND BALANCE

Physiologic monitoring of the critically ill patient provides crucial information for clinical decision-making. Studies by Bland, Shoemaker,

and Shabot[34] have shown that the customary use of traditional variables, including mean arterial pressure (MAP), heart rate, central venous pressure (CVP), pulmonary capillary wedge pressure (PCWP), and cardiac output, is not sufficient in predicting outcome or as goals of therapy in the critically ill patient population. In a large series of high-risk postoperative patients, these variables were restored to normal in 75% of the survivors as compared with 76% of nonsurvivors. In other words, restoration of normal values did not improve survival.

Hemodynamic measurements, laboratory values, and calculated oxygen transport variables must be linked together to evaluate the adequacy of oxygen delivery and tissue utilization of oxygen. A properly placed pulmonary artery catheter is necessary in order for this to be accomplished. Rather than normalizing each individual parameter to the standard textbook norm, the goal in critical care is to balance oxygen delivery with the individual patient's tissue oxygen requirements. If the tissue demands exceed supply, a loss of membrane permeability will occur, followed by loss of vital organ function. Restoration of oxygen supply/demand is of utmost importance in preventing MSOF in the critically ill patient.[35] This may focus on maximizing the peripheral transport of oxygen or on minimizing the metabolic oxygen demands.[2] A recent report by Russell et al[4] indicated a strong inverse relationship between oxygen delivery and the development of MSOF in patients with ARDS. Accordingly, the study showed a greater oxygen delivery and oxygen consumption in survivors than in nonsurvivors. The greater oxygen delivery in survivors was due to a greater cardiac index, which was related to ejection of a greater stroke volume index from a greater end-diastolic volume. The investigators theorized that the greater end-diastolic volume was due to increased ventricular compliance[4] (see Chapter 10). Actual ventricular dilatation has also been suggested as a possible source of greater end-diastolic volume.[15]

In order for oxygen supply/demand balance to be maintained or restored, clinical evaluation of the patient must include assessment of tissue oxygenation. This goes beyond blood gas analysis to include calculation of oxygen transport, oxygen consumption, and the oxygen extraction ratio. In some situations, monitoring the $S\bar{v}O_2$ may be beneficial.

---

*References 2, 5, 16, 20, 31-33.

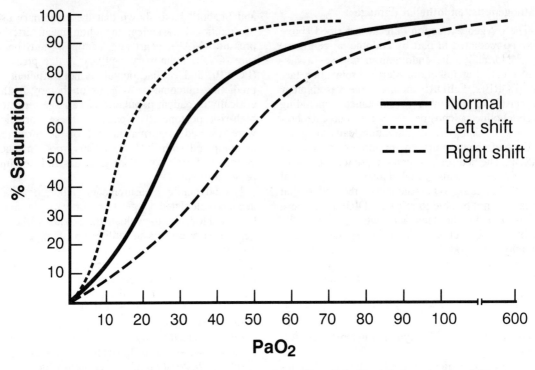

Fig. 6-3 Oxyhemoglobin dissociation curve. (From Mims BC. Physiologic rationale of $S\bar{v}o_2$ monitoring. Crit Care Nurs Clin North Am 1989;1:623.)

Partial pressure of oxygen (Pao₂)

The Pao_2 is the partial pressure exerted by oxygen dissolved in the plasma of arterial blood. The normal value is 80 to 100 mm Hg for a young, healthy person breathing room air at sea level. The Pao_2 reflects useful information about lung function and the adequacy of arterial oxygenation, but in isolation it does not reflect the adequacy of tissue oxygenation.[36]

Arterial oxygen saturation (Sao₂)

The saturation of hemoglobin with oxygen in the arterial blood (Sao_2) is the amount of hemoglobin combined with oxygen divided by the total amount of hemoglobin available. An Sao_2 of 90% or greater is generally considered acceptable from an oxygen transport standpoint.[37] The saturation rarely exceeds 98%, because venous blood from the bron-chial, pleural, and thebesian circulations flows directly into the left side of the heart.

The Sao_2 is determined primarily by the Pao_2. The relationship between the Pao_2 and Sao_2 is expressed in the oxyhemoglobin dissociation curve (Fig. 6-3). On the steep portion of the curve, small changes in Pao_2 will significantly alter the Sao_2. This occurs in the Pao_2 range from 0 to 60 mm Hg. On the flat portion, above a Pao_2 of 60 mm Hg, even large changes in Pao_2 produce minimal changes in Sao_2.

The classic oxyhemoglobin dissociation curve is constructed with a temperature of 37° C, a $Paco_2$ of 40 mm Hg, and a pH of 7.40. Under these conditions, a normal adult will have an Sao_2 of 50% with a Pao_2 of 26.6 mm Hg. This is termed P_{50}, or the Pao_2 at which 50% of the hemoglobin is saturated with oxygen.[36] If the P_{50} is above 26.6

mm Hg, the curve has shifted to the right. The affinity of hemoglobin for oxygen decreases, resulting in a lower saturation for a given partial pressure. Factors shifting the curve to the right include increased $PaCO_2$, decreased pH, increased temperature, and increased levels of 2,3-DPG (diphosphoglycerate). As blood moves from the lungs to the tissue bed, the CO_2 increases and pH decreases, which shifts the curve to the right and facilitates the dissociation of oxygen from hemoglobin.

When the P_{50} is less than 26.6 mm Hg, the curve shifts to the left. The affinity of hemoglobin for oxygen increases, which impedes the dissociation of oxygen from hemoglobin and creates a higher saturation for a given partial pressure. Factors shifting the curve to the left include decreased $PaCO_2$, increased pH, decreased body temperature, and decreased levels of 2,3-DPG. Banked blood is deficient in 2,3-DPG, so massive transfusions may shift the curve to the left.

Arterial oxygen content (CaO_2)

Arterial oxygen content is defined as the actual quantity (mL) of oxygen in each 100 mL of arterial blood. It is determined by the partial pressure of oxygen in arterial blood (PaO_2), the saturation of hemoglobin with oxygen in arterial blood (SaO_2), and the hemoglobin (Hgb) level. The relationship between these determinants is illustrated in the following formula[38]:

$$CaO_2 = (Hgb \times 1.39 \times SaO_2) + (0.003 \times PaO_2)$$

Each gram of hemoglobin is capable of carrying 1.39 mL of oxygen (this value varies in the literature from 1.34 to 1.39).[39] Therefore:

$$\text{Oxygen-carrying capacity} = Hgb \times 1.39$$

To determine the amount of oxygen actually carried on the hemoglobin, the oxygen-carrying capacity is multiplied by the SaO_2:

$$Hgb \times 1.39 \times SaO_2$$

Most of the oxygen is carried in combination with hemoglobin. The small quantity of oxygen that is carried dissolved in the plasma of arterial blood can be determined by multiplying the solubility coefficient for oxygen, 0.003, by the PaO_2.[40] With a normal PaO_2 of 100 mm Hg, there is only 0.3 mL of oxygen dissolved in the plasma of 100 mL of arterial blood:

$$0.003 \times 100 \text{ mm Hg} = 0.3 \text{ ml } O_2$$

Since the amount of oxygen dissolved in the plasma is so small, it is usually acceptable to use the abbreviated formula for oxygen content in clinical practice[40-42]:

$$CaO_2 = Hgb \times 1.39 \times SaO_2$$

When a high FiO_2 is administered and results in a high PaO_2, the amount of dissolved O_2 may be significant, and the entire formula should be used. By working with the formula, the relative importance of Hgb, PaO_2, and SaO_2 becomes obvious. Although PaO_2 is important because it determines SaO_2, it has less effect on oxygen content than does Hgb or SaO_2. As long as the PaO_2 is above 60 mm Hg, the SaO_2 will be 90% or greater[42] if the curve is not shifted severely to the right. In this range, changes in PaO_2 will result in negligible changes in oxygen content. If PaO_2 is the only value assessed to determine arterial oxygenation, serious errors can occur.

Cardiac output/cardiac index

Although the cardiac output is the major determinant of oxygen transport,[43] its role is frequently underestimated. Unless the arterial blood is delivered in adequate quantities to the systemic capillary bed, the tissues will be deprived of oxygen.

The cardiac index (CI) is the cardiac output divided by the body surface area (BSA).[44] The BSA is obtained by inserting the patient's height and weight into a nomogram. The cardiac index is a more precise parameter than cardiac output because it takes into account the patient's body size. The normal CI is 2.5 to 4.0 L/min/m^2.

Many of the formulas that are used in evaluating tissue oxygenation include cardiac output. Substituting cardiac index increases the meaning of the value calculated with the formula because the patient's total body surface area is taken into account.

Oxygen delivery (DO_2)

The oxygen delivery (DO_2) is the amount of oxygen delivered to the tissues each minute. This is an extremely important parameter, since the overall goal of all cardiopulmonary function is to deliver adequate oxygen to meet the tissue demands. The oxygen delivery is determined by the amount of oxygen in the blood (CaO_2) and the amount of blood delivered to the tissues (CO/CI). When oxygen transport is reduced, it may be due to decreased oxygen content (decreased hemoglobin, PaO_2, or SaO_2) or to decreased cardiac output. Oxygen delivery may be calculated as follows[38]:

$$Do_2 = \underset{\text{(CO)}}{\text{cardiac output}} \times \underset{\text{(CaO}_2\text{)}}{\text{arterial O}_2 \text{ content}} \times 10$$

The formula may be modified to include the cardiac index in place of the cardiac output.[45] As previously described, this takes into account the patient's body surface area, which increases the usefulness of the calculated value. The formula would then be:

$$Do_2I = \underset{\text{(CI)}}{\text{cardiac index}} \times \underset{\text{(CaO}_2\text{)}}{\text{arterial O}_2 \text{ content}} \times 10$$

The normal oxygen transport is approximately 640 to 1400 mL/min,[38] or 500 to 600 mL/min/m^2.[45] Common causes of inadequate oxygen delivery include ventilatory failure, failure of arterial oxygenation, profound anemia, hypovolemia, and myocardial dysfunction. A recent study identified oxygen delivery, along with the alveolar-arterial oxygen gradient, as the two most important determinants of survival in patients with ARDS.[46] The data showed that optimization of Do_2 and the alveolar-arterial oxygen gradient may promote resolution of ARDS, prevent MSOF, and improve survival. These data may apply to all critically ill patients, such as those with medical conditions.

Oxygen consumption (Vo_2)

The oxygen consumption is the amount of oxygen used by the tissues each minute. It reflects the sum of all oxidative metabolism as well as the adequacy of the circulatory system.[47] The most common reason that Vo_2 varies is a change in metabolic demands, either increased or decreased. Only in certain pathologic states is Vo_2 supply dependent. In critical illness, sufficient Do_2 to promote adequate Vo_2 is maintained by such compensatory mechanisms as increased heart rate, increased cardiac output, and increased oxygen extraction. Failure of the compensatory mechanisms is reflected in the decrease in oxygen consumption and ultimately in the death of the patient.

Measurements of oxidative metabolism are the most sensitive of all monitored cardiorespiratory variables for acute circulatory failure.[47,48] Calcu-

lation of oxygen consumption may be performed using the following formula[44]:

$$Vo_2 = CO \times Hgb \times 13.9 \times (SaO_2 - S\bar{v}o_2)$$

If the cardiac index is used, the formula is:

$$Vo_2I = CI \times Hgb \times 13.9 \times (SaO_2 - S\bar{v}o_2)$$

The normal oxygen consumption is approximately 180 to 280 mL/min,[37] or 110 to 160 mL/min/m^2.[45]

Decreased oxygen consumption is usually due to inadequate oxygen delivery. Shoemaker et al[47] demonstrated that mortality could be decreased by optimizing oxygen consumption. This requires maintenance of blood volume, cardiac index, and oxygen delivery. It has been shown that increasing cardiac output with fluid challenges results in increased oxygen consumption in patients with hypovolemic and septic shock.[49]

If oxygen consumption is calculated and found to be increased, it does not guarantee that the patient's metabolic needs have been met. It may be increased as a reflection of the patient's increased metabolic rate. MSOF is a hypermetabolic state associated with increases in oxygen consumption as part of the normal inflammatory response to tissue injury. Fever, increased heart rate, acute phase protein synthesis, muscle catabolism, and the maintenance of cellular osmotic integrity all contribute to increased tissue oxygen demands in MSOF.[50-52] In order to determine whether the oxygen requirements of the tissues are being met at the calculated value for oxygen consumption, an empiric trial of therapy is appropriate. If the cardiac index, oxygen transport, and oxygen consumption increase with therapy, it is likely that an oxygen debt existed.[47]

Oxygen extraction ratio

The oxygen extraction ratio is defined as

$$\frac{CaO_2 - C\bar{v}o_2}{CaO_2}$$

where CaO_2 and $C\bar{v}o_2$ represent the arterial and mixed venous oxygen contents, respectively. The normal oxygen extraction ratio ranges from 22% to 30%.[38] When oxygen transport decreases, the extraction ratio normally increases to meet the tissue demands for oxygen. In cases of pathologic supply dependency, such as patients with ARDS, the oxygen extraction ratio does not increase ap-

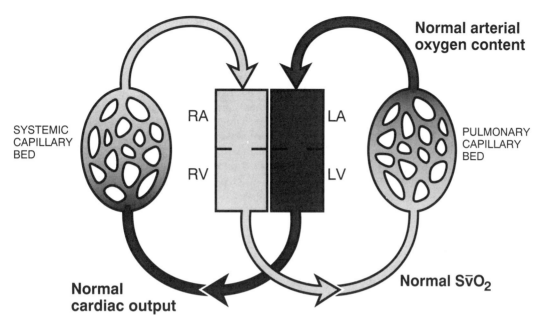

Fig. 6-4   Normal circulation. Abbreviations: *LA,* left atrium; *LV,* left ventricle; *RA,* right atrium; *RV,* right ventricle; *S$\bar{v}o_2$,* mixed venous oxygen saturation. (From Mims BC. Physiologic rationale of S$\bar{v}o_2$ monitoring. Crit Care Nurs Clin North Am 1989;1:620.)

propriately in response to decreased oxygen transport. A failure of the extraction ratio to increase is the hallmark of a pathologic oxygen supply dependency.[6] In addition, the fact that the extraction ratio does not increase explains why the mixed venous oxygen parameters (Pvo_2 and S$\bar{v}o_2$) do not reflect oxygen supply/demand imbalances in patients with a pathologic supply dependency.

Mixed venous oxygen saturation (S$\bar{v}o_2$)

The continuous monitoring of mixed venous oxygen saturation (S$\bar{v}o_2$) is used to provide ongoing evidence of the balance between oxygen supply and demand.[53] Since maintenance and/or restoration of oxygen supply/demand balance is central to averting MSOF in the critically ill patient, S$\bar{v}o_2$ can be quite useful. However, it should be noted that once sepsis, ARDS, or MSOF results in a pathologic oxygen supply dependency, the S$\bar{v}o_2$ will no longer reflect the balance between oxygen supply and demand.

Circulatory anatomy. A schematic representation of the circulatory system is depicted in Fig. 6-4. Once blood passes through the lungs and be-comes oxygenated, it flows into the left side of the heart, which then pumps blood to the systemic capillary bed. The amount of blood pumped by the heart each minute (cardiac output) depends on both heart rate and stroke volume, with the normal cardiac output being 4 to 8 L/min.[54] Once blood reaches the systemic capillary bed, oxygen is extracted from the blood and used in aerobic metabolism. The amount of oxygen extracted from the blood depends on the tissue oxygen demands, the affinity of hemoglobin for oxygen, and the absence of any cellular defects preventing oxygen utilization.[44]

Upon leaving the systemic capillary bed, venous blood flows into the right atrium. Several structures contribute venous return to the right atrium, including the superior vena cava, inferior vena cava, and coronary sinus. This blood mixes, passes through the tricuspid valve into the right ventricle, and is ejected into the pulmonary artery. This blood is termed "mixed venous blood," which implies an aggregate of venous drainage from all perfused body parts. By using a special pulmonary artery catheter that has a fiberoptic bundle, the percent saturation of hemoglobin with oxygen in mixed venous blood can be continuously monitored.[54]

Determinants of $S\bar{v}O_2$

Oxygen content. Several factors determine the saturation of hemoglobin in mixed venous blood. First, if there is a pathologic lung condition that impairs oxygen transfer across the alveolocapillary membrane, there will be less oxygen than normal in the blood as it leaves the lungs and enters the left side of the heart. Likewise, a hemoglobin deficiency reduces the oxygen-carrying capacity of the blood, resulting in a lower-than-normal oxygen content in the blood entering the left side of the heart. When this blood circulates through the left side of the heart and arrives at the systemic capillary bed, there is less oxygen than normal in the blood passing through the arterioles. If the amount of blood arriving at the systemic capillaries (cardiac output) has not increased and the cells extract the usual amount of oxygen, then the amount of oxygen in the blood will be decreased when the blood circulates back through the right side of the heart and into the pulmonary artery. This is reflected in a decreased $S\bar{v}O_2$. Therefore the oxygen content, as determined by the PaO_2, SaO_2, and hemoglobin level, is an important determinant of $S\bar{v}O_2$ (Fig. 6-5).

Cardiac output. In Fig. 6-6, the amount of oxygen in the arterial blood (arterial oxygen content) is normal, but the cardiac output is low. Less blood than normal arrives at the systemic capillary bed each minute. In order for the cells to use normal amounts of oxygen, since they receive less blood than normal, more than the usual amount of oxygen must be extracted from each 100 mL of blood that is delivered. When the blood circulates back through the right side of the heart and enters the pulmonary artery, the $S\bar{v}O_2$ will be decreased.

Tissue oxygen demands. In Fig. 6-7, both oxygen content and cardiac output are normal, but the tissue oxygen demands are exceptionally high. This may occur with fever, seizures, shivering, and other hypermetabolic conditions. The tissues extract an increased amount of oxygen, and the blood circulating back through the right side of the heart and into the pulmonary artery has a lower-than-normal $S\bar{v}O_2$. Thus, rather than indicating a specific clinical event, $S\bar{v}O_2$ reflects the balance between oxygen supply and demand.[55]

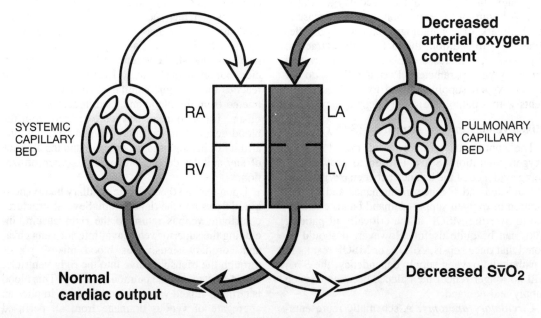

Fig. 6-5 Low arterial oxygen content. Abbreviations: *LA,* left atrium; *LV,* left ventricle; *RA,* right atrium; *RV,* right ventricle; *S$\bar{v}$o$_2$,* mixed venous oxygen saturation. (From Mims BC. Physiologic rationale of S$\bar{v}$o$_2$ monitoring. Crit Care Nurs Clin North Am 1989;1:620.)

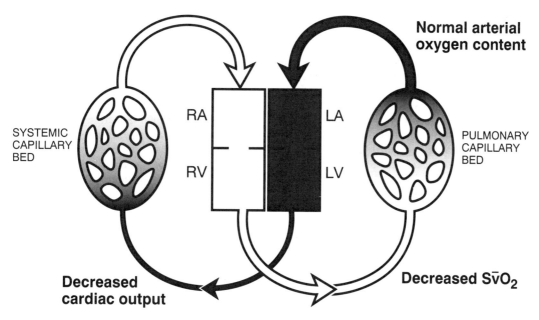

Fig. 6-6 Low cardiac output. Abbreviations: *LA*, left atrium; *LV*, left ventricle; *RA*, right atrium; *RV*, right ventricle; $S\bar{v}o_2$, mixed venous oxygen saturation. (From Mims BC. Physiologic rationale of $S\bar{v}o_2$ monitoring. Crit Care Nurs Clin North Am 1989;1:621.)

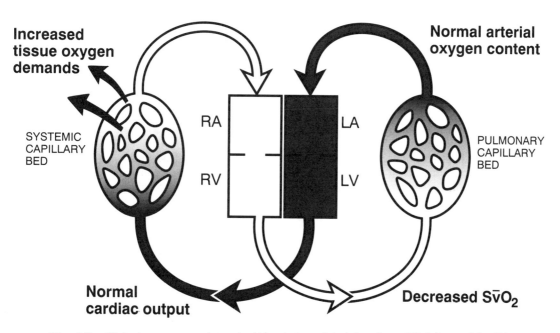

Fig. 6-7 High tissue oxygen demand. Abbreviations: *LA*, left atrium; *LV*, left ventricle; *RA*, right atrium; *RV*, right ventricle; $S\bar{v}o_2$, mixed venous oxygen saturation. (From Mims BC. Physiologic rationale of $S\bar{v}o_2$ monitoring. Crit Care Nurs Clin North Am 1989;1:621.)

Decreased ***S$\bar{v}$O$_2$.*** The normal range of S$\bar{v}$O$_2$ is 60% to 80%.[56,57] An S$\bar{v}$O$_2$ below 60% reflects an imbalance between oxygen supply and demand and use of the venous oxygen reserve. A decreased S$\bar{v}$O$_2$ is a nonspecific finding, and further investigation is required to identify the exact cause of the imbalance. This point must be appreciated, or the utility of S$\bar{v}$O$_2$ as a monitoring parameter is negated. The S$\bar{v}$O$_2$ may fall when oxygen supply (D$_O2$) decreases or when oxygen demand increases. Common causes of decreased S$\bar{v}$O$_2$ include decreased cardiac output, decreased arterial oxygenation, and anemia.[53] A steady, gradual decline of S$\bar{v}$O$_2$ may indicate occult blood loss in the postoperative patient.[58] A decreased S$\bar{v}$O$_2$ may also occur when tissue oxygen demand goes up as with pain, fever, anxiety, shivering, seizures, physical activity, or increased work of breathing.

Increased ***S$\bar{v}$O$_2$.*** Several possibilities exist when the S$\bar{v}$O$_2$ is higher than normal. First, the tip of the pulmonary artery catheter may be wedged. Since the balloon obstructs forward flow of blood, blood stagnates distal to the balloon. This creates a high ventilation to perfusion (V/Q) ratio, and oxygen is absorbed from the surrounding alveoli,[54] yielding a high saturation at that point.

An increased S$\bar{v}$O$_2$, especially when coupled with a decreased oxygen consumption, is frequently an early indication of sepsis.[58] In sepsis, even though the metabolic needs of the tissues are high, tissues are not able to extract and use oxygen. This may be due to shortened capillary transit time, peripheral arteriovenous shunting, or a cellular defect, which prevents the mitochondria from being able to extract and use oxygen. Since the oxygen is not used, the S$\bar{v}$O$_2$ is high, but the calculated oxygen consumption is low. Anaerobic metabolism occurs; lactate is produced; and acidosis follows.

Cyanide poisoning secondary to excessive administration of nitroprusside may also result in an increased S$\bar{v}$O$_2$. Intracellular respiration is disrupted by the reaction of cyanide with the iron in cytochrome *c* oxidase. Although the Pa$_O2$, Sa$_O2$, Ca$_O2$, and oxygen transport are all normal, the cells cannot use oxygen for aerobic metabolism.[59] The patient develops lactic acidosis, yet the blood returning to the right side of the heart and pulmonary artery has an abnormally high S$\bar{v}$O$_2$.

When oxygen transport is normal, decreased tissue oxygen demand (hypothermia, anesthesia, or pharmacologic paralysis) can result in an increased S$\bar{v}$O$_2$.[54] Less oxygen is used by the tissues, so more oxygen than normal remains in the venous blood as it travels from the systemic capillary bed back to the right side of the heart and on into the pulmonary artery. An intracardiac left-to-right shunt, such as that which occurs with an atrial septal defect, ventricular septal defect, anomalous pulmonary venous return, or patent ductus arteriosus, will also increase the S$\bar{v}$O$_2$ in the pulmonary artery.[60]

Interpretation ***of "normal"*** ***S$\bar{v}$O$_2$.*** When the S$\bar{v}$O$_2$ is in the normal range of 60% to 80%, it usually indicates that oxygen transport is meeting the tissue oxygen demands. That is, the cardiac output, arterial oxygenation, and hemoglobin are adequate to meet the tissue oxygen demands without the use of the venous oxygen reserve. However, if a compensatory mechanism such as an increased cardiac output is in use, a normal S$\bar{v}$O$_2$ does not ensure that all of the components of the oxygen supply/demand axis are normal. If compensation is required to maintain oxygen supply/demand balance, further increases in oxygen requirements may result in serious consequences.

Summary. The S$\bar{v}$O$_2$ may not reflect the imbalance between oxygen supply/demand that occurs in sepsis, ARDS, and MSOF. As previously described, there is a linear relationship between oxygen transport and oxygen consumption in these clinical situations.[12] That is, as oxygen transport falls, less oxygen is extracted and used by the tissues. The oxygen extraction ratio does not increase, and venous oxygen remains high even though tissue oxygen demands are not met.[61,62] Therefore a normal S$\bar{v}$O$_2$ may not reflect normal tissue oxygenation in patients with a pathologic oxygen supply dependency. When an elevated S$\bar{v}$O$_2$ level is observed in a critically ill patient, the possibility of sepsis or other causes of a pathologic supply dependency should be considered. Further, it should be noted that S$\bar{v}$O$_2$ does not reflect the tissue P$_O2$ level.

Assessing O$_2$ supply/demand in splanchnic organs

Although calculation of oxygen transport and oxygen consumption provides valuable information regarding overall aerobic metabolism, neither reflects the balance between oxygen use and actual tissue oxygen demands.[1] Furthermore, since different organs react differently during shock and critical illness, measurements of total body Do_2 and Vo_2 do not reflect adequacy of tissue oxygenation in each individual organ.

As previously mentioned, the adequacy of tissue oxygenation in the splanchnic organs is of great importance. The ability to assess the balance between oxygen delivery and tissue needs in the splanchnic organs of the critically ill patient would be extremely valuable. This has been done experimentally using the fiberoptic Swan-Ganz catheter to measure O_2 content of portal venous and hepatic venous blood. This is technically difficult, however, and the results may be affected by increased tissue oxygen extraction and by tissue hypoxia. Another technique that has been used is indirectly measuring gastrointestinal intramucosal pH by tonometry.[63] This involves placing a small expanded polytetrafluoroethylene balloon attached to a thin catheter into the gut lumen. The balloon is a micropermeable membrane that allows free transfer of gases. By measuring the Pco_2 in the gut lumen, the intramural (gut wall) pH can be estimated using the Henderson-Hasselbalch equation. Low pH values of the gut mucosa may reflect an oxygen supply/demand imbalance of the mucosal tissue. In the future, this may provide useful information regarding which patients are likely to develop complications of mucosal disruption, such as infections and MSOF.[64]

CLINICAL IMPLICATIONS
Goals of care

A central goal in critical care involves the prevention of MSOF by maintaining a balance between oxygen delivery and tissue oxygen requirements. Volume loading, blood transfusion, inotropic and vasoactive drug administration, and ventilatory support are used to ensure adequate oxygen transport. Steps should also be taken to minimize undue oxygen demands. Fever, increased work of breathing, anxiety, shivering, seizures, and agitation all increase the metabolic rate. Controlling excessive fever can assist in restoring oxygen supply/demand balance. Acetaminophen is the agent of choice because antipyretics such as aspirin that inhibit prostaglandin synthesis can decrease renal blood flow. Hypothermia units should rarely be used since they can cause shivering and thus increase oxygen demands. The patient's tempera-

ture should not be reduced below 37° C because this can shift the oxyhemoglobin dissociation curve to the left and impair the oxygen extraction ability of the tissues.[8] Mechanical ventilation with ample sedation or neuromuscular blockade may also be used to minimize tissue oxygen requirements.

Supranormal values as endpoints

Although normal values for oxygen delivery and oxygen consumption are appropriate for normal, unstressed resting subjects, critically ill patients may require supranormal values because of increased metabolic and hemodynamic needs. Shoemaker et al[65-68] and Hankeln et al[69] propose that the empirically determined cardiorespiratory patterns of surviving patients are the appropriate goals of therapy for critically ill postoperative patients.

Proposed goals of therapy, some of which are controversial, consistent with this include the following:

*1. Cardiac index 50% in excess of normal
*2. Blood volume 500 mL greater than normal, provided that this could be attained without exceeding PCWP of 20 mm Hg
*3. Oxygen delivery (Do_2) greater than 600 mL/min/m²
*4. Oxygen consumption (Vo_2) greater than 170 mL/min/m²
 5. Normal blood pressure
*6. PVRI less than 250 dyne/sec/cm⁵/m²
 7. Metabolic and nutritional support

To achieve these therapeutic goals, Shoemaker et al propose vigorous volume loading while maintaining a PCWP no greater than 18 mm Hg. Colloids are used by this group, since they have found that colloids expand the plasma volume without an undue increase in interstitial water. Once fluid loading has been achieved, the next step in Shoemaker's therapeutic plan involves administering an inotrope, such as dobutamine, beginning with 2 µg/kg/min. The dosage is titrated to achieve the best cardiac index, Do_2, and Vo_2. If the MAP and systemic vascular resistance index are high, a vasodilator such as nitroglycerin or nitroprusside is added. The vasodilator is titrated to improve cardiac index without causing hypotension (keep MAP > 80 mm Hg, systolic

*Controversial.

blood pressure > 110 mm Hg). If the combination of fluids, inotropes, and vasodilators is ineffective in reaching the therapeutic goals, then a vasopressor such as dopamine is added in small doses to maintain the MAP at 80 mm Hg and systolic pressure at 110 mm Hg.[47]

Patients with severe trauma, sepsis, stress, and hypercatabolic states may demonstrate an increased V_{O_2} and yet still have unmet metabolic needs. If a trial of therapy as described above raises cardiac output and V_{O_2}, it is likely that therapy opened up additional microcirculatory channels that perfused relatively hypoxic tissues, which then extracted more O_2. If V_{O_2} increases after a fluid challenge, then it must be inferred that an O_2 debt had been present. It should be noted that this therapeutic regimen is aimed at supporting the patient's normal compensatory mechanisms and maintaining an optimal hemodynamic state, thus preventing the development of tissue hypoxia from blood volume, hemodynamic, and O_2 transport deficits.

Hemoglobin or hematocrit should be maintained at or near normal in the patient with potential D_{O_2} problems. However, the increased blood viscosity associated with a hematocrit $>45\%$ may result in decreased blood flow to vital organs.[7]

CONCLUSION

An imbalance in oxygen supply and demand plays a major role in the pathophysiology of MSOF. Hypoxic tissue damage is extremely difficult to reverse, so prevention and early recognition of an oxygen supply/demand imbalance are of utmost importance in critical illness. This requires hemodynamic monitoring, arterial blood gas analysis, and calculation of oxygen transport, oxygen consumption, and the oxygen extraction ratio. Continuous on-line monitoring of $S\bar{v}_{O_2}$ may be helpful in detecting oxygen supply/demand imbalances, but not in cases of pathologic oxygen supply dependency. Restoring oxygen supply and demand balance may require volume loading, inotropic support, optimization of Hgb, ventilatory support, and control of the patient's tissue oxygen requirements. Supranormal values for cardiorespiratory values have been proposed by some as goals of treatment in many critically ill patients. However, optimal clinical endpoints are not well defined, and further research is indicated.

REFERENCES

1. Haglund U, Fiddian-Green RG. Assessment of adequate tissue oxygenation in shock and critical illness: Oxygen transport in sepsis. Bermuda, April 1 and 2, 1989. Intens Care Med 1989;15:475-477.
2. Gutierrez G, Lund N, Bryan-Brown CW. Cellular oxygen utilization during multiple organ failure. Crit Care Clin 1989;5(2):271-287.
3. Schumacker PT, Samsel RW. Oxygen delivery and uptake by peripheral tissues: Physiology and pathophysiology. Crit Care Clin 1989;5:255-269.
4. Russell JA et al. Oxygen delivery and consumption and ventricular preload are greater in survivors than in nonsurvivors of the adult respiratory distress syndrome. Am Rev Respir Dis 1990;141:659-665.
5. Dantzker D. Oxygen delivery and utilization in sepsis. Crit Care Clin 1989;5:81-98.
6. Schumacker PT, Cain SM. The concept of a critical oxygen delivery. Intens Care Med 1987;13:223-229.
7. Weg JG. Oxygen transport in adult respiratory distress syndrome and other acute circulatory problems: Relationships of oxygen delivery and oxygen consumption. Crit Care Med 1991;19:650-657.
8. Schumacker PT, Samsel RW. Oxygen supply and consumption in the adult respiratory distress syndrome. Clin Chest Med 1990;11:715-722.
9. Bersten A, Sibbald WJ. Circulatory disturbances in multiple systems organ failure. Crit Care Clin 1989;5:233-254.
10. Bihari D et al. The effects of vasodilation with prostacyclin on oxygen delivery and uptake in critically ill patients. N Engl J Med 1987;317:397-403.
11. Cain SM, Curtis SE. Experimental models of pathologic oxygen supply dependency. Crit Care Med 1991;19:603-612.
12. Mohsenifar Z et al. Relationship between O_2 delivery and O_2 consumption in the adult respiratory distress syndrome. Chest 1983;84:267-271.
13. Shibutani K, Komatsu T, Kubal K. Critical level of oxygen delivery in anesthetized man. Crit Care Med 1983;11:640-643.
14. Tenney SM. A theoretical analysis of the relationship between venous blood and mean tissue oxygen pressures. Respir Physiol 1974;20:283-296.
15. Parillo JE et al. Septic shock in humans: Advances in the understanding of pathogenesis, cardiovascular dysfunction, and therapy. Ann Intern Med 1990;113:227-242.
16. Tuchschmidt J, Oblitas D, Fried JC. Oxygen consumption in sepsis and septic shock. Crit Care Med 1991;19:664-671.
17. Hyers JM, Gee M, Andreadis NA. Cellular interactions in the multiple organ injury syndrome. Am Rev Respir Dis 1987;135:952-953.
18. Cain SM. Supply dependency of oxygen uptake in ARDS: Myth or reality. Am J Med Sci 1984;288:119-124.
19. Groeneveld AB et al. Relation of arterial blood lactate to oxygen delivery and hemodynamic variables in human shock states. Circ Shock 1987;22:35-53.
20. Gutierrez G. The rate of oxygen release and its effect on capillary O_2 tension: A mathematical analysis. Respir Physiol 1985;63:79-96.
21. Gutierrez G, Pohil RJ, Strong R. Effect of flow on O_2 consumption during progressive hypoxemia. J Appl Physiol 1988;65:601-607.

22. Astiz M et al. Oxygen delivery and consumption in patients with hyderdynamic septic shock. Crit Care Med 1987;15:26-28.

23. Kaufman BS, Rackow EC, Falk JL. The relationship between oxygen delivery and consumption during fluid resuscitation of hypovolemic and septic shock. Chest 1984;85:336-340.

24. Gutierrez G, Pohil RJ. Oxygen consumption is linearly related to O_2 supply in critically ill patients. J Crit Care 1986;1:45-53.

25. Nelson DP et al. Pathologic supply dependence of O_2 uptake during bacteremia in dogs. J Appl Physiol 1987;63:1487-1492.

26. Furchgott RF. The role of endothelium in the responses of vascular smooth muscle to drugs. Annu Rev Pharmacol Toxicol 1984;24:175-197.

27. Palmer RM, Ferrige AG, Moncada S. Nitric oxide release accounts for the biological activity of endothelium-derived relaxing factor. Nature 1987;327:524-526.

28. Shepro D, D'Amore PA. Physiology and biochemistry of the vascular wall endothelium. In: Renkin EM, Michel CC, eds. Handbook of Physiology. Section 2. The cardiovascular system. Baltimore: Williams and Wilkins, 1984.

29. Grisham MB, Everse J, Janssen HF. Endotoxemia and neutrophil activation in vivo. Am J Physiol 1988;254:H1017-H1022.

30. Korthius RJ, Grisham MB, Granger DN. Leukocyte depletion attenuates vascular injury in postischemic skeletal muscle. Am J Physiol 1988;254:H823-H827.

31. Gilbert EM et al. The effect of fluid loading, blood transfusion, and catecholamine infusion on oxygen delivery and consumption in patients with sepsis. Am Rev Respir Dis 1986;134:873-878.

32. Bronsveld WA et al. Regional blood flow and metabolism in canine endotoxin shock before, during, and after infusion of glucose-insulin-potassium (GIK). Circ Shock 1986;18:31-42.

33. Houtchens BA, Westenskow DR. Oxygen consumption in septic shock: Collective review. Circ Shock 1984;13:361-384.

34. Bland R, Shoemaker WC, Shabot MM. Physiologic monitoring goals for the critically ill patient. Surg Gynecol Obstet 1978;147:833-841.

35. Cain FB et al. Hepatic dysfunction in multiple systems organ failure as a manifestation of altered cell-cell interaction. Prog Clin Biol Res 1989;308:563-573.

36. Fromm, Jr. RE et al. The craft of cardiopulmonary analysis. In: Snyder JV, Pinsky MR, eds. Oxygen transport in the critically ill. St. Louis: Mosby–Year Book, 1987.

37. Nearman HS, Sampliner JE. Respiratory monitoring. In: Berk JL, Sampliner JE, eds. Handbook of critical care. 3rd ed. Boston: Little, Brown, & Company, 1990.

38. Varon AJ, Civetta JM. Hemodynamic monitoring. In: Berk JL, Sampliner JE. Handbook of critical care. Boston: Little, Brown & Company, 1990.

39. Albert RK. Physiology and management of failure of arterial oxygenation. In: Fallat RJ, Luce JM, eds. Clinics in critical care medicine: Cardiopulmonary critical care management. New York: Churchill Livingstone, 1988.

40. Barone JE, Snyder AB. Treatment strategies in shock: Use of oxygen transport measurements. Heart Lung 1991;20:81-86.

41. Schweiss JF. Mixed venous hemoglobin saturation: Theory and application. Int Anesthesiol Clin 1987;25:113-136.

42. Snyder JV. Assessment of systemic oxygen transport. In: Snyder JV, Pinsky MR, eds. Oxygen transport in the critically ill. St. Louis: Mosby–Year Book, 1987.

43. Ahrens TS. Concepts in the assessment of oxygenation. Focus Crit Care 1987;14:36-44.

44. Mims BC, ed. Case studies in critical care nursing. Baltimore: Williams & Wilkins, 1990.

45. Marino PL. The ICU book. Philadelphia: Lea & Febiger, 1991.

46. Cryer HG et al. Oxygen delivery in patients with adult respiratory distress syndrome who undergo surgery: Correlation with multiple-system organ failure. Arch Surg 1989;124:1378-1384.

47. Shoemaker WC, Bland RD, Appel PL. Therapy of critically ill postoperative patients based on outcome prediction and prospective clinical trials. Surg Clin North Am 1985;65:811-833.

48. Buran MJ. Oxygen consumption. In: Snyder JV, Pinksy MR, eds. Oxygen transport in the critically ill. St. Louis: Mosby–Year Book, 1987.

49. Halfman-Franey M. Current trends in hemodynamic monitoring in patients in shock. Crit Care Nurs Q 1988;11:9-18.

50. Cerra FB. Hypermetabolism, organ failure and metabolic support. Surgery 1987;101:1-14.

51. Dahn MS et al. Splanchnic and total body oxygen consumption differences in septic and injured patients. Surgery 1987;101:69-80.

52. Stoner HB. Metabolism after trauma and in sepsis. Circ Shock 1986;19:75-87.

53. Mims BC. Physiologic rationale of SvO_2 monitoring. Crit Care Nurs Clin North Am 1989;1:619-628.

54. Briones TL. SvO_2 monitoring: Part I. Clinical case application. Dimen Crit Care Nurs 1988;7:70-78.

55. Stewart FM. SvO_2 monitoring: Part II. Nursing research applications. Dimen Crit Care Nurs 1988;7:79-82.

56. Kersten LD. Comprehensive respiratory nursing. Philadelphia: WB Saunders, 1989.

57. White KM. Continuous monitoring of mixed venous oxygen saturation: A new assessment tool in critical care nursing-Part I. Cardiovasc Nurs 1987;23:1-6.

58. White KM. Continuous monitoring of mixed venous oxygen saturations (SvO_2): A new assessment tool in critical care nursing-Part II. Cardiovasc Nurs 1987;23:7-12.

59. Clemmer TP, Orme JF, Thomas FO. Physiology and management of failure of oxygen transport and utilization. In: Fallat RJ, Luce JM, eds. Clinics in critical care medicine: Cardiopulmonary critical care management. New York: Churchill Livingstone, 1988;61-87.

60. Gore JM, Sloan K. Use of continuous monitoring of mixed venous saturation in the coronary care unit. Chest 1984;86:757-761.

61. Bone RC. Respiratory monitoring. In: Fallat RJ, Luce J, eds. Clinics in critical care medicine: Cardiopulmonary critical care management. New York: Churchill Livingstone, 1988.

62. Rashkin MC, Boskin C, Baughman RP. Oxygen delivery in critically ill patients: Relationship to blood lactate and survival. Chest 1985;87:580-584.

63. Gutierrez G. Cellular energy metabolism during hypoxia. Crit Care Med 1991:19:619-626.

64. Fiddian-Green RG, Nelson MG. Transient episodes of sigmoid ischemia and their relation to infection from intestinal organisms after abdominal aortic operation. Crit Care Med 1987;15:835-839.

65. Shoemaker WC et al. Prospective trial of supranormal values of survivors as therapeutic goals in high-risk surgical patients. Chest 1988;94:1176-1186.

66. Shoemaker WC. Relation of oxygen transport patterns to the pathophysiology and therapy of shock states. Intens Care Med 1987;13:230-243.

67. Shoemaker WC, Appel PL, Kram HB. Tissue oxygen debt as determinant of lethal and nonlethal postoperative organ failure. Crit Care Med 1988;16:1117-1120.

68. Shoemaker WC. Oxygen transport measurements to evaluate tissue perfusion and titrate therapy: Dobutamine and dopamine effects. Crit Care Med 1991;19:672-688.

69. Hankeln KB et al. Evaluation of prognostic indices based on hemodynamic and oxygen transport variables in shock patients with respiratory distress syndrome. Crit Care Med 1987;15:1-7.

7 Alterations in Metabolism

Joy Davis Kimbrell

The insults and complications that precede multisystem organ failure (MSOF) are complex, multifactorial, challenging syndromes that provoke alterations in the normal metabolic response. Specific clinical conditions associated with the evolution of the metabolic response include injured or necrotic tissue, inflammation, sepsis, and perfusion deficits.[1] Alterations in metabolism are initially compensatory mechanisms aimed at meeting the body's increased needs. Over time, however, metabolic changes may result in significant detrimental effects on the patient's prognosis and duration of illness.[2]

Neuroendocrine responses are at least partially responsible for the alterations of protein, carbohydrate, and lipid metabolism that occur following a major insult. Other possible contributing factors to the metabolic response are less clearly understood and remain under investigation. Activation of cellular mediators, such as interleukin-1, discussed in Chapter 3, may play a pivotal role.[3,4]

Because there are major alterations in metabolism with marked increases in resting energy expenditure (REE) and catabolism of lean body mass and visceral organs, nutritional and metabolic support serves as a primary adjunctive therapeutic tool in managing the patient with MSOF. For this reason, knowledge of current methods of metabolic assessment and support with parenteral and enteral nutrition is essential.

PATHOPHYSIOLOGY OF METABOLIC RESPONSE

Altered metabolic regulation typical of major insults such as trauma and sepsis includes a neuroendocrine response mediated primarily by the sympathetic nervous system[5,6] (Fig. 7-1). This response serves as a compensatory mechanism to provide substrate for increased energy demands, and it is characterized by hypermetabolism, hyperglycemia, and hypercatabolism. Initially, the "ebb phase," normally lasting 48 to 72 hours, occurs with little change or slight depression in the metabolic response.[7] At the end of this period of relative metabolic rate stability, the "flow phase" begins,[7] characterized by hypermetabolism. The classic features seen in the hypermetabolic response include an increase in the resting energy expenditure (170% to 200% of baseline), increase in cardiac output, increase in oxygen consumption, and increase in carbon dioxide production.[8]

With the initiating stress, the sympathetic nervous system is stimulated and, in turn, stimulates the adrenal medulla to release the catecholamines epinephrine and norepinephrine. Epinephrine release increases cardiac output, blood pressure, pulse, and rate and depth of respirations. Epinephrine also stimulates hepatic glycogenolysis (breakdown of glycogen to re-form glucose) and gluconeogenesis (formation of glucose from amino acids and fat). In addition, epinephrine inhibits insulin secretion and the uptake of glucose in the peripheral tissues and stimulates the hydrolysis (breakdown) of fat. The other catecholamine released, norepinephrine, also increases metabolic activity and fat hydrolysis and stimulates peripheral vasoconstriction.[6,9]

Following stress or insult, the hypothalamus becomes excited and releases corticotropin releasing hormone (CRH), which stimulates the anterior pituitary gland to secrete adrenocorticotropic hormone (ACTH). ACTH stimulates the adrenal cortex to release cortisol,[6,9] a glucocorticoid with a powerful ability to alter metabolism, primarily increasing the production of glucose. Cortisol stimulates the mobilization and transport of amino acids from muscle stores to be used by the liver to produce glucose (gluconeogenesis). In addition, cortisol

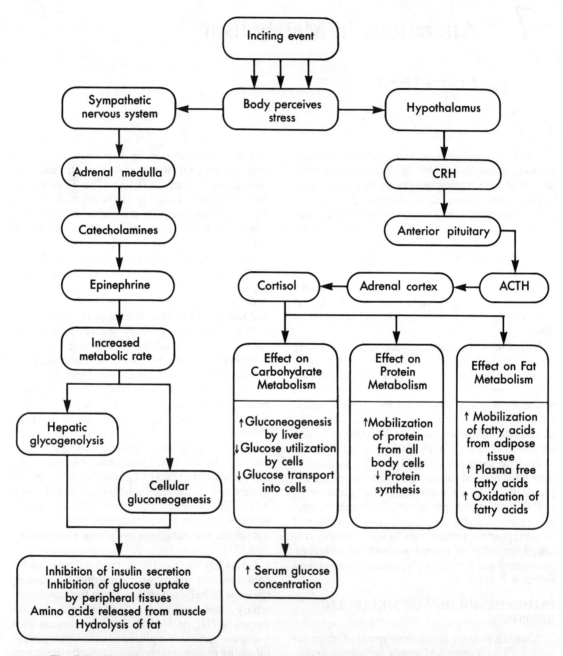

Fig. 7-1 Neuroendocrine effects on metabolism. As the body perceives stress or insult, neuro-endocrine compensatory mechanisms are triggered to provide more energy to meet the body's needs. *CRH*, Corticotropin releasing hormone; *ACTH*, adrenocorticotropic hormone.

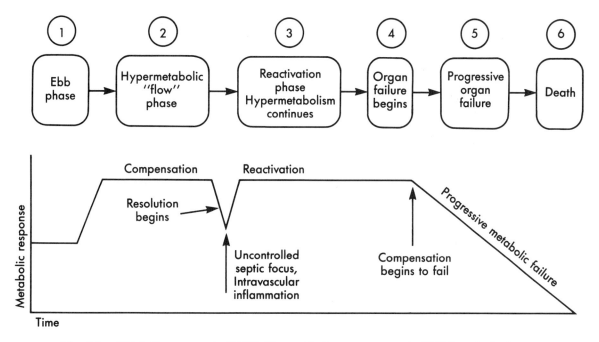

Fig. 7-2 Metabolic response in MSOF. The metabolic response seen in MSOF can be broken down into six steps. The multileveled horizontal line in the center of the graph represents the increases and decreases in metabolism that occur as the patient progresses through the steps. The patient may recover at any point with the metabolism returning to near normal. (From Kimbrell JD. In Huddleston VB. Multisystem Organ Failure: A Pathophysiologic Approach. Boston, 1991;23.)

stimulates an increase in the enzymes required to convert amino acids to glucose.[10]

In many stress states other than MSOF, the hypermetabolic "flow" phase normally peaks in 48 to 72 hours and abates completely in 7 to 10 days. With MSOF, forces such as uncontrolled intravascular inflammation or a continued septic focus trigger a "reactivation" phase.[11] Hypermetabolism then continues until the source of inflammation or sepsis is controlled or the organ failure stage begins.[12] With organ failure, the liver, kidney, and other organs progressively fail, and the body may not be able to continue manufacturing substrates for energy. Metabolism then plummets as decompensation occurs, leading to progressive cellular damage and irreversible injury.[13] If the inflammation or uncontrolled septic focus continues unabated, the ultimate outcome is death (Fig. 7-2). Whether metabolic failure is the *cause* of MSOF or the *outcome* of sepsis, inflammation, and multiple organ damage remains to be determined.

Carbohydrate metabolism

The metabolic response preceding actual organ failure includes a significant alteration in carbohydrate metabolism. In conditions of simple starvation, the initial primary source of energy is glucose in the form of glycogen. Glycogen stores are limited (about 1200 kcal)[14] and after these are depleted, the body energy substrate source changes to fatty acids and ketones derived from fat. With superimposed stress states and organ failure, there is mixed substrate oxidation (the breakdown of a substance, often for the purpose of energy production). The fraction of energy obtained from glucose is significantly reduced while the fraction obtained from oxidation of amino acids and fat rises.

Altered metabolism in stress states is reflected by changes in the respiratory quotient (RQ), the ratio of carbon dioxide production to oxygen consumption. The RQ varies depending on the substrate metabolized.[15] In simple starvation states, the RQ would be 0.70, reflecting metabolism of fat stores for energy. In hypermetabolic states, the RQ may be 0.8 to 0.85, reflecting oxidation of mixed substrates of fat, carbohydrate, and amino acids for energy.[8] This reflects the increased reliance on amino acids during stress states.

In stress states, after the initial stores of glycogen are depleted (about 6 to 12 hours), the liver converts amino acids to glucose (gluconeogenesis). The body catabolizes skeletal muscles to obtain these amino acids (proteolysis). Catabolism results in a mild-to-moderate hyperglycemia, which is mediated by increased secretion of epinephrine and cortisol. In addition, epinephrine inhibits insulin secretion and promotes the development of insulin resistance.[16] Other poorly defined mechanisms may also contribute to insulin resistance. The compensatory attempt to keep the blood glucose elevated is thought to occur in part because of the body's preference for glucose as the substrate for wound repair[17] and also because glucose is necessary to supply the needs of the brain, red and white blood cells, bone marrow, and cardiac muscle.

As the hypermetabolic response progresses, lactic acid is produced from muscle glycogen oxidation and carried to the liver, where it is converted back to glucose. As organs fail and the liver becomes dysfunctional, plasma lactate rises. Some tissues, such as myocardium, can use lactate as an energy substrate by allowing direct entry of the lactate into mitochondria.[8] However, most tissues, such as the central nervous system, are glucose dependent and are unable to use lactate as an energy source. Lactic acidosis usually results as lactate production increases and ATP breaks down and is not recycled. With further progression of hypermetabolism and a continued need for increased energy, substrate stores are exhausted or the body is unable to use them, and the mitochondria fail to produce ATP for energy. Without energy available to carry out their functions, organs progressively fail.[13] The compensatory mechanisms to produce substrates for fuel are made useless. Hypoglycemia will be evident as the liver becomes unable to produce glucose through gluconeogenesis in the late stages of MSOF.[8] This hypoglycemia is considered by many clinicians to be an ominous sign and often heralds the onset of liver failure and death.

Lipid metabolism

Injury and sepsis, as well as other conditions that incite organ failure, produce significant alterations in lipid metabolism.[18,19] With increased catecholamine secretion and decreased insulin levels, triglycerides are catabolized to free fatty acids and ketone bodies for energy sources. There is increased turnover and oxidation of medium- and long-chain fatty acids that can meet the energy needs of cardiac and skeletal muscles. In this manner, up to 80% of the body's energy needs can be provided for the tissues that are not solely glucose-dependent. Glucose is spared for use by the tissues that can only use glucose for energy such as the central nervous system. Specific processes such as cell-mediated immune activity and wound healing are also exclusively dependent on glucose for energy. This alteration in lipid metabolism may actually help to conserve protein by signaling muscle tissue to minimize the release of amino acids during prolonged stress and sepsis.[6]

As the organ failure syndrome progresses, there is an increase in hepatic lipogenesis reflected by a progressive rise in the RQ, which eventually exceeds 1.0.[20] Triglyceride clearance decreases, and a spontaneous lipemia or hypertriglyceridemia may occur secondary to increased hepatic lipogenesis and decreased fat uptake by the peripheral adipose tissue. Both tumor necrosis factor and interleukin-1 have been implicated in these alterations of fat metabolism.[21,22] The alteration in fat metabolism contributes to weight loss and depletion of subcutaneous fat stores and may contribute to acidosis.[6]

Protein metabolism

Protein, in the form of amino acids, becomes an important energy source during stress.[6] Amino acids are used as the fuel for hepatic conversion to glucose during gluconeogenesis. Unfortunately, the primary site for obtaining amino acids is skeletal muscle, connective tissue, and the unstimulated gut.[20] This mechanism causes autocannibalism with rapid loss of skeletal muscle mass as the body breaks down muscle protein to provide energy substrate. As skeletal muscle mass is depleted, catabolism of visceral proteins occurs to provide amino acids to the liver. Autocannibalism causes decreased muscle strength and serious compromise of the respiratory system and limits amino acids available for protein synthesis, immune system function, and wound healing. Eventually, as the visceral stores are catabolized, organ function may be impaired, leading to progressive organ failure.[23]

As muscles are broken down, a relative deficiency of essential amino acids, particularly branched-chain amino acids (BCAA), develops. This occurs because there is an elevation in the oxidation of BCAA during stress states; BCAA are used as an energy source by skeletal muscles and as substrate for gluconeogenesis by the liver.[6]

A measure to quantify the degree of stress and protein breakdown is urea nitrogen excretion. Nitrogen, a by-product of protein breakdown and gluconeogenesis, is converted to urea in the liver (ureagenesis). The amount of nitrogen lost from protein breakdown can be measured in the urine as urea nitrogen and is proportional to the degree of stress. Thus the clinician can measure the degree of protein catabolism for a specific patient. The measurement and quantification of stress will be discussed further in "Assessment of Metabolic Requirements."

As MSOF progresses, total body and hepatic protein synthesis fails and amino acid clearance decreases, particularly aromatic amino acids. The body is unresponsive to exogenous amino acid administration. With poor hepatic clearance, plasma levels of all amino acids increase, including BCAA. There is continued catabolism, and urine urea nitrogen output rises.[24] The failing kidneys are unable to excrete the excess amino acids, resulting in prerenal azotemia and further damage.[8,21]

Consequences of alterations in metabolism

The metabolic response described above is a compensatory mechanism for maintaining organ viability by producing energy for metabolic reactions. However, it is intended to be a short-term response. Prolonging the hypermetabolic response by the reactivation that occurs in MSOF and its associated conditions can produce the rapid detrimental effects of excessive catabolism and protein-calorie malnutrition. Lean body mass can become significantly depleted in as little as 7 days,[23] so early measures must be initiated to meet metabolic requirements. In MSOF, excessive catabolism of protein and fat stores and a decrease in overall body protein synthesis cause negative nitrogen balance with multiple adverse effects.

Weight loss, fatigue, and overall muscle weakness occur. The ability to turn, cough, and deep breathe is dramatically affected, and ventilatory reserves are decreased. Protein-calorie malnutrition decreases the body's ability to mount an immune response, and the alterations in metabolism may adversely affect wound healing, although the latter is a current area of controversy.

Overall, malnutrition resulting from the metabolic response and subsequent failure is associated with delayed recovery,[25-27] increased susceptibility to infection,[28,29] and increased morbidity and mortality.[30]

METABOLIC SUPPORT
Benefits of metabolic support

Metabolic support refers to nutritional support and monitoring of the critically ill patient. Although the hypermetabolic response cannot be prevented, providing adequate metabolic support can preserve lean body mass, prevent visceral malnutrition, and control nutrient deficiencies.[16,20] Even though nutritional repletion is difficult or impossible during periods of extreme stress, maintenance of bodily stores can be achieved,[2] emphasizing the importance of beginning metabolic support at the earliest possible opportunity.

Cerra[31] has outlined the principles or goals for metabolic support when managing critically ill patients, particularly those who have developed hypermetabolism and MSOF. His principles are:
1. Do no harm.
2. Prevent substrate-limited metabolism.
3. Support organ structure and function.
4. Attempt to alter the disease course.
5. Attempt to reduce morbidity and mortality.

Assessment of metabolic requirements

From the discussion of metabolic alterations and later negative consequences, it is clear that the judicious use of metabolic support is an important adjunctive tool in supporting the patient at risk for MSOF. It is prudent to point out that a clinician cannot determine the exact degree of catabolism and risk for malnutrition just by looking at the patient. Delivering too many calories may produce many respiratory and hepatic complications as well as detrimental effects on metabolism, organ structure, and function. Therefore it is extremely important to accurately determine the patient's calorie and protein needs and to estimate the degree of hypermetabolism for each patient. This is best accomplished by a complete metabolic assessment.[32]

The most logical approach to a comprehensive metabolic assessment is multidisciplinary.[5,33] If available, the metabolic or nutrition support team

COMPONENTS OF A COMPREHENSIVE NUTRITIONAL ASSESSMENT

1. Review of medical, social, and dietary history
2. Clinical assessment
3. Anthropometric measurements to provide information about muscle and fat stores
4. Visceral protein measurements (Table 7-1)
   a. Serum albumin
   b. Serum transferrin
   c. Prealbumin
   d. Retinol-binding protein
5. Tests of immune competence
   a. Total lymphocyte count = (% lymphocytes × WBC) ÷ 100

      Normal = >2000/mm³
      Mild depletion = 1200 to 2000/mm³
      Moderate depletion = 800 to 1199/mm³
      Severe depletion = <800/mm³

   b. Cell-mediated immunity—tested by administering common skin test antigens and measuring reactions:

      Normal = Ability to react to one or more antigens

6. Nitrogen balance study—24-hour urine collection to monitor nitrogen losses
   a. Nitrogen balance = Nitrogen intake minus total urinary nitrogen minus insensible losses minus gastrointestinal losses
   b. Positive balance is indicative of an anabolic state
   c. Negative balance is indicative of a catabolic state

      Mild = −5 to −10 g/day
      Moderate = −10 to −15 g/day
      Severe = >−15 g/day

7. Determination of caloric needs
   a. Estimation of total caloric needs:
      1) Estimation of basal energy expenditure (BEE) is most frequently calculated by using Harris-Benedict equation
         FEMALE: BEE = 655 + (9.56 × W) + (1.85 × H) − (4.7 × A)
         MALE: BEE = 66 + (13.75 × W) + (5.00 × H) − (6.75 × A)
         (W = Weight in kg; H = Height in cm; A = Age in years)

      2) Estimation of activity factor and injury factor:[30]

         Activity factor: Confined to bed = 1.2
         Ambulatory = 1.3
         Injury factor:

Surgery		**Trauma**	
Minor = 1.1		Skeletal = 1.35	
Major = 1.2		Head = 1.6	
		Blunt = 1.35	
Infection		**Burns**	
Mild = 1.2		40% = 1.5	
Moderate = 1.4		100% = 1.95	
Severe = 1.8			

      3) Estimation of total caloric needs:
         BEE × Activity factor × Injury factor = Calorie needs for 24 hours
   b. Measured energy expenditure
      1) Indirect calorimetry (metabolic cart studies)—Calculated energy expenditure by measurement of oxygen consumed and CO_2 produced. Based on the assumption that oxygen consumed (V_{O_2}) and carbon dioxide produced (V_{CO_2}) represent intracellular metabolism.
      2) This method requires expensive, bulky equipment and trained operators and is currently not widely available. However, preliminary evidence points to the fact that there may actually be a significant cost *savings* with this method because of the associated lower caloric needs reported, compared to the Harris-Benedict equation, which is an estimate. Many clinicians believe indirect calorimetry will improve patient care and become more widely used in the next decade.

8. Determination of protein needs
   a. Calculated on ideal body weight
   b. Estimated protein needs:

      Healthy adult = 0.8 g/kg/day
      Moderate stress = 1.5 g/kg/day
      Severe stress = 1.5 to 2.5 g/kg/day
      Peritoneal/hemodialysis = 1.2 to 2.5 g/kg/day
      Burns = 1.5 to 3.0 g/kg/day

   c. Factors to consider
      1) Visceral protein status—reflects internal organ mass (see Table 7-1)
      2) Protein losses—drains, wounds, diarrhea, or fistulas
      3) Disease status—hepatic and renal function
      4 Urinary nitrogen losses

Table 7-1 Visceral Proteins

Name	Normal range Half-life	Function	Notes	Significance of abnormalities
Serum albumin	>3.5g/dL 20 days	Maintains plasma oncotic pressure Carrier protein	Long half-life does not reflect acute protein status changes Values affected by hydration status	Mild depletion 3.0 to 3.5 g/dL Moderate depletion 2.4 to 2.9 g/dL Severe depletion <2.4 g/dL
Serum transferrin	>200 mg/dL 8 to 10 days	Carrier protein for iron	Shorter half-life more sensitive indicator of protein status	Mild depletion 150 to 200 mg/dL Moderate depletion 100 to 150 mg/dL Severe depletion <100 mg/dL
Prealbumin	20 mg/dL 2 to 3 days	Carrier protein for retinol-binding protein	Very sensitive to acute changes in protein status	Mild depletion 10 to 15 mg/dL Moderate depletion 5 to 10 mg/dL Severe depletion <5 mg/dL
Retinol-binding protein	3 to 5 mEq/dL 10 to 18 hours	Carrier protein for retinol	Extremely sensitive to acute changes in protein synthesis	

should be consulted early in the clinical course. The registered dietitian on the team is equipped with the education and experience necessary to conduct a comprehensive nutritional assessment and collaborate with the physician on disease-specific enteral and parenteral formulas. The registered nurse offers input concerning gut function and fluid and electrolyte status and monitors the patient's tolerance of nutritional support. Important components of a comprehensive nutritional assessment are described in the accompanying box.[34]

Methods of metabolic support: enteral vs. parenteral

Deciding on the proper route is a complex process and requires careful collaboration between the nurse, physician, dietitian, and pharmacist. The decision tree in Fig. 7-3 may be used as a tool to assist with this process. For the critically ill, hypermetabolic patient, metabolic support should be initiated at the earliest possible opportunity.

Enteral Route

Advantages. The use of the enteral route for metabolic support has received renewed interest because it is simpler, safer, and cheaper.[35,36] Also, nutrients delivered through the enteral route are used more efficiently by the body and serve to maintain structural and functional integrity of the bowel.[37]

Several investigators[31,38-41] have concluded that enteral nutrition has a role in preserving the gut mucosal barrier and preventing translocation of bacteria, thus ultimately decreasing sepsis and enhancing the immune response. This phenomenon is discussed comprehensively in Chapter 9.

In addition, Barracos et al[42] found that enteral feedings eliminate problems of biliary sludge and cholestasis in many patients. The enteral route also provides improved nitrogen retention when compared to identical solutions given intravenously,[43,44] and enteral feedings can successfully prevent stress ulcerations without adding other stress prophylaxis therapies.[45,46] One group of investigators[47] even

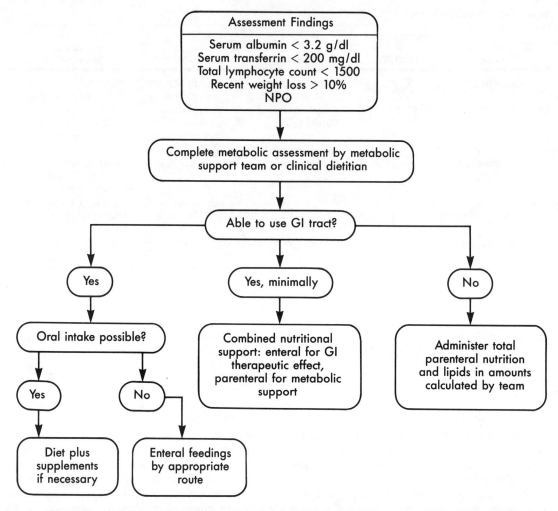

Fig. 7-3 Decision tree for enteral and parenteral nutrition. Decision tree to assist in determining the appropriate route of metabolic support for a particular patient. *GI,* Gastrointestinal.

demonstrated improved survival rates in an animal burn model when one group received early enteral feedings vs. total parenteral nutrition in the other group, although extrapolation of these conclusions to human populations is controversial.[48]

Complications. Even though there are many potential benefits, the use of the enteral route in the critically ill population has been hampered by the problems of ileus, diarrhea, obstruction of feeding tubes, and aspiration pneumonia.

Ileus. The gut is often overlooked as a route for providing early metabolic support because of the inherent problem of ileus associated with critical illnesses. However, several studies[49-51] indicate that most of the atony occurs in the stomach and colon and that the small bowel is resistant to the development of ileus. Small intestinal motility usually returns within the first 24 hours following an insult.[50,51] Cerra et al[49] also found that even when an ileus is present, nutrient absorption occurs in the small bowel without increasing the rate of diarrhea. Therefore feeding tubes placed distal to the pylorus into the duodenum or jejunum can be successfully used for early enteral metabolic support. These tubes may be placed either surgically, fluoroscopically, or endoscopically or passed at the bedside with the position confirmed by radiography.

Diarrhea. Several studies have shown that the most frequent complication of enteral feedings is diarrhea.[52,53] Although there is no standard definition of diarrhea, many researchers have investigated the problem. Flynn, Norton, and Fisher[52] found that 60% of studied patients experienced diarrhea for an average 2.6 days. This finding does not surprise any nurse who has cared for patients receiving enteral feedings. Diarrhea causes great concern for critical care practitioners because it can initiate multiple complications, many of which may be life-threatening to critically ill patients.[53] Complications of diarrhea include dehydration, electrolyte imbalances, skin breakdown, and, ultimately, sepsis. Severe diarrhea may cause fluid losses of 5 to 10 L/day,[54] and losses of this magnitude exacerbate poor perfusion of vital organs and maintenance of blood pressure.[55]

Recognizing that diarrhea may be a major problem with enteral feedings, nurse researchers have studied many of the possible contributing factors. Two researchers have studied the effects of formula temperature on the incidence of diarrhea. When Williams and Walike[56] compared delivery of cold, room-temperature, and warm enteral formulas in rhesus monkey models, they found that temperature variations in the formula caused only brief and inconclusive effects on gastric motility. They concluded that the temperature of the formula does not contribute to diarrhea.

Kagawa-Busby et al[57] used human subjects to investigate differences in cold, room-temperature, and warm enteral formulas and development of diarrhea. Their results again showed no significant difference between the temperature of enteral feedings and gastric motility and diarrhea.

The implication for practice from these findings is that temperature of the enteral formula is not a significant factor in the incidence of diarrhea. Some[53] have suggested that feedings may be refrigerated after opening and administered without rewarming the formula. This practice has the advantage of being potentially time-saving for the nurse and thus cost-effective for the hospital.

Heitkemper et al[58,59] studied the effects of formula rate and volume on gastrointestinal symptoms in their human subjects. They studied bolus feeding and found that the rate of formula delivery had little effect on mean gastric motility or return time of motility. Therefore when delivering bolus tube feedings, moderate rates such as 60 mL/min are recommended to decrease the subjective feelings of discomfort.[53] Others have suggested that when delivering continuous tube feedings, the rate should be increased slowly, followed by an increased concentration of formula over 4 to 7 days.[60,61]

Researchers have studied the incidence of diarrhea with intermittent vs. continuous administration of enteral formulas, and they report conflicting results. Hiebert et al[62] compared continuous and intermittent feedings in adult burn patients. They found significantly fewer stools and subjective complaints of abdominal discomfort with continuous tube feedings. They also found that the time required to reach calculated nutritional goals was significantly reduced in the continuously fed group. This study supports the current practice of delivering enteral formulas by continuous drip.

Keohane et al[63] investigated the relationship between osmolality of enteral feeding and gastrointestinal side effects. In the investigation, 118 subjects were given either hypertonic, isotonic, or hypotonic formula by continuous nasogastric infusion. Results showed that diarrhea is not related to the administration of full-strength hypertonic enteral feedings. The investigators further concluded that using diluted formula as a starter or using isotonic formulas decreased nutrient intake and nitrogen balance and did not reduce diarrhea. This conclusion remains controversial and is an area of continued research.

Bacterial contamination of enteral products and/or delivery sets as a cause of diarrhea also has been studied.[64-66] Implications for practice from these studies show that containers and tubing should be changed on a daily basis to avoid bacterial contamination.[67]

Tube obstruction. A major advance in enteral metabolic support was the advent of the small-bone, pliable, weighted feeding tube. These small tubes are much more comfortable for the patient, and their weighted ends facilitate passage into the small bowel. One of the disadvantages of using these tubes is that they often become occluded.

Replacement leads to increased costs related to additional nursing and physician time, exposure to radiation for position confirmation, and trauma for the patient. Marcuard and Perkins[68] studied frequently used major formulas to see if the type of formula used contributed to obstruction of the feeding tubes. Obstruction was observed in all tubes in which intact protein formulas were being delivered. The formula that caused the most obstruction was Pulmocare, followed by Ensure Plus and Osmolite. Diluting these formulas to half-strength helped decrease obstruction. The researchers concluded that the acidity of the stomach contents led to precipitation of certain proteins and was an important factor in tube obstruction. They offered the following suggestions to prevent obstruction of feeding tubes:

1. Flush the feeding tube before and after aspirating for gastric residuals to eliminate acid precipitation of formula in the feeding tube.
2. Advance the feeding tube into the duodenum (pH in the duodenum is higher and less likely to cause precipitation).
3. Avoid mixing enteral products with liquid medications having a pH value of 5.0 or less.[68]

Nurses have tried many innovative, creative methods to unclog feeding tubes. Meat tenderizer, warm coffee, cola products, and cranberry juice are a few of those frequently mentioned. The use of these methods has come under scrutiny, particularly the use of meat tenderizer, since it has been associated with significant complications such as electrolyte imbalances. Metheny, Eisenberg, and McSweeney[69] studied the effectiveness of three irrigant fluids (cranberry juice, cola, and water) in preventing tube obstruction. Their results demonstrated that water and cola were consistently superior to cranberry juice as irrigating fluids, with no difference between water and cola noted. They also investigated tube material and found that polyurethane tubes were consistently superior to silicone tubes in preventing tube obstructions. Finally, they found that tube diameter had no effect on the incidence of obstruction.

Treating feeding tube obstructions with activated pancreatic enzyme has been identified as a successful method when water fails to clear the obstructions. Marcuard and Stegall[70] found that injecting activated pancreatic enzyme into the obstructed feeding tube was 96% successful in

clearing the obstruction when formula clotting was identified as the cause of the obstruction.

Aspiration. Aspiration pneumonia is a potentially fatal complication of enteral feeding, and much of patient care focuses on its prevention. One group of researchers found that the incidence of aspiration in patients fed with nasogastric tubes was five times greater than those fed with nasointestinal tubes.[71] Tubes can also be placed accidentally in the lung or become dislodged from the stomach by coughing, vomiting, and movement. Traditionally, correct position of the nasoenteral tube is initially confirmed by radiograph (an extremely accurate method). However, follow-up confirmation on an intermittent basis is usually accomplished by aspirating stomach or intestinal contents or by auscultating for noise while insufflating bursts of air through the tube. Both of these methods may be very deceiving and lead to false assurances of tube position.[72] Recognizing this, Metheny et al[73] studied the effectiveness of pH readings in differentiating between gastric and intestinal placement. They also found that it was possible to aspirate enough fluid for pH testing in more than 90% of both nasogastric and nasointestinal tubes. They found that in cases when they were unable to obtain enough fluid to test for pH, insufflation of small bursts of air through the tubes facilitated aspiration of fluid through the syringe, reportedly by forcing the ports away from the mucosa. Tubes in the stomach had aspirate pH values ranging from 1 to 4, and those in the small bowel had values of 6 or greater. Tubes that had inadvertently been placed in the lung had aspirates with alkaline pH.[73] This method of tube position confirmation seems to hold promise and deserves further study; it may prove to be an acceptable nursing practice.

Metheny et al[71] studied the incidence of aspiration pneumonia in tube-fed patients and found that 5.7% of the group studied demonstrated pulmonary aspiration directly related to the tube feedings. Most of those who aspirated had their feeding tubes in the stomach rather than in the small bowel. It is also interesting that 83% of the group that aspirated had the head of the bed lowered at some point near the aspiration event. Two researchers have also investigated the practice of elevating the head of the patient's bed to protect the patient from aspiration pneumonia. Both concluded that although this practice is recommended, it is not consistently practiced in the clinical setting.[52,71] This inconsistency may contribute to the incidence of aspiration pneumonia.

Flynn, Norton, and Fisher[52] also investigated practices associated with enteral tube feedings in the acutely ill population and found that only 15% of the study group had a nutritional assessment completed before or during the period they were being fed. They reported that most of the patients were being fed in hypocaloric concentrations when they calculated the patients' caloric needs. They also found that a standard protocol was not used in most of these patients. This again demonstrates the need for consultation with a nutrition support team to calculate a specific patient's calorie needs and to provide guidance for developing standard protocols.

Formulas. A wide variety of enteral formulas is available on the market, including many organ- and disease-specific formulas. Research examining the efficacy of these formulas is ongoing and is promising. Development and refinement of these formulas are constantly changing; therefore selecting the proper formula is a very complicated process that involves many variables. A report by Eisenberg[74] offers an excellent review of indications, formulas, and delivery techniques, as well as a sample protocol. It is strongly recommended that collaboration with a clinical dietitian or metabolic support team occurs when selecting the appropriate formula for a specific patient with organ failure.

Parenteral route

The enteral route is not always appropriate or available for use because of problems with bowel obstruction or the need for bowel rest. When this occurs, the parenteral route is indicated for metabolic support.

Advantages. The use of the parenteral route to deliver total parenteral nutrition (TPN) has improved drastically over the past 15 years. The ability to precisely deliver a prescribed daily intake of calories, carbohydrates, fat, protein, vitamins, and minerals is very desirable in the critically ill patient. In addition, with TPN, the clinician has the ability to infuse high osmolar solutions and therefore minimize the volume while optimizing rapid caloric delivery.

Complications. The complications associated with using TPN are often related to technical problems with the vascular access—pneumothorax, arterial laceration, venous thrombosis, air embolism,

and cardiac dysrhythmias. Other complications and the nursing measures aimed at their identification and prevention—such as fluid overload, electrolyte imbalances, hyperglycemia, and septic complications—are discussed extensively in the literature and will not be reviewed here.

In the beginning, metabolic support through TPN was accomplished primarily with glucose-based solutions. This type of support produced many detrimental effects, including increased resting energy expenditure, increased CO_2 production, elevated RQ with resulting increased ventilatory demand, fatty liver syndrome, hyperglycemia, hyperosmolar states, increased body fat mass, stimulation of catecholamine release, elevated lactate formation, bowel distention, and increased gas production.* These problems have been attributed to delivering excess calories or excess glucose calories.

Investigators have reported that when more than 5 mg/kg/min of glucose is infused, only 50% to 70% of the glucose is directly oxidized for energy.[77] Others have reported that glucose in excess of 7 mg/kg/min is metabolized to fat and leads to fatty infiltrates of the liver and derangement of hepatic enzymes.[78] Duncan, Bistrian, and Blackburn[2] also reported that the body can oxidize infused glucose up to 4 to 5 mg/kg/min (400 to 500 g of glucose/day for a 70-kg adult). Excess infused glucose is converted to fat. The lipogenesis from glucose produces large quantities of water and CO_2. This may exacerbate pulmonary dysfunction, so limitation of excessive glucose administration is recommended.[2]

To prevent the described problems of overfeeding, it is extremely important to deliver only the number of calories needed by the individual patient. This goal may be accomplished by calculating the patient's needs based on the techniques discussed under "Assessment of Metabolic Requirements."

One solution to delivering too many glucose calories is to meet calorie needs by supplementing with intravenous fat emulsions. These fat emulsions are produced from soybean and/or safflower oil. The solutions not only serve to prevent essential fatty acid deficiency but also may be used as a calorie source. Animal studies with septic models show better preservation of lung architecture, surfactant composition, and pulmonary function with

---

*References 8, 24, 31, 75, and 76.

the use of fat emulsions.[8] In addition, Nordenstrom et al[79,80] and Askanazi et al[81] compared the effects of TPN delivered as a "glucose system" (all nonprotein calories supplied as carbohydrates) vs. a "lipid system" (nonprotein calories supplied as equal amounts of glucose and fat). All patients were given equal amounts of protein. The investigators compared nitrogen balance studies in the two groups and found no difference between them, but they did demonstrate that the "lipid system" group had a lower metabolic response and lower levels of norepinephrine excretion.[79-81]

Cerra[8] concluded that standard TPN with caloric loads greater than 50 kcal/kg caused increased organ failure resulting from increased CO_2 production, increased minute ventilation, ventilatory failure, hepatic steatosis, suboptimal nitrogen retention, hyperglycemia with hyperosmolar problems, and elevations in resting energy expenditure.

From these findings it is recommended that TPN be delivered as a mixed substrate solution of carbohydrate, fats, and protein in the form of amino acids. However, it is also recommended that no more than 30% to 40% of nonprotein calories be delivered as fat calories.[82] It is very important to monitor lipid clearance by way of serum triglyceride levels when providing calories in this manner. Overfeeding fat sources may block reticuloendothelial activity and thus impair overall immune function, but this theory is controversial.[2] In organ failure, determining the exact mix of the three major substrates depends on the individual patient's needs and the specific organs involved. Research and improved TPN usage in organ failure is ongoing, and consultation with a metabolic support team or clinical dietitian is critical when choosing care for an individual patient with organ failure. An excellent review of composition and administration of formulas, vascular access, and care of the patient with TPN has been reported by Worthington and Wagner.[83]

Disease- and organ-specific formulas. Areas of ongoing research in TPN delivery to patients with organ failure include the following:

Hepatic failure. Some researchers suggest that, with fulminant hepatic failure, TPN solutions should contain only the branched-chain amino acids and decreased aromatic amino acids. They propose that this will help reduce endogenous protein breakdown without increasing encephalopathy because the aromatic amino acids have been iden-

tified as the culprits in contributing to encephalopathy.[84,85] Fischer[86] and Freund et al[87] found that branched-chain solutions given to patients with hepatic encephalopathy were well tolerated and caused no worsening of the hepatic encephalopathy. However, these formulas are very expensive, and their efficacy is questioned by many practitioners; more research is indicated.

Renal failure. Studies indicate the mortality rate in acute renal failure may be decreased if nutritional status is maintained,[88] but careful manipulation of fluid, electrolytes, and proteins is required. Specialized formulas for renal failure include Aminosyn-RF, Nephramine, and RenAmin. Aminosyn-RF has only essential amino acids plus arginine. Nephramine contains only essential amino acids. RenAmin contains more nonessential amino acids. For renal failure patients not on dialysis, 250 mL of these solutions may be mixed with 500 mL of 70% dextrose and administered in volumes equal to 1 L/day. Patients on dialysis may tolerate rates of 2 to 2.5 L/day.[89] There are also reports of using continuous arteriovenous hemofiltration in conjunction with metabolic support. In this case, aggressive metabolic support may be done without worry of protein and fluid loads adversely affecting BUN and creatinine levels.[90]

Cardiopulmonary failure. Adequate metabolic support is essential to maintain adequate cardiopulmonary function, maintain host defenses against pulmonary infections, and provide energy to recover from ventilatory failure. As described earlier, calories from carbohydrates must be limited and calorie needs met through an appropriate mix of carbohydrates and fats.[89,90]

Monitoring of metabolic support

Table 7-2 indicates recommendations for monitoring parenteral and enteral nutrition. Specific timeframes and components monitored vary from institution to institution.

INVESTIGATIONAL THERAPIES
Growth hormone

While studying the effects of growth hormone on metabolic support, Manson, Smith, and Wilmore[91] found that growth hormone favored nitrogen retention and protein synthesis when a hypocaloric parenteral glucose solution was given. Another study demonstrated improved nitrogen retention when growth hormone was given with

Table 7-2 Monitoring for Parenteral and Enteral Nutrition

Parameter	Parenteral nutrition	Enteral nutrition
Weight	Daily	Daily
Intake and output	Every shift	Every shift
Electrolytes	Daily	Daily until stable, then as indicated
CBC	First day, then Mondays and Thursdays	First day, then Mondays and Thursdays
Nitrogen balance	Weekly	Weekly
Nutritional assessment	Weekly	Weekly
Fingerstick glucose monitoring	q4-6h (or more if unstable)	q4-6h until stable, then daily
Urine glucose and acetone	q6h	q6h
Tube position	n/a	q4h
Transferrin	Weekly	Weekly
SMA12	First day, then Mondays and Thursdays	First day, then Mondays and Thursdays
Magnesium	Weekly	Weekly
Vitamin levels	As indicated by metabolic support team	As indicated by metabolic support team

TPN.[92] Promising research is ongoing in the area of combining growth hormone with metabolic support.

Glutamine

The major amino acid in the plasma and cells is glutamine. The kidneys and small intestine are the major organs that use glutamine. Patients receiving TPN with glutamine demonstrated a significantly lower loss of nitrogen than did control patients.[93] Souba[94] demonstrated that animals fed glutamine-supplemented diets had a significantly lower incidence of bacterial translocation of the gut and speculated that glutamine may support intestinal metabolism, structure, and function.

Other areas of research

Research is ongoing to determine more precisely the caloric needs and ideal substrate mix for the MSOF patient. Indirect calorimetry provides vital information in this area. Research is also promising in the area of combined enteral and parenteral nutrition for the patient whose gut cannot support the entire nutritional requirement but for whom the therapeutic effect of gut stimulation is advantageous.

CONCLUSION

The metabolic alterations and ultimate metabolic failure seen in patients with multisystem organ failure are not yet clearly defined. The hypermetabolic state is a compensatory mechanism initially triggered to help meet short-term increased energy needs. In the MSOF syndrome, continued hypermetabolism places tremendous demands on the skeletal muscle mass, the liver, and other organs. Whether this overwhelming demand is the *cause* of progressive organ failure or whether the ongoing hypermetabolic response is the *result* of other mechanisms triggered by failing organs remains to be elucidated. Clearly, no matter what the cause-and-effect relationship that nutrition and metabolism play, aggressive metabolic support is a *vital* adjunctive tool in the arsenal of treatment modalities currently available for patients suffering from or at risk for MSOF.

REFERENCES

1. Lekander BJ, Cerra FB. The syndrome of multiple organ failure. Crit Care Nurs Clin North Am 1990;2:331-342.
2. Duncan JL, Bistrian BR, Blackburn GL. Septic stress: Nutritional management of the patient. Consultant 1982; 22:235-247.
3. Pomposelli JJ, Flores EA, Bistrian BR. Role of biochemical mediators in clinical nutrition and surgical metabolism. JPEN 1988;12:212-218.
4. Dinarello CA. Interleukin-1 and the pathogenesis of the acute phase response. N Engl J Med 1984;311:1413-1418.
5. Buckner MM. Perioperative nutrition problems: Nursing management. Crit Care Nurs Clin North Am 1990;2:559-566.
6. Leupold C. Critical care–stress, trauma, burns, and sepsis. In: Kennedy-Caldwell C, Guenter P, eds. Nutrition support nursing, core curriculum. 2nd ed. Silver Spring: ASPEN, 1988:413-453.

7. Cuthbertson DP. Post-shock metabolic response. Lancet 1942;1:433-437.

8. Cerra FB.Hypermetabolism, organ failure, and metabolic support. Surgery 1987;101:1-14.

9. Guyton AC. Textbook of Medical Physiology. 8th ed. Philadelphia: WB Saunders, 1991.

10. Johnson D. Metabolic and endocrine alterations in the multiply injured patient. Crit Care Nurs Q 1988;11(2):35-41.

11. Barton R, Cerra FB. The hypermetabolism multiple organ failure syndrome. Chest 1989;96:1153-1160.

12. Cerra FB. Hypermetabolism-organ failure syndrome: A metabolic response to injury. Crit Care Clin 1989;5(2):289-302.

13. Gutierrez G, Lund N, Bryan-Brown CW. Cellular oxygen utilitzation during multiple organ failure. Crit Care Clin 1989;5:271-287.

14. Barrocas A, Webb G, St. Romain C. Nutritional considerations in the critically ill. South Med J 1982;75:848-851.

15. Kovacerich D. Nutritional alterations in illness: Pulmonary. In: Kennedy-Caldwell C, Guenter P, eds. Nutrition support nursing core curriculum. 2nd ed. Silver Spring: ASPEN, 1988.

16. Kinney JM. Nutrition in the intensive care patient. Crit Care Clin 1987;3:1-10.

17. Wilmore DW et al. The gut: a central organ after surgical stress. Surgery 1988;104:917-923.

18. Heath DF, Stone HB. Studies on the metabolism of shock: Non-esterified fatty acid metabolism in normal and injured rats. Br J Exp Pathol 1968;49:168-169.

19. Babgy GJ et al. Lipoprotein lipase-suppressing mediator in serum of endotoxin-treated rats. Am J Physiol 1986; 251:E470-E476.

20. Cerra FB. Hypermetabolism-organ failure syndrome: A metabolic response to injury. Crit Care Clin 1989;5:289-302.

21. Cerra FB et al. Autocannibalism, a failure of exogenous nutritional support. Ann Surg 1980;192:570-574.

22. Lindholm M, Rossner S. Rate of elimination of the intralipid fat emulsion from the circulation in ICU patients. Crit Care Med 1983;10:740.

23. Lekander BJ, Cerra FB. The syndrome of multiple organ failure. Crit Care Nurs Clin North Am 1990;2(2):331-342.

24. Cerra FB. The syndrome of multiple organ failure. In: Cerra FB, Bihari D, eds. New Horizon Series: Cell injury and organ failure. Fullerton: Society of Critical Care Medicine, 1988.

25. Hill GL et al. Malnutrition in surgical patients: An unrecognized problem. Lancet 1977;1(8013):689-692.

26. Woolfson AMJ. Artificial nutrition in the hospital. Br Med J 1983;287:1004-1006.

27. Dempsey DT, Mullen JL, Buzby GP. The link between nutritional status and clinical outcome: Can nutritional intervention modify it? Am J Clin Nutr 1988;47:352-356.

28. Law DK, Dudrick SJ, Abdou NI. The effects of protein-calorie malnutrition on immune competence of the surgical patient. Surg Gynecol Obstet 1974;139:257-266.

29. Stoddart JC. Multiorgan failure and its management in the intensive therapy unit. Br Med Bull 1988;44:475-498.

30. Kuhn MM. Nutritional support for the shock patient. Crit Care Nurs Clin North Am 1990;2:201-220.

31. Cerra FB. The hypermetabolism organ failure complex. World J Surg 1987;11:173-181.

32. Littleton MT. Pathophysiology and assessment of sepsis and septic shock. Crit Care Nurs Q 1988;11(1):30-47.

33. Champagne MT, Ashley ML. Nutritional support in the critically ill elderly patient. Crit Care Nurs Q 1989;12(1):15-25.

34. Curtis S. Nutritional assessment. In: Kennedy-Caldwell C, Guenter P, eds. Nutrition Support Nursing Core Curriculum. 2nd ed. Silver Spring: ASPEN, 1988:29-42.

35. Silk DBA. Enteral nutrition. Postgrad Med J 1984;60:779-790.

36. Cataldi-Betcher E et al. Complications occurring during enteral nutrition support: A prospective study. JPEN 1983; 7:546-552.

37. Levine GM et al. Role of oral intake in maintenance of gut mass and disaccharide activity. Gastroenterology 1974;67:975.

38. Andrassy RJ. Practical rewards of enteral feeding for the surgical patient. Contemp Surg 1989;35(5-A):20-23.

39. Kever AJH et al. Prevention and colonization of infection in critically ill patients: A prospective, randomized study. Crit Care Med 1988;16:1087-1094.

40. Kripke SA et al. Stimulation of mucosal growth with intracolonic butyrate infusion. Surg Forum 1987;38:47-49.

41. Alverdy JC. The GI tract as an immunologic organ. Contemp Surg 1989;35(5-A):14-19.

42. Barracos V, Rodemann HP, Dinarello C. Stimulation of muscle protein degradation on PGE2 release by leukocyte pyrogen. N Engl J Med 1983;308:553-558.

43. Allardyce DB, Groves AC. A comparison of nutritional gains resulting from intravenous and enteral feedings. Surg Gynecol Obstet 1974;139:180-184.

44. Hindmarch JT, Clark RG. The effects in intravenous and intraduodenal feeding on nitrogen balance after surgery. Br J Surg 1973;60:589-594.

45. Pingleton SK, Harmon GS. Nutritional management in acute respiratory failure. JAMA 1987;257:3094-3099.

46. Saito H, Trock O, Alexander J. Comparison of immediate postburn enterval vs. parenteral nutrition. [Abstract]. ASPEN Clinical Congress 1985.

47. Cerra FB et al. Branched chain metabolic support. Ann Surg 1984;199:286-291.

48. Cerra FB et al. Enteral nutrition does not prevent multiple organ failure syndrome (MOFS) after sepsis. Surgery 1988;104:727-733.

49. Cerra FB et al. Enteral feeding in sepsis: A prospective, randomized, double-blind trial. Surgery 1985;98:632-639.

50. Rothnie NG, Harper RAK, Catchpole BN. Early postoperative gastrointestinal activity. Lancet 1963;2:64-67.

51. Wells C et al. Postoperative gastrointestinal motility. Lancet 1964;1:4-10.

52. Flynn KT, Norton LC, Fisher RL. Enteral tube feeding: Indications, practices and outcomes. Image 1987;19(1):16-19.

53. Zimmaro DM. Diarrhea associated with enteral nutrition. Focus Crit Care 1986;13(5):58-63.

54. Groer M, Shekleton M. Basic pathology: A conceptual Approach. St Louis: Mosby–Year Book, 1979.

55. Walike BC et al. Patient problems related to tube feeding. Commun Nurs Res 1975;7:89-112.

56. Williams KR, Walike BC. Effect of the temperature of tube feeding on gastric motility in monkeys. Nurs Res 1975;24:4-9.

57. Kagawa-Busby K et al. Effects of diet temperature on tolerance of enteral feedings. Nurs Res 1980;29:276-280.

58. Heitkemper M, Hanson R, Hansen B. Effects of rate and volume of tube feeding in normal human subjects. Commun Nurs Res 1977;10:71-89.

59. Heitkemper M et al. Rate and volume of intermittent enteral feeding. JPEN 1981;5:125-129.

60. Hersh R, Rudman D. Nasogastric hyperalimentation through a polyethylene catheter. Am J Clin Nutr 1979; 32:1112-1120.

61. Hoover HC, Ryan JA, Anderson EJ, Fischer JE. Nutritional benefits of immediate post-operative jejunal feeding of an elemental diet. Am J Surg 1980;139:153-159.

62. Hiebert J, Brown A, Anderson RG, Halfacre S, Rodeheaver G, Edlich R. Comparison of continuous vs. intermittent tube feedings in adult burn patients. JPEN 1981;5:73-75.

63. Keohane PP et al. Relation between osmolality of diet and gastrointestinal side effects in enteral nutrition. Br Med J 1984;288:678-680.

64. Hosteller C et al. Bacterial safety of reconstituted continuous drip tube feeding. JPEN 1982;6:232-235.

65. Scheimer RL et al. Environmental contamination of continuous drip feedings. Pediatrics 1979;63:232-237.

66. Schroeder P et al. Microbial contamination of enteral feeding solutions in a community. JPEN 1983;7:364-367.

67. Koruda MJ, Guenter P. Enteral nutrition in the critically ill. Crit Care Clin 1987;3:133-153.

68. Marcuard SP, Perkins AM. Clogging of feeding tubes. JPEN 1988;12:403-405.

69. Metheny N, Eisenberg P, McSweeney M. Effect of feeding tube properties and three irrigants on clogging rates. Nurs Res 1988;37:165-169.

70. Marcuard S, Stegall K. Unclogging feeding tubes with pancreatic enzyme. JPEN 1990;14:198-200.

71. Metheny N, Eisenberg P, Spies M. Aspiration pneumonia in patients fed through nasoenteral tubes. Heart Lung 1986; 15:256-261.

72. Kohn CL, Keithley JK. Enteral nutrition: Potential complications and patient monitoring. Nurs Clin North Am 1989; 24:338-353.

73. Metheny N et al. Effectiveness of pH measurements in predicting feeding tube placement. Nurs Res 1989;38:280-285.

74. Eisenberg P. Enteral Nutrition: Indications, formulas, and delivery techniques. Nurs Clin North Am 1989;24:315-338.

75. Shaw JHF, Wolfe RR. Glucose and urea kinetics in patients with early and advanced gastrointestinal cancer: The response to glucose infusion, parenteral feeding, and surgical resection. Surgery 1987;101:181-191.

76. White RH et al. Hormonal and metabolic responses to glucose infusion in sepsis studies by the hyperglycemic clamp technique. JPEN 1987;11:345-353.

77. Wolfe BR, Allsop JR, Burke JF. Glucose metabolism in man: Response to intravenous glucose infusion. Metabolism 1979;28:210.

78. Sheldon GF, Peterson SC, Sanders R. Hepatic dysfunction during hyperalimentation. Arch Surg 1978;113:504-508.

79. Nordenstrom J, Jeevanandam J, Elwyn DH. Increasing glucose intake during total parenteral nutrition increases norepinephrine excretion in trauma and sepsis. Clin Physiol 1981;1:525-534.

80. Nordenstrom J et al. Nitrogen balance during total parenteral nutrition: Glucose vs. fat. Ann Surg 1983;197:27-33.

81. Askanazi J et al. Influence of total parenteral nutrition of fuel utilization in injury and sepsis. Ann Surg 1980;191:40-46.

82. Macho J, Luce J. Rational approach to management of multisystems organ failure. Crit Care Clinics 1989; 5:379-392.

83. Worthington PH, Wagner BA. Total parenteral nutrition. Nurs Clin North Am 1987;24:355-371.

84. Wahren J, Davis J, Desurmont P. Is intravenous administration of branched chain amino acids effective in the treatment of hepatic encephalopathy? A multicentre study. Hepatology 1983;3:294-304.

85. Millikan WJ, Henderson JM, Warren WD. Total parenteral nutrition with F080 in cirrhosis with subclinical encephalopathy. Ann Surg 1983;3:294-304.

86. Fischer JE. Portasystemic encephalopathy. In: Wright R et al, eds. Liver and biliary disease: Pathophysiology, diagnosis, management. Philadelphia: WB Saunders, 1979:973-1001.

87. Freund H et al. Infusion of branched-chain enriched amino acid solution in patients with hepatic encephalopathy. Ann Surg 1982;196:209-220.

88. Baek SM et al. The influence of parenteral nutrition on the course of acute renal failure. Surg Gynecol Obstet 1975;141:405-408.

89. Baue AE. Multiple organ failure: Patient care and prevention. St. Louis: Mosby–Year Book, 1990:390.

90. Bessey PQ. Nutritional support in critical illness. In: Deitch E, ed. Multiple organ failure: Pathophysiology and basic concepts of therapy. New York: Thieme Medical Publishers, 1990:126-149.

91. Manson JM, Smith RJ, Wilmore DW. Growth hormone stimulates protein synthesis during hypocaloric parenteral nutrition: Role of hormonal-substrate environment. Ann Surg 1988;208:143-149.

92. Ziegler TR et al. Metabolic effects of recombinant human growth hormone in patients receiving parenteral nutrition. Ann Surg 1988;208:6-16.

93. Hammarqvist F et al. Addition of glutamine to total parenteral nutrition after elective abdominal surgery spares free glutamine in muscle, counteracts the fall in muscle protein synthesis, and improves nitrogen balance. Ann Surg 1989;84:224-230.

94. Souba WW. The gut—a key metabolic organ following surgical stress. Contemp Surg 1989;35(5-A):5-13.

Organ Involvement and Clinical Presentation

As pathophysiologic changes continue, organ dysfunction occurs, often remote from the initial site of injury or inflammation. The organs do not fail in isolation but within the entire presentation of multisystem organ failure. Organ ischemia and damage further stimulate the overwhelming inflammatory/immune response and contribute to the failure of other organs. As each additional organ fails, morbidity and mortality escalate.

8 Hepatic Dysfunction and Kupffer Cell Activity

Jo-ell M. Lohrman

The liver plays an integral role in the MSOF syndrome. The liver, a vital organ performing more than 400 functions, affects virtually every other organ system in both its healthy and pathophysiologic states. Any alteration in liver function from sepsis or injury can greatly affect the overall immune response, since the liver contains approximately 85% of the reticuloendothelial system (RES) in the form of fixed macrophages.[1]

The liver plays an active role in the MSOF process much earlier than has been previously suggested. Liver involvement may be present even before clinical markers such as elevated liver enzymes or depressed RES activity are evident.[2] Many clinicians believe the stages of MSOF parallel liver dysfunction and failure.[3-6]

ANATOMY OF THE LIVER

The critical care nurse must have a basic understanding of liver anatomy to fully comprehend and integrate the liver's role in MSOF. The liver is located in the right upper quadrant (RUQ) of the abdomen. It is divided into two lobes, with the right lobe being larger than the left. The liver contains 50,000 to 100,000 lobules, the functional unit of the liver[7] (Fig. 8-1).

Blood supply

The liver receives a dual blood supply—from both the hepatic artery and the portal vein. The hepatic artery provides 30% of the blood supply and delivers oxygen-rich blood. The portal vein delivers the remaining 70% and contains nutrients as well as bacterial and particulate matter from the gastrointestinal system. Blood from both vessels enters the lobule sinusoids, where numerous exchanges of oxygen, nutrients, and foreign material

take place. The total blood flow from the hepatic artery and portal vein is about 1450 mL/min, or a little less than one third of the resting cardiac output.[7]

The blood leaves the liver lobule by way of the central vein. The central veins drain into the hepatic veins, which empty into the inferior vena cava. This completes the circuit of blood flow through the liver.

Portal circulation

The portal circulation terminates in the portal vein, which is responsible for draining the venous blood from the majority of the gastrointestinal tract. The splenic vein, coronary (gastric) vein, superior mesenteric vein, and inferior mesenteric vein drain venous blood from their respective organs within the gastrointestinal system into the portal vein (Fig. 8-2).

Cell types

The two main cell types located in each liver lobule are hepatocytes and Kupffer cells. The hepatocytes perform most of the liver's functions. Adjacent to the hepatocytes are the bile canaliculi, which are tiny bile ducts that drain bile produced by the hepatocytes. These connect to form the biliary radicles and right and left hepatic ducts. The Kupffer cells, as tissue macrophages of the reticuloendothelial system, phagocytize bacteria and other foreign matter delivered by the portal vein.

LIVER FUNCTION AND PHYSIOLOGY
Vascular function

The major functions of the liver are classified into three categories: vascular, metabolic, and secretory.[7,8] The vascular functions include blood

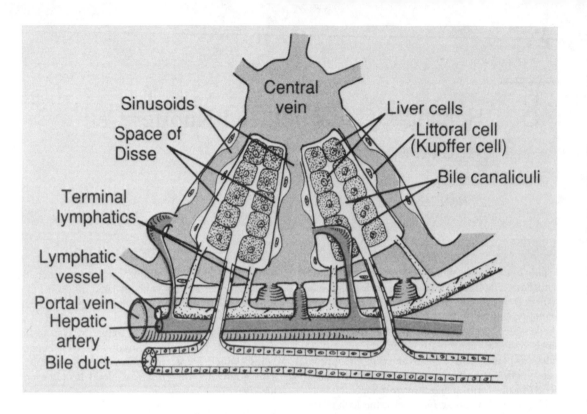

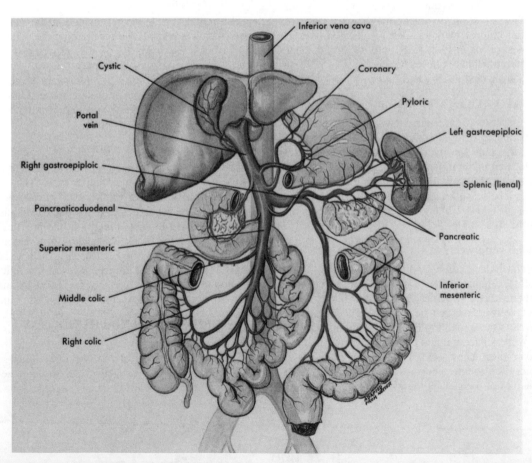

Fig. 8-1 Basic structure of a liver lobule displaying the dual blood supply, the cellular components (hepatocytes and Kupffer cells), and the bile-collecting system. (From Guyton AC. Textbook of medical physiology, 8th ed. Philadelphia: WB Saunders, 1991;772.)

Fig. 8-2 The portal circulation. (From Thibodeau GA, Anthony CP, eds. Structure and function of the body. 8th ed. St. Louis: Mosby–Year Book, 1988;268.)

storage, lymph formation, and filtration of foreign debris. In the normal physiologic state, the liver contains approximately 450 mL, or 10%, of the total blood volume; however, the liver is capable of expanding and storing 0.5 to 1.0 L of extra blood.[7] Thus the liver serves as a reservoir of blood and is capable of shunting excess blood into the systemic circulation when needed. This is a valuable reserve, especially in the setting of hypovolemic shock.[8]

More than one half of the body's total lymphatic fluid is formed in the liver. The liver sinusoids are very permeable and allow large quantities of fluid and protein to cross over into the space of Disse (space surrounding the hepatocytes) and drain into the lymphatic channels. Even slight increases in hepatic venous pressure can lead to increased movement of fluid into the space of Disse as well as through the outer surface of the liver capsule. This free fluid accumulation in the abdominal cavity is known as ascites.

The Kupffer cells filter foreign debris and particulate matter from the blood as the blood moves through the liver. The Kupffer cells have highly efficient phagocytic properties to remove bacteria and foreign matter received from the intestines through the portal vein. Under physiologic conditions, fewer than 1% of the bacteria in the portal circulation pass into the systemic circulation.[7]

Metabolic function

Carbohydrate metabolism. The liver coordinates much of the body's carbohydrate, lipid, and protein metabolism. In carbohydrate metabolism, the liver plays a crucial role in regulating normal serum glucose. This is achieved by the storage of simple sugars as glycogen (glycogenesis). This reserve of glycogen can be reconverted to glucose (glycogenolysis) when the serum glucose concentration falls. If the glycogen stores are depleted or carbohydrate intake is inadequate, the liver is ca-

pable of converting amino acids and fats into glucose (gluconeogenesis). All of these processes work together to maintain a normal serum glucose level.

Lipid metabolism. Lipid metabolism occurs in individual body cells; however, principal aspects of lipid metabolism take place primarily in the liver. The liver breaks down fat to provide another source of energy to meet body demands. In addition to fat catabolism, the liver converts excess carbohydrates and proteins into fat to be stored in the adipose tissue for later use.

The liver is also responsible for the synthesis of cholesterol and phospholipids. The majority of the cholesterol formed is converted into bile salts and subsequently secreted into the bile. The other portion of the cholesterol, and the phospholipids generated by the liver, are used elsewhere in the body for other cellular functions. The cholesterol and phospholipids are transported by circulating lipoproteins, which are also synthesized by the liver.

Protein metabolism. Although the liver plays an important role in carbohydrate and fat metabolism, its role in protein metabolism is the most crucial to host survival. Death is imminent in a few days without proper protein metabolism by the liver.[7] The three most important areas of protein metabolism performed by the liver are deamination of amino acids, ureagenesis, and plasma protein synthesis. Deamination of amino acids refers to the removal of an amino group (NH_2) so that the amino acids can be used as an energy source. Deamination is also necessary before the amino acids can be converted into fat or carbohydrates. It is important to mention that not only does deamination of amino acids occur, but the liver is also capable of synthesizing amino acids and forming other compounds from these amino acids.

Ureagenesis is the process whereby the liver converts ammonia to urea. Ammonia is formed as a by-product of deamination of amino acids and is

COMMON DRUGS METABOLIZED BY THE LIVER*

Antibiotic

Aztreonam (Azactam)
Cefoperazone (Cefobid)
Cefotaxime (Claforan)
Ceftriaxone (Rocephin)
Cephalothin (Keflin)
Chloramphenicol
Clindamycin (Cleocin)
Erythromycin
Isoniazid (INH)
Metronidazole (Flagyl)
Nafcillin (Nafcil)
Rifampin (Rifadin)
Co-trimoxazole (Bactrim or Septra)
Tetracycline (Sumycin)

Analgesic

Acetaminophen (Tylenol)
Meperidine (Demerol)
Methadone
Morphine
Pentazocine (Talwin)
Propoxyphene (Darvon)

Antiepileptic

Carbamazepine (Tegretol)
Phenobarbital (Luminal)
Phenytoin (Dilantin)
Valproic acid (Depakene)

Antipyretic/Antiinflammatory

Acetylsalicylic acid (aspirin)
Dexamethasone (Decadron)
Fenoprofen (Nalfon)
Ibuprofen (Motrin)
Indomethacin (Indocin)
Naproxen (Naprosyn)
Phenylbutazone (Butazolidin)
Prednisolone

Cardiovascular

Digitoxin
Digoxin (Lanoxin)
Disopyramide (Norpace)
Labetalol (Trandate or Normodyne)
Lidocaine
Methyldopa (Aldomet)
Metoprolol (Lopressor)
Nifedipine (Procardia)
Pindolol (Visken)
Prazosin (Minipress)
Procainamide (Pronestyl)
Propranolol (Inderal)
Quinidine
Tocainide (Tonocard)
Verapamil (Calan)

Diuretic

Furosemide (Lasix)
Spironolactone (Aldactone)
Triamterene/HCTZ (Dyazide)

Sedative/Hypnotic

Amobarbital (Amytal)
Chlordiazepoxide (Librium)
Diazepam (Valium)
Lorazepam (Ativan)
Midazolam (Versed)
Oxazepam (Serax)
Pentobarbital (Nembutal)
Primidone (Mysoline)
Temazepam (Restoril)

Others

Chlorpromazine (Thorazine)
Cimetidine (Tagamet)
Diphenhydramine (Benadryl)
Fentanyl (Sufenta)
Ranitidine (Zantac)
Theophylline (Theo-Dur)
Thiopental (Pentothal Sodium)
Tolbutamide (Orinase)
Warfarin (Coumadin)

*This list is not meant to be comprehensive. Modified from Arns PA, Wedlund PJ, Branch RA. Adjustment or medications in liver failure. In Chernow B. The pharmacologic approach to the critically ill patient. 2nd ed. Baltimore: Williams & Wilkins, 1988: 85-111.

also formed by bacteria in the gastrointestinal system. If ureagenesis is impaired, the serum ammonia level can rise, producing coma and ultimately death.[7,8]

The hepatocytes synthesize the majority of plasma proteins. There are three proteins of particular importance: albumin, fibrinogen, and globulins. Albumin is found within the vascular space and is responsible for maintaining the colloid oncotic pressure. Fibrinogen is crucial for blood coagulation. Globulins function as cellular enzymes and transporters of other proteins.

The liver is also responsible for the production of acute-phase reactants. These products are plasma proteins whose selective production increases in the setting of tissue injury or infection. The following are the major acute-phase reactants: C-reactive protein, fibrinogen, alpha$_1$-antitrypsin, transferrin, and alpha$_2$-macroglobulin.[1] C-reactive protein receives the most attention since it is paramount in cellular migration and activation of the complement system.

Miscellaneous functions. Besides the complex metabolic functions (carbohydrate, fat, and protein-metabolic) of the liver, there are equally important miscellaneous metabolic functions, including synthesis and removal of coagulation components; detoxification of drugs, hormones, and other circulating substances; and vitamin storage. The liver produces most of the clotting factors necessary for the coagulation cascade: fibrinogen, prothrombin (Factor II), Factors V, VII, VIII, IX, X, and accelerator globulin. The liver also removes many of these factors after they have been activated.

Detoxification of drugs, hormones, and other products further demonstrates the liver's diverse metabolic activities. The liver breaks down these substances for excretion into the bile or urine. Some of the drugs metabolized by the liver include diazepam, acetaminophen, quinidine sulfate, and Dilantin (see box on p. 146). In addition, the liver metabolizes and excretes numerous hormones such as estrogen, testosterone, aldosterone, cortisol, and thyroxine into the bile. The liver also assists in removing calcium through bile production and excretion in the stool.

Secretory function

Bile production. In addition to its vascular and metabolic functions, the liver serves a secretory function. There are two important secretory functions: bile production and bilirubin metabolism. The bile is produced by the hepatocytes and is composed of bile salts, bile pigments, and cholesterol. The liver produces cholesterol that is converted into bile salts, which are necessary for fat digestion in the intestines. After the bile is produced by the hepatocytes, it is drained through the bile canaliculi into the hepatic ducts. The bile then continues to the gallbladder, where it is concentrated and stored.

Bilirubin metabolism. Bilirubin forms as a byproduct of red blood cell destruction. When a red blood cell is destroyed, hemoglobin is released. After releasing its iron, the heme portion is converted to bilirubin, which combines with circulating albumin and is transported to the liver. This type of bilirubin is called free, indirect, or unconjugated. Once in the liver, the bilirubin is combined with other substances, forming conjugated or direct bilirubin. Conjugated bilirubin is excreted in the bile into the intestines. A small portion of conjugated bilirubin reenters the sinusoidal blood and is cleared by the kidneys and excreted in the urine.

Storage reservoir

The liver also plays a role as a storage reservoir for blood, glucose, fat, vitamins, and minerals. Vitamins stored include A, D, and B$_{12}$. A large percentage of total body iron is stored as ferritin and is released when the body supply is low.

The liver performs a wide range of functions that have a tremendous impact on total body function (see box on p. 148). Small derangements in liver functioning can sequentially alter the homeostatic milieu.

HYPERMETABOLISM, LIVER FUNCTION, AND THE PROGRESSION TO MSOF

When the patient experiences a primary insult such as severe inflammation, shock, tissue injury, or ischemia, the patient mounts a metabolic response. If this response continues unabated, the patient will enter a stage of extensive hypermetabolism. This is often heralded by the onset of pulmonary dysfunction and progression to ARDS.[3,9,10]

This period of hypermetabolism and increased body requirements affects the liver significantly. The liver's major role in normal metabolism places it in a key role in the development and progression of the hypermetabolic state. In order to meet the body's increasing demands, the liver increases the

FUNCTIONS OF THE LIVER

Vascular

Blood storage
Lymph formation
Blood filtration

Metabolic

Carbohydrate metabolism
 Regulation of serum glucose by
  glycogenesis
  glycogenolysis
  glyconeogenesis
Fat metabolism
 Fat catabolism
 Conversion of carbohydrates and proteins into
  fat for storage in the adipose tissue
 Synthesis of cholesterol and phospholipids
Protein metabolism
 Deamination of amino acids
 Ureagenesis
 Synthesis of plasma proteins
 Production of acute-phase reactants
Synthesis and removal of coagulation compo-
 nents
Detoxification of drugs, hormones, and calcium
Vitamin storage

Secretory

Bile production
Bilirubin metabolism

From Keith, JS. Hepatic failure: Etiologies, manifestations, and management. Crit Care Nurse 1985;5(1):60-86.

rate of gluconeogenesis with simultaneous increases in protein catabolism and ureagenesis.[11] The urinary excretion of nitrogen is subsequently increased. This process is not affected or inhibited by the exogenous administration of glucose substances. There is an increase in calories obtained from amino acids, accompanied by a decrease in calories obtained from glucose and fat. The amino acids that are used for energy are the branched-chain amino acids taken from the muscle. Moyer et al[12] have found that low levels or depletion of branched-chain amino acids affects liver function. They discovered that these low levels impair hepatic protein synthesis and actually produce liver dysfunction.

The stage of hypermetabolism may last a few days to 3 weeks. Either the patient's condition im-

proves or the patient deteriorates to the organ failure phase. This ongoing hypermetabolism represents a change from an enhanced metabolic regulation into a disorganized and unregulated phase that signifies the presence of the organ failure syndrome. This transition to MSOF is hallmarked by an increasing serum bilirubin and evidence of hepatic failure. As a preterminal event, metabolism may become blocked or completely fail.*

A close examination of the metabolic derangements occurring in the liver as the progression to organ failure occurs is important (Fig. 8-3). Increased glycogenolysis and gluconeogenesis continue, and an inability to convert lactate to glucose develops; thus lactate clearance decreases as failure progresses. Eventually, the liver is unable to maintain a baseline level of glucose, and hypoglycemia ensues.[15]

Lipid metabolism is altered because increased lipolysis and lipogenesis occur. Feingold and Grunfeld[16] discovered that tumor necrosis factor (TNF) released by the rat macrophage causes the hepatocyte to increase lipogenesis. In conjunction with this increased triglyceride production there is also decreased peripheral triglyceride clearance. Lipemic serum levels are evident. Initially, lipids are converted to ketones for energy; however, as the process continues, the hepatocyte cannot use the ketones as before.

The derangement in protein metabolism is significant. The liver's ability to extract or clear amino acids is decreased. Ureagenesis continues to increase, leading to elevated plasma urea levels, especially in the setting of renal failure. There are elevated levels of the aromatic amino acids (phenylalanine and tyrosine); however, there are decreased levels of the branched-chain amino acids.[17] Some clinicians have indicated that the accumulation of the aromatic acids is the culprit that causes hepatic encephalopathy.[18,19]

Hepatic protein synthesis is also reduced, specifically albumin and transferrin. This reduction in albumin affects the circulating volume, since albumin plays an important role in plasma oncotic pressure. It is interesting that exogenous administration of albumin is ineffective and does not improve the oncotic pressure. If albumin is administered, it is quickly broken down and catabolized.[1]

*References 3, 6, 9, 10, 13, and 14.

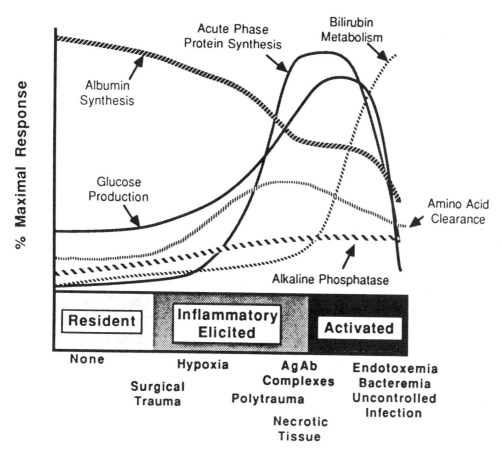

Fig. 8-3 Postulated hepatocellular dysfunction from early hypermetabolism to MSOF. (From Cerra FB. Hypermetabolism-organ failure syndrome: A metabolic response to injury. Crit Care Clin 1989;5:297.)

Keith[8] notes that there is an associated poor prognosis in liver failure when the albumin is less than 3.0 g/dL.

As a rule, protein synthesis is diminished; however, the production of acute-phase reactants is increased following an insult. This is thought to be in response to infection or tissue injury and necessary for survival.[13] Thus, as the process continues, there is progressive failure in the metabolic, immune, and synthetic properties of the liver. Cerra,[3] Clowes et al,[20] and Pearl et al[21] indicate the liver's inability to clear amino acids and synthesize proteins is a major determinant of mortality in MSOF.

As liver failure progresses, detoxification of drugs, toxins, and hormones diminishes. Judicious use of hepatotoxic drugs is paramount. Since reg-

ulation of hormones is affected, uncontrolled increases in aldosterone and antidiuretic hormone (ADH) contribute to complications, such as hepatorenal syndrome, development of ascites, and poor blood pressure regulation.

In addition to the metabolic derangements occurring in liver failure, the immune system continues to be burdened. Kupffer cells are unable to phagocytize bacteria properly. Fibronectin is partially synthesized by the liver under homeostatic conditions and is depleted during stress or infection. Its main role is to enhance phagocytosis. Without the presence of fibronectin, the bacteria are more mobile and difficult to phagocytize.[15]

The liver is affected by multiple factors as the body mounts a metabolic response to injury. This hypermetabolic response may continue unabated and uncontrolled and subsequently leads to MSOF. All facets of carbohydrate, lipid, and protein metabolism are deranged, and normal detoxification and immune functions are impaired. All these factors afflict an already overburdened system.

MECHANISM OF LIVER DAMAGE SUSTAINED IN THE MSOF PROCESS
Hypoperfusion

Differences in opinion exist among well-known clinicians concerning the mechanism of hepatic insufficiency and damage in MSOF. Baue[1] states that the liver's role in MSOF is related to changes that occur in sepsis, although the exact mechanism is not completely understood. During sepsis there is inadequate circulation to the liver, resulting in ischemia. As a result, the Kupffer cells and hepatocytes are incapable of optimal function. In addition, several mediators present during sepsis have been implicated in liver damage. These include superoxides, fibrinolysin, fibronectin depletion, elastase, lysosomal by-products, and permeability factors.[1] Another consideration in hypoperfusion is the decreased substrate delivery to the liver. Without the necessary carbohydrate, protein, and lipid, further alterations in metabolism occur. Thus Baue believes hepatic hypoperfusion is the major factor.

Although it is obvious that low-flow states such as shock and arrest situations could lead to hepatic ischemia and tissue damage, it is less clear why decreased flow has also been noted during hyperdynamic states. It has been suggested that following complement activation, neutrophils aggregate and release oxygen-derived free radicals and proteases. The ensuing vascular permeability, obstruction, and damage not only hinder flow but incite platelet activation and fibrin deposition. Activated platelets release thromboxane, which is a potent vasoconstrictor. The action of these inflammatory mediators along with vascular and tissue damage contributes to the development and progression of hepatic damage.[22,23]

Kupffer cell activity

Another popular theory of liver involvement in MSOF is related to macrophages and monokines. Keller et al[24,25] have noted that hepatic failure is not always precipitated by an episode of hypoperfusion. They believe hypoperfusion and associated

hypoxia cannot solely cause the liver damage observed in these patients. The liver dysfunction can result from a Kupffer cell–mediated response.*

The hypothesis states that the Kupffer cells are stimulated by endotoxin or other inflammatory mediators from the initial insult or secondary complications, such as shock and sepsis. The Kupffer cells then release toxic mediators, including TNF, interleukin-1 (IL-1), oxygen-derived free radicals, lysosomal enzymes, and arachidonic acid metabolites. Since the Kupffer cells and hepatocytes are in close proximity, these released mediators (specifically a monokine such as IL-1) act upon the hepatocytes, altering hepatocyte function but not causing cellular death (Fig. 8-4). The hepatocyte carries out many of the major functions of the liver, such as protein synthesis, metabolic activities, bilirubin conjugation, and detoxification. Therefore hepatocellular damage, whether a result of ischemia, hypoperfusion, or Kupffer cell activation and subsequent mediator release, leads to major alterations in liver function.

If the Kupffer cell–mediated response actually occurs, two important problems surface: the liver's ability to recover from the damage sustained and the liver's ability to synthesize the necessary proteins and substrates for recovery.[26] Both present major challenges that the body must overcome for survival.

Contributing factors

Not only is a perfusion deficit or ischemia implicated in hepatic damage, but persistent inflammatory foci such as injured or necrotic tissue may also contribute to hepatic dysfunction. Schirmer et al[33] and Seibel et al[34] noted that wounds associated with fractures release products that alter hepatocellular function.

The presence of preexisting fibrotic liver disease predisposes patients to hepatic involvement in MSOF and must be considered in their evaluation and treatment. These patients already suffer abnormalities in hepatocyte structure and function and are frequently malnourished. Thus any additional burden on an already compromised organ could hasten liver dysfunction and failure.

In summary, factors operating in both theories (hypoperfusion and the Kupffer cell response)

---

*References 3, 4, 14, and 24-32.

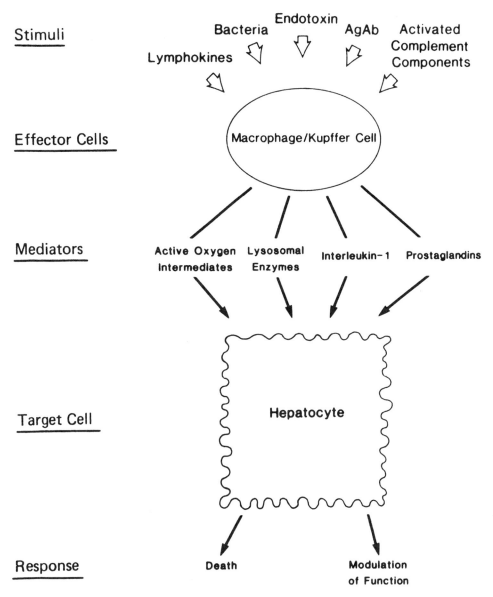

Fig. 8-4 The Kupffer cell–mediated alteration of hepatocyte function. (From Keller GA et al. Macrophage-mediated modulation of hepatic function in multiple-system failure. J Surg Res 1985;39:560.)

probably play a role in the development of liver failure in the MSOF setting, along with additional contributing factors. Hypoperfusion, microcirculatory changes, Kupffer cell activation, and direct mediator damage all have the potential to greatly affect hepatic oxygen uptake, energy use, and organ function.

CLINICAL PRESENTATION AND ASSESSMENT

It is obvious that during hypermetabolism liver involvement occurs before clinical markers appear. Usually hepatic dysfunction will be evident several days after the clinical picture of hypermetabolism and the hyperdynamic phase has occurred.[35] Clinicians do not agree on a specific set and range of laboratory values or clinical markers, but general values commonly used are listed in the box below.

The single clinical marker consistently mentioned is an elevated serum bilirubin. The elevation indicating liver dysfunction is variously described as greater than 2 or 3 mg/dL.[10,11] Other causes of hyperbilirubinemia must be ruled out, such as transfusion reaction, resorption of a large hematoma, or common bile duct blockage.

Theoretically, hyperbilirubinemia is caused by free or indirect bilirubin entering the hepatocyte and becoming conjugated. However, because of a possible hepatocellular excretory defect, intrahepatic cholestasis occurs. Conjugated or direct bilirubin is absorbed back into the vascular system, causing an elevation in the plasma. Therefore the elevation in the total bilirubin is usually reflective of an increase in the conjugated form.[35,36]

Elevated bilirubin levels are implicated as predictors of mortality. Sarfeh and Balint[36] state that on the fourth day the bilirubin levels are lower for survivors (1.6 mg/dL ± 0.3) than for patients who do not survive (3.6 mg/dL ± 0.6). Cerra et al[37] discovered that survivors have a bilirubin of 2.2 mg/dL ± 0.6, and patients who die as a result of MSOF and other forms of critical illness have a bilirubin of 8.5 mg/dL ± 2.2.

Hyperbilirubinemia must not be looked at in isolation, but in conjunction with other clinical markers. Fry[11] and Baue[1] both state the importance of obtaining hepatic enzyme levels to determine liver involvement. Fry specifically states that the serum glutamic-oxaloacetic transaminase (SGOT) and lactic dehydrogenase (LDH) must be double the normal value.

Walvatne and Cerra[35] have emphasized plasma phenylalanine levels to identify liver failure in conjunction with an elevated bilirubin. A level greater than 100 μmol/L is considered clinically significant. Phenylalanine is an amino acid that elevates in the plasma secondary to faulty liver metabolism. When the bilirubin is greater than 3.0 g/dL and the phenylalanine is greater than 100 μmol/L, the SGOT, SGPT, and alkaline phosphatase may only be slightly elevated or normal.[36] Thus there is a direct correlation between elevated phenylalanine, bilirubin elevation, degree of hepatic dysfunction, and mortality.[37-39]

The presence of jaundice is also considered significant, although no specific assessment guidelines are mentioned in the literature except that jaundice is seen with an elevated bilirubin as the patient moves into MSOF with liver involvement. The bilirubin must be at least 1.5 mg/dL (three times normal level) before jaundice appears in the skin,[7] although jaundice is not consistently seen until a level of 3.5 mg/dL. Therefore jaundice is often a late indicator of hepatic involvement.

Another clinical marker is hepatic encephalopathy. Elevated levels of certain amino acids, specifically phenylalanine and tyrosine, contribute to hepatic encephalopathy by altering cerebral neurotransmission.[17-19] This is difficult to evaluate in the critically ill patient because other variables are present that alter mental function. Sleep deprivation and medications commonly affect the assessment of cerebral function.

Liver involvement is present by the time the clinical markers appear. The excretory functions of the liver are characteristically affected before its synthetic functions. An early diagnostic marker of

---

CLINICAL MARKERS OF HEPATIC INVOLVEMENT IN MSOF

Elevated serum bilirubin (>2 or 3 mg/dL)
Elevated SGOT and LDH (double the normal
    value)
Elevated plasma phenylalanine levels
    (>100 μmol/L)
Decreased serum albumin
Decreased serum transferrin
Jaundice
Hepatic encephalopathy

hepatic dysfunction would be helpful and may involve injecting a substance into the bloodstream to be picked up by the hepatocytes and successfully excreted in the bile.[35] In the MSOF setting, the substance would not be excreted properly by the hepatocyte, indicating cellular dysfunction. To avoid misdiagnosis, ultrasound would be used to rule out extrahepatic biliary obstruction, which may have similar clinical findings.

IMPACT OF LIVER FAILURE ON THE MSOF PROCESS

The liver not only is damaged by the insult and MSOF process but in turn affects the progression of the syndrome. MSOF is not a series of isolated failures, but rather involves a constant interplay between the major organ systems. This interplay is one reason the process is so overwhelming and has an associated high mortality. As additional organs fail, mortality increases significantly.

The center of liver involvement rests with the Kupffer cells. Many of the circulating mediators in the MSOF process stimulate the Kupffer cells to produce toxic products. The products can directly enter the venous circulation and perpetuate the problem. The venous blood supply leaving the liver quickly enters the pulmonary circulation. These toxic products cause further damage to the pulmonary endothelium and continue to activate the pulmonary macrophages.[40,41]

As hepatic dysfunction continues, the normal clotting process is altered (Fig. 8-5). Simple bruising, obvious bleeding, and a prolonged prothrombin time are evident. The synthesis of clotting factors is decreased, as is the liver's ability to remove the clotting factors once activated. Patients with these symptoms are predisposed to the development of DIC.[15,17] This only compounds an already complicated and potentially fatal clinical course.

The liver also interacts closely with the gastrointestinal system. The liver receives blood supply from the portal circulation, which may contain bacteria translocated from the gut. Because the gastrointestinal tract is a reservoir of potentially damaging pathogens that may enter the portal circulation,[42] the gut continually puts the liver "to the test" to clear bacteria and other foreign matter.

Liver failure continues to compound the problem of MSOF treatment. It becomes a major impediment in the patient's recovery, since the normal ability to clear and detoxify metabolites is upset.

Without this ability, many general MSOF treatment methods are unsuccessful or contraindicated.

THERAPEUTIC MANAGEMENT
General therapy

In general, treatment for MSOF focuses on three main goals: source control, maintenance of oxygen transport, and nutritional support.[6,10,14,17] Whenever possible, the source of inflammation, ischemia, or infection must be removed. A persistent inflammatory focus guarantees a higher mortality.[6,10] Generic therapies to maximize oxygen delivery, such as fluid resuscitation, inotropes, and mechanical ventilation, are used. Oxygen consumption and serum lactate levels are evaluated to determine the effectiveness of these therapies. Nutritional support is paramount since malnutrition is clearly present in MSOF.[6,10] It is important to keep the whole picture in mind and not focus solely on treatment for an individual organ. This philosophy rests on two premises: (1) the complex interaction between organ systems is not completely understood, and (2) an individual treatment for one organ system may hinder other organ systems, thus perpetuating MSOF.[42]

Therapy for liver dysfunction

Tissue perfusion. Three areas specifically targeted for the patient suffering liver dysfunction in MSOF are adequate tissue perfusion, sufficient nutritional support, and judicious use of hepatotoxic, pharmacologic agents. Adequate tissue perfusion of the liver is essential to provide an environment where cell regeneration can occur. This may be assisted by administering low-dose dopamine to increase hepatic blood flow.[1,17] However, with inadequate fluid resuscitation or higher doses, dopamine will decrease hepatic and splanchnic perfusion. The use of dopamine must be examined in concert with other therapies to ensure a consistent and collective treatment plan.

Nutritional support. Nutritional support is the mainstay of hepatic support, and most of the literature focuses on its role. As previously discussed, the metabolism of carbohydrate, fat, and protein is altered in hepatic dysfunction. The goal of nutritional support is to avoid the administration of excess carbohydrates and fats and to provide amino acids for nitrogen balance.

Specialized nutritive sources may be helpful. The administration of branched-chain amino acids

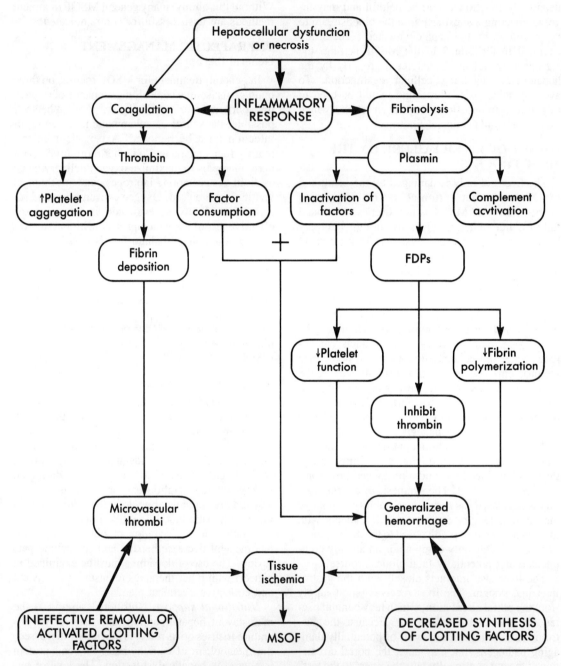

Fig. 8-5   The impact of liver dysfunction on the development and progression of DIC. Alterations occurring in hepatic damage are activation of the inflammatory response, ineffective removal of activated clotting factors, and decreased synthesis of clotting factors. Abbreviations: *FDP*, fibrin degradation products; *MSOF*, multisystem organ failure. (Modified from Huddleston VB. Multisystem organ failure: A pathophysiologic approach. Boston, 1991;16.)

(BCAA)—leucine, isoleucine, and valine—is one source.[1,35,43] The formulas available that are high in branched-chain amino acids and low in the aromatic amino acids (phenylalanine and tyrosine) include HepatAmine, FreAmine HBC, and Branchamine. These formulas supplement the low BCAA levels while simultaneously avoiding those aromatic amino acids that are already elevated and hepatotoxic.

The benefit of use of these formulas is threefold. They achieve nitrogen retention, support hepatic protein synthesis, and decrease ureagenesis.[10,14,35] Another attractive benefit is that their metabolism occurs in peripheral muscle and not in the liver. Thus they provide energy and nutrition without depending on normal liver metabolism.[1] At present, these benefits are theoretical, and no proven difference in outcome has been demonstrated among patients with MSOF.

This nutritional information is related to the patient's overall prognosis. Baue[1] states that as the patient enters the late stages of liver involvement in MSOF, even the initially low levels of BCAA

will rise. This suggests a poor availability of substrate for metabolism and carries a poor prognosis. Cerra et al[44] also documented a higher mortality in patients unable to maintain protein synthesis in response to exogenous amino acid administration.

Nutrition may also play a role in treatments aimed at mediator cells. Fish oil, containing ω-3 polyunsaturated fatty acids, is capable of entering cell membranes and altering inflammatory mediators. Billiar et al[45] state that a Kupffer cell stimulated by endotoxin will alter its release of TNF and IL-1 in the presence of ω-3 fatty acids. This carries important ramifications in the prevention of the postulated hepatocyte damage caused by the release of Kupffer cell mediators. This remains an area for future exploration and research.

Hepatotoxic agents. The third area in the treatment of liver failure and MSOF is the judicious use of hepatotoxic pharmacologic agents. Several factors must be evaluated for continued drug use, such as the necessity and availability of a similar nonhepatotoxic agent and the level of renal dysfunction (see box on p. 156 and Table 8-1).

Table 8-1 Considerations for Drug Dosage Adjustments in Liver Disease Patients

Extent of change in drug dose	Conditions or requirements to be satisfied
No change or minor change in dose	1. Mild liver disease 2. Extensive elimination of drug by kidneys and no renal dysfunction 3. Elimination by pathways of metabolism spared by liver disease 4. Drug is enzyme-limited and given acutely 5. Drug is flow/enzyme-sensitive and only given acutely by IV 6. No alteration in drug sensitivity
Decrease in dose up to 25%	1. Elimination by liver does not exceed 40% at the dose; no renal dysfunction 2. Drug is flow-limited and given by IV, with no large change in protein binding 3. Drug is flow/enzyme-limited and given acutely by mouth 4. Drug has a large therapeutic ratio
Decrease in dose of greater than 25%	1. Drug metabolism is affected by liver disease; drug administered chronically 2. Drug has a narrow therapeutic range; protein binding altered significantly 3. Drug is flow-limited and given orally 4. Drug is eliminated by kidneys and renal function severely affected 5. Altered sensitivity to drug as a result of liver disease

From Arns PA, Wedlund PJ, Branch RA. Adjustment or medications in liver failure. In: Chernow B. The pharmacologic approach to the critically ill patient. 2nd ed. Baltimore: Williams & Wilkins, 1988:85-111.

DRUGS THAT SHOULD BE USED WITH CAUTION OR NOT AT ALL IN LIVER DISEASE PATIENTS

Group I: Drugs capable of causing hepatic damage

Acetaminophen
Acetylsalicylic acid
Chlorpromazine
Erythromycin estolate
Methotrexate
Methyldopa

Group II: Drugs that can compromise liver functions

Anabolic and contraceptive steroids
Prednisone (in acute viral hepatitis)
Tetracycline

Group III: Drugs that make complications of liver disease worse

Cyclooxygenase inhibitors (indomethacin)
Diuretics
Meperidine and other CNS depressants
Morphine
Pentazocine
Phenylbutazone

From Arns PA, Wedlund PJ, Branch RA. Adjustment or medications in liver failure. In: Chernow B. The pharmacologic approach to the critically ill patient. 2nd ed. Baltimore: Williams & Wilkins, 1988:85-111.

CONCLUSION

Unfortunately, there is no *early* sensitive clinical marker of poor hepatic microcirculation or hepatocellular dysfunction in MSOF. Hepatic failure usually heralds the transition into true MSOF with much of MSOF paralleling liver failure.* The more severe the liver failure, the more severe the overall MSOF. Several studies have indicated that the presence of liver failure, not the pulmonary or renal indices, differentiates survivors from patients who do not survive. Even when oxygenation is supported, liver failure may be the common pathway leading to death in MSOF.[23] Once liver failure is established in the setting of MSOF, mortality approaches 90% to 100%.†

---

*References 3-6, 9, 10, 14, and 21.
†References 10, 11, 14, 35, and 46.

Current treatment principles emphasize supportive care and avoiding further harm. Primary therapies include removing inflammatory stimuli, modulating an overzealous immune response, and finding suitable exogenous protein replacements.

REFERENCES

1. Baue AE. Multiple organ failure: Patient care and prevention. St. Louis: Mosby–Year Book, 1990:323-329.
2. Wang P, Hauptman JG, Chaudry IH. Hepatocellular dysfunction occurs early after hemorrhage and persists despite fluid resuscitation. J Surg Res 1990;48:464-470.
3. Cerra FB. Hypermetabolism, organ failure, and metabolic support. Surgery 1987;101:1-14.
4. Cerra FB et al. Hepatic dysfunction in multiple systems organ failure as a manifestation of altered cell-cell interaction. Prog Clin Biol Res 1989;308:563-573.
5. Huddleston VB. Multisystem organ failure: A pathophysiologic approach. Boston, 1991.
6. Lekander BJ, Cerra FB. The syndrome of multiple organ failure. Crit Care Nurs Clin North Am 1990;2:331-342.
7. Guyton AC. Textbook of Medical Physiology. 8th ed. Philadelphia: WB Saunders, 1991:771-776.
8. Keith JS. Hepatic failure: Etiologies, manifestations, and management. Crit Care Nurse 1985;5(2):60-86.
9. Cerra FB. Hypermetabolism–organ failure syndrome: A metabolic response to injury. Crit Care Clin 1989;5:289-302.
10. Cerra FB. Multiple organ failure syndrome. Perspect Crit Care 1988;1:1-22.
11. Fry DE. Multiple system organ failure. Surg Clin North Am 1988;68(1):107-122.
12. Moyer E et al. Multiple systems organ failure: VII. Reduction in plasma branched-chain amino acids—correlations with liver failure and amino acid infusion. J Trauma 1981, 21:965-969.
13. Bailey PM. The metabolic response to injury: Overview and introduction to multiple system organ failure. Trauma Q 1991;7(2):1-11.
14. Barton R, Cerra FB. The hypermetabolism–multiple organ failure syndrome. Chest 1989;96:1153-1160.
15. DeCamp MM, Demling RH. Posttraumatic multisystem organ failure. JAMA 1988;260:530-534.
16. Feingold KR, Grunfeld C. Tumor necrosis factor-alpha stimulates hepatic lipogenesis in the rat in vivo. J Clin Invest 1987;80:184-190.
17. Collins AS. Gastrointestinal complications in shock. Crit Care Nurs Clin North Am 1990;2:269-277.
18. Fischer JE, Baldessarini RJ. False neurotransmitters and hepatic failure. Lancet 1971;2:75-79.
19. Shils M, Young VT. Modern nutrition in health and disease. Philadelphia: Lea & Febiger, 1988:1186-1188.
20. Clowes GHA et al. Survival from sepsis: The significance of altered protein metabolism regulated by proteolysis-inducing factor, the circulating cleavage product of interleukin-1. Ann Surg 1985;202:446-458.
21. Pearl RH et al. Prognosis and survival as determined by visceral amino acid clearance in severe trauma. J Trauma 1985;25:777-783.
22. Fry DE. Splanchic perfusion and sepsis. Prog Clin Biol Res 1989;299:9-17.

23. Schwartz DB et al. Hepatic dysfunction in the adult respiratory distress syndrome. Chest 1989;95:871-875.

24. Keller GA et al. Macrophage-mediated modulation of hepatic function in multiple-system failure. J Surg Res 1985;39:555-563.

25. Keller GA et al. Modulation of hepatocyte protein synthesis by endotoxin activated Kupffer cells. Ann Surg 1985;201:87-95.

26. Carrico CM et al. Multiple-organ-failure syndrome. Arch Surg 1986;121:196-208.

27. Cerra FB et al. Role of monokines in altering hepatic metabolism in sepsis. Prog Clin Biol Res 1989;286:265-277.

28. Cerra FB et al. Hypermetabolism organ failure: The role of the activated macrophage as a metabolic regulator. Prog Clin Biol Res 1988;264:27-42.

29. Mazuski JE et al. Direct effects of endotoxin on hepatocytes. Arch Surg 1988;123:340-344.

30. West MA et al. Endotoxin modulation of hepatocyte secretory and cellular protein synthesis is mediated by Kupffer cells. Arch Surg 1988;123:1400-1405.

31. West MA et al. Further characterization of Kupffer cell/macrophage-mediated alterations in hepatocyte protein synthesis. Surgery 1986;100:416-423.

32. West MA et al. Hepatocyte function in sepsis: Kupffer cells mediate a biphasic protein synthesis response in hepatocytes after exposure to endotoxin or killed *Escherichia coli*. Surgery 1985;98:388-395.

33. Schirmer WM et al. Femur fracture with associated soft-tissue injury produces hepatic ischemia. Arch Surg 1988;123:412-415.

34. Seibel R et al. Blunt multiple trauma (ISS 36), Femur traction, and the pulmonary failure-septic state. Ann Surg 1985;202:283-295.

35. Walvatne C, Cerra FB. Hepatic dysfunction in multiple organ failure. In: Deitch EA, ed. Multiple organ failure. New York: Thieme Medical Publishers, 1990:241-260.

36. Sarfeh IJ, Balint JA. The clinical significance of hyperbilirubinemia following trauma. J Trauma 1978;18:56-62.

37. Cerra FB et al. Multiple organ failure syndrome: Patterns and effect of current therapy. Update in Intensive Care and Emergency Medicine. Vol II. 1990.

38. Fath JJ et al. Alterations in amino acid clearance during ischemia predict hepatocellular ATP changes. Surgery 1985;98:396-404.

39. Becker W et al. Plasma amino acid clearance as an indicator of hepatic function and high-energy phosphate in hepatic ischemia. Surgery 1987;102:777-783.

40. Border JR. Hypothesis: Sepsis, multiple systems organ failure, and the macrophage (Editorial). Arch Surg 1988;123:285-286.

41. Matuschak GM, Rinaldo JE. Organ interactions in the adult respiratory distress syndrome during sepsis: Role of the liver in host defense. Chest 1988;94:400-406.

42. Pinsky MR, Matuschak GM. A unifying hypothesis of multiple systems organ failure: Failure of host defense homeostasis. J Crit Care 1990;5:108-114.

43. Chiarla C et al. Inhibition of posttraumatic septic proteolysis and ureagenesis and stimulation of hepatic acute-phase protein production by branched-chain amino acid TPN. J Trauma 1988;28:1145-1172.

44. Cerra FB et al. Septic autocannibalism: A failure of exogenous nutritional support. Ann Surg 1980;192:570-580.

45. Billiar TR et al. Fatty acid intake and Kupffer cell function: Fish oil alters eicosanoid and monokine production to endotoxin stimulation. Surgery 1988;104:343-349.

46. Matuschak GM, Martin DJ. Influence of end-stage liver failure on survival during multiple systems organ failure. Transplant Proc 1987;19(4):40-46.

9 Gastrointestinal System: Target Organ and Source

Pamela Lash O'Neill

There is an increasing body of evidence that suggests the gut, long thought to be quiescent in critical illness, may play a pivotal role in the MSOF syndrome. The hypothesis that the gut may be a major mediator in MSOF is not a new one. In 1923, Cannon[1] proposed that the gut is a source of the development of profound, irreversible shock. In the 1960s, Fine[2] proposed that bacteria and endotoxin escaping from the gut were the source for systemic infection. These theories, however, fell into disfavor, in part because of contradictory data published by other investigators.[3] Now, some 20 years later, an increasing body of evidence suggests the gut is indeed a vital organ in the MSOF syndrome.

This chapter will discuss GI anatomy and physiology as it relates to MSOF and the pathophysiologic derangements specific to the gut in the MSOF process. Clinical evidence of failure and the impact of the GI tract on MSOF will be discussed, and, finally, treatment specific to the GI tract will be presented.

ANATOMY AND PHYSIOLOGY

In addition to its role in nutrient absorption, the GI system has important metabolic, immunologic, endocrine, and barrier functions. In particular, alterations in the barrier and immunologic capabilities affect gut integrity, and many of the derangements seen in MSOF are the result of, or compounded by, the breakdown of these normal physiologic defense mechanisms.

General morphology

Throughout the GI tract there are four morphologic layers of the luminal walls: the mucosa, submucosa, muscularis, and serosa (Fig. 9-1). The mucosal layer is of primary importance in MSOF.

The mucosa is further subdivided into three components: the epithelium, the lamina propria, and the muscularis mucosa, which consists of a thin smooth-muscle layer. The epithelium may form glands that extend into the lamina propria or the submucosa. In other regions, the epithelium may project into the lumen as fingerlike projections (villi) or folds (rugae or plicae) that enhance the effective surface area of the gut tremendously.

The lamina propria contains abundant quantities of lymphocytes and is a major site for gut immunologic responsiveness.[4] The mucosa differs considerably in different regions of the GI tract and will be addressed in greater detail when the functional anatomy of each individual site is discussed.

Vascular physiology

The GI tract receives approximately 15% to 20% of the cardiac output in a resting person. The mucosa of the hollow organs receives the highest blood flow in the GI tract, and the muscle layer receives the lowest blood flow (Fig. 9-2). This flow distribution is, in part, related to the mucosa's high metabolic demands during digestion, absorption, and secretion. Various factors regulate the blood flow to the GI tract (Fig. 9-3). Of particular interest are the blood-borne substances and local vascular factors.

Neurohumoral substances are released from the kidney, adrenal medulla, and other organs in response to stress, low-flow states, and other conditions associated with critical illness. Catecholamines (epinephrine and norepinephrine) and vasoactive peptides (angiotensin II) cause selective splanchnic vasoconstriction and compromise mucosal blood flow. The vasodilator metabolites, on the other hand, are released in response to increased

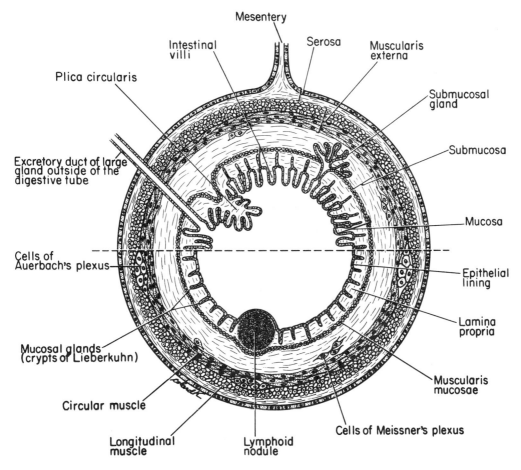

Mesentery

Intestinal villi

Plica circularis

Serosa

Muscularis externa

Submucosal gland

Submucosa

Excretory duct of large gland outside of the digestive tube

Mucosa

Cells of Auerbach's plexus

Epithelial lining

Lamina propria

Mucosal glands (crypts of Lieberkuhn)

Muscularis mucosae

Circular muscle

Cells of Meissner's plexus

Longitudinal muscle

Lymphoid nodule

Fig. 9-1 Overall histologic organization of the digestive tract—the stomach through the large intestine. (From Bloom W, Fawcett DW. A textbook of histology. 10th ed. Philadelphia: WB Saunders, 1975;599.)

Fig. 9-2 Detail of submucosal arteries. Note the arterial network of the mucosa. (From Larsen KR, Moody FG. In: Abramson PI, Dobrin PB, eds. Blood vessels and lymphatics in organ systems. New York: Academic Press, 1983;412.)

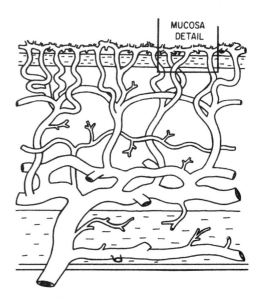

MUCOSA DETAIL

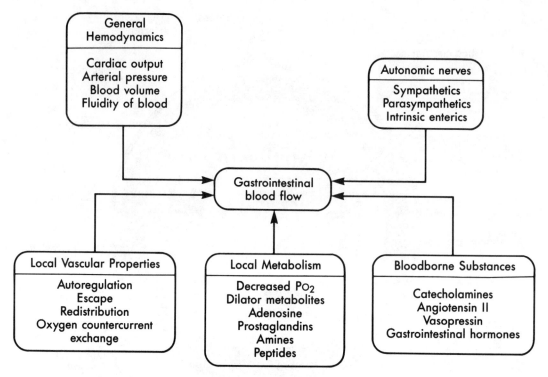

Fig. 9-3   Factors that regulate gastrointestinal blood flow. (From Jacobsen ED. In: Johnson LR, ed. Gastrointestinal physiology. 4th ed. St Louis: Mosby–Year Book, 1991;144.)

organ function, such as ingestion and digestion of food. The local vascular properties of the GI tract include autoregulation, escape, redistribution, and the oxygen countercurrent exchange system.[5]

Autoregulation. *Autoregulation* is the ability of an organ system to maintain steady blood flow despite fluctuations in systemic blood pressure. Organ systems that exhibit autoregulation include the brain, heart, liver, kidney, and intestines. In general, systolic pressures from 80 to 160 mm Hg are sufficient to maintain the autoregulatory capacity within the GI tract. Any abrupt change in organ flow can cause autoregulation to fail, further compromising mucosal blood flow.

Escape. *Escape* is similar to autoregulation. Although autoregulation protects the gut from changes in systemic flow, the phenomenon of escape involves the blood-borne substances, such as the catecholamines and angiotensin II, that act directly on the splanchnic resistance vessels. Although a transient fall in gut blood flow occurs with this infusion, blood flow returns to normal within minutes because of an intrinsic escape mechanism that is not fully understood.[5]

Redistribution. *Redistribution* is a phenomenon that occurs secondary to sympathetic stimulation. In essence, blood flow is redistributed from the mucosa to the muscular layer of the gut. Mucosal ischemia occurs, although total organ flow remains constant. The clinical significance of redistribution is that although blood flow through the superior mesenteric artery appears angiographically normal, the mucosa may be ischemic.[5]

Oxygen countercurrent exchange mechanism. An oxygen countercurrent exchange mechanism exists in the intestinal villi. Oxygen is progressively shunted from the arterial blood to the venule without going through the villus tip capillaries, thereby creating an oxygen gradient between the base and the tip of the villus (Fig. 9-4). Under steady-state conditions and with normal flow, the decrease in oxygen to the villus tip does not represent a sig-

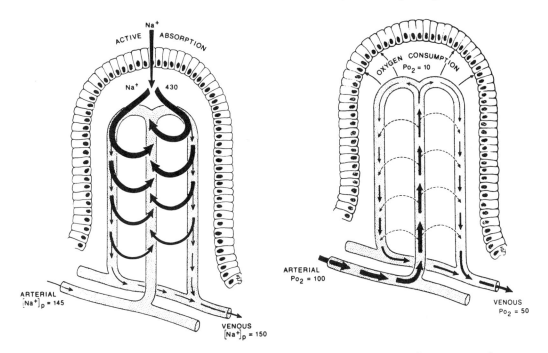

Fig. 9-4 The oxygen countercurrent exchange mechanism. On the left, sodium concentration increases at the villus tip during active absorption. On the right, a low partial pressure of oxygen at the villus tip caused by the short-circuit transfer of oxygen from the arteriole to the venule. (From Davenport H. Physiology of the digestive tract. 4th ed. St Louis: Mosby–Year Book, 1977;71.)

nificant problem. In low-flow states, however, the reduction in perfusion can lead to destruction of the luminal walls, with necrosis beginning at the villus tip and moving into deeper layers of the gut wall.

Stomach

Functional anatomy. The stomach receives and stores ingested material, alters the composition of the material to facilitate discharge into the duodenum, and delivers the processed material (chyme) to the duodenum. The chyme is continually degraded until the particulate matter size is approximately 1 mm. It is then suspended as a liquid and moved through the pylorus.[6] In addition to its role in ingestion and digestion of food, the stomach's acidic juices destroy ingested bacteria.

The capacity of the average stomach is 1 to 1.5 L. It is divided into the cardia, fundus, body, antrum, and pylorus. The pylorus regulates the pas-

sage of chyme into the duodenum, and the motility at the gastroduodenal junction functions as a barrier against reflux of duodenal contents into the stomach.

Blood supply. Blood supply to the stomach is derived primarily from the celiac trunk. This gives rise to the splenic, left gastric, and hepatic branches (Fig. 9-5). Increased blood flow to the stomach causes the rugae to fill and the mucosa to swell. In addition, secretion is enhanced because adequate flow is required for the stomach to secrete its digestive juices.

Secretory role. In the stomach, the mucosal surface is composed of columnar cells and contains individual glands that secrete pepsinogen, hydrochloric acid, or mucus. These secretory products are necessary for the digestion of ingested matter and the protection of the stomach.

Pepsinogen is converted to pepsin by hydrochloric acid or pepsin. Pepsin hydrolyzes protein

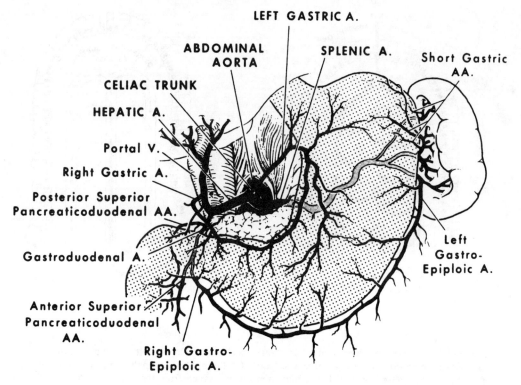

Fig. 9-5 Blood supply to the stomach and duodenum. (From Grendell JH, Ockner RK. In: Sleisenger MH, Fordtran JS, eds. Gastrointestinal disease: Pathophysiology, diagnosis, management. Vol. 2 Philadelphia: WB Saunders, 1989;1903.)

to proteases and peptides. The optimal pH for pepsin activity is 1.2 to 2.4.[7] Thus the relative acidity of the stomach is necessary for effective digestive activity. By lowering the pH, hydrochloric acid increases pepsinogen conversion to pepsin, and in conjunction with the pepsin, converts the ingested food to chyme. In addition, hydrochloric acid kills bacteria.

Mucus production in the stomach is stimulated by any irritation of the mucosa, such as the ingestion of food. The mucous layer provides lubrication and a mucosal barrier from luminal acids. This barrier function will be explored in greater detail later in this chapter as an essential defense mechanism within the GI tract. Hydrochloric acid, pepsinogen, and mucus sterilize and break down ingested material and then facilitate its transport to the duodenum for absorption.

Small intestine

Functional anatomy. The small intestine is divided into the duodenum, jejunum, and ileum; its primary function is to absorb nutrients. It also plays a role in the continued movement of ingested substances along the intestinal tract for the purpose of elimination once nutrient absorption has occurred.

Blood supply. Arterial supply to the small intestines is derived from the celiac artery and the superior and inferior mesenteric arteries. The celiac artery supplies blood to the midduodenum, and the superior mesenteric artery supplies blood from the mid-duodenum to the distal third of the transverse colon. The inferior mesenteric artery supplies blood from the distal third of the transverse colon to the anal canal (Figs. 9-5 and 9-6).

Secretory role. The digestive enzymes of the small intestine are not secreted but are integral parts

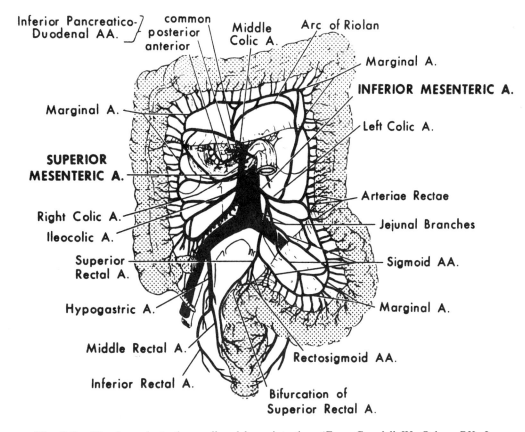

Fig. 9-6 Blood supply to the small and large intestine. (From Grendell JH, Ockner RK. In: Sleisenger MH, Fordtran JS, eds. Gastrointestinal disease: Pathophysiology, diagnosis, management. Vol. 2 Philadelphia: WB Saunders, 1989;1904.)

of the brush border. The mucosal layer of the small bowel is covered with villi (Fig. 9-1) that contain glands. On the surface of the villi are hundreds of microvilli. Like the stomach, the mucosal layer of the small intestine receives the major portion of the blood supply. The mucosal folds and villi are less prominent in the distal part of the small intestine. In fact, almost half of the total mucosal surface occurs in the first quarter of the small bowel, which is the predominant site of nutrient absorption.

Colorectum

Functional anatomy. The divisions of the colorectum include the cecum and appendix; the ascending, transverse, descending, and sigmoid co-lon; and the rectum. The functions of the colon are related to absorption and final elimination of intestinal contents. The colon reabsorbs water and secretes mucus to facilitate elimination of feces. The muscularis of the colon is divided into longitudinal bands that assist in elimination. The colon contains abundant quantities of lymphoid tissue that assist in maintaining stability in the presence of pathogenic bacteria.

Blood supply. The superior mesenteric artery supplies the cecum, right colon, and transverse colon to the splenic flexure. The inferior mesenteric artery feeds the descending colon and the proximal portion of the rectum. The hypogastric artery gives rise to the middle and rectal arteries that supply blood to the distal rectum (Fig. 9-6).

Mucosa. The mucosa of the large intestine differs in that villi do not occur below the ileocecal valve. The colonic mucosa consists of crypts and surfaces between the crypts, which are covered by epithelial cells. The crypts and epithelial lining contain an abundant supply of mucus-producing cells. The minimal fluid secreted by the colon is highly alkaline and neutralizes fecal material. The outermost layer of mucus desquamates onto the fecal material, which facilitates fecal movement and eventual elimination from the body.[8]

GUT DEFENSES

A variety of mechanisms exist within the GI tract to aid in overall gut integrity. The mucous barrier plays an essential role and protects the body by preventing translocation of gut flora to extraintestinal sites. Motility assists in the mechanics of digestion and absorption while maintaining flora within their proper environments. Gut immunity and acidity protect the gut against invasion by external pathogens and protect it from profound immunologic reactions against the normal gut flora. The flora present within the intestines assists in absorption and elimination. In MSOF, these mechanisms are altered by both pathologic mechanisms and therapeutic modalities that allow bacteria and their toxins access into and out of the GI lumen.

Gut barrier

Throughout the GI system, a barrier exists that is both physical and chemical. This barrier maintains GI integrity by protecting the wall of the gut from foreign and/or toxic substances. Potential pathogens normally found in the GI tract must be retained within the gut lumen. The barrier includes the tight junctions between the cells of the epithelial layer, the rapid turnover of the epithelial cells, and the mucous layer.

Epithelial cells. Tight junctions between the epithelium are essentially impervious to large antigenic molecules. The proliferative epithelium replaces itself at a very rapid rate, thus ensuring the integrity of the gastrointestinal luminal walls and minimizing adherence of the normal flora.

Mucus production. The mucous-bicarbonate barrier of the stomach protects the underlying epithelium from luminal acids. This function is accomplished by the exclusion of hydrogen ions from back diffusion along a gradient between the lumen

and the mucosal interstitium. Secreted bicarbonate is maintained within this layer and forms a barrier of alkalinity between the epithelium and the luminal acid.[9]

Despite the efficiency of the mucous barrier, some back diffusion of acid to the mucosal layer does occur. Bicarbonate is supplied by the microvasculature to assist in the neutralization of these hydrogen ions. Increased hydrogen-ion concentration within the gastric lumen stimulates increased blood flow to the mucosa. Since bicarbonate is present in the microvascular circulation, the increased flow provides additional bicarbonate to neutralize the hydrogen ions.[10]

Mucus-producing cells are present in large numbers in the duodenum. Mucus secreted by the small intestine functions to lubricate the lumen and act as a mechanical barrier by maintaining a neutral fluid layer against the mucosa. This mucous barrier is especially important in the duodenum, where influx of gastric acid is most likely to occur.

In the colon, the mucus is alkaline, and its production is stimulated by any irritation to the mucosa. In addition to protecting the intestinal wall from excoriation and providing the material for holding fecal matter together, the mucus protects the intestinal wall from bacterial activity within the feces. The alkalinity of the mucus provides a barrier that prevents acids formed within the feces from attacking the colonic wall.

Motility

Motility within the GI tract aids in the digestion and absorption of nutrients. In addition, it prevents bacteria in the distal small bowel and colon from migrating proximally into the sterile small intestine and stomach. The flushing action constantly keeps bacteria from adhering to the luminal wall, where penetration and translocation could occur.

In the stomach, motility maintains gut integrity by two mechanisms. If the ingested contents of the stomach are toxic, the vomiting center in the medulla is stimulated, and expulsion of the toxic contents ensues. If the ingested substance is suitable for onward passage, gastric motility determines the form and speed at which the material is emptied into the duodenum. The motility at the gastroduodenal junction functions as a barrier against reflux of duodenal contents back into the stomach.

In the small intestine, contractions mix ingested

food with digestive secretions, ensure contact of all intestinal contents with the mucosa, and facilitate transport to the colon. Both neural and gastrointestinal peptides control the motility of the small intestine.[11]

Colonic motility is designed for absorption and elimination of fecal matter. The importance of colonic motility as a defense mechanism is well established. The colon can move pathogens and potential carcinogens out of the body. In addition, normal motility ensures an even distribution of pressure along the colonic lumen and assists in protecting the integrity of the colonic wall.

Gut Immunity

The gut is a reservoir of potentially pathogenic bacteria and, as such, has an extremely complicated immune system that assists in recognizing pathogens and destroying them. This system also neutralizes the body's response to the toxins that are normally present in the distal small bowel and colon.

Dispersed aggregates of nonencapsulated lymphoid tissue, known as Gut-Associated Lymphoid Tissue (GALT), are found in the submucosa of the GI tract. The lymphoid cells appear as either clusters or diffuse aggregates and accumulate in the lamina propria of the intestinal wall or in Peyer's patches.[12]

A large number of the B lymphocytes of the lamina propria bear surface IgA. In addition, the Peyer's patches contain a large number of B lymphocytes that are dedicated to the synthesis of IgA antibody.[13] Secretory IgA plays a major role in preventing attachment of luminal bacteria to mucosal cells. It predominates in the gut secretions and is extremely resistant to enzymatic degradation.

After synthesis, secretory IgA is delivered to mucous-membrane epithelial cells. Secretory IgA binds to bacteria and prevents bacteria from binding to mucous cells. It works in conjunction with the normal flora of the gut, which also bind to the mucous membrane cells. Here the resident bacteria consume nutrients and release metabolites that are toxic to pathogenic bacteria.

The stomach's bactericidal activity includes digestion of bacteria and the secretory IgA/bacterial complex. Food ingestion stimulates secretions of the salivary glands and stomach. These secretions support the growth of commensal bacteria and assist in keeping the oropharynx and esophagus clean. Food ingestion also stimulates the growth and replication of GALT and enterocytes, which are the mucus-secreting cells.[14]

Although the tight junctions of the GI epithelium are essentially impervious to large antigenic molecules that may be introduced into the system, some antigens may still be ingested and absorbed. Macrophages of the lamina propria assist in phagocytizing and removing these antigens. Also, local synthesis of antibodies in the GALT and the evolution of a non–complement-fixing immunoglobulin isotype ensure that the reaction is minimized. Suppression of tissue-damaging immune responses is well developed in the mucosa.

During immunosuppressed states, it appears that an intact gut mucosa is an effective barrier against transepithelial migration of luminal contents.[15] This mucosal barrier suggests that the cell-mediated immunity of the GI tract may play a secondary role in the maintenance of overall GI integrity.

Gastric acid

In the healthy human stomach, intragastric pH varies widely, but studies have recorded gastric pH levels of 1 to 2 for extended periods.[16] The acidity in the stomach is essential in protecting the stomach from ingested bacteria and toxins. The acidity also plays an important role in intestinal defense since it prevents bacteria and/or pathogens from entering the small bowel. After ingestion of food, gastric pH may rise transiently, but as digestion continues, pH drops back below 4, which is generally sufficient to kill bacteria.[17] The importance of gastric acidity as a gut defense is evident in studies that have demonstrated increased gastric and jejunal colonization in patients with impaired gastric acid secretion.[18-20]

Commensal bacteria

The gut flora is highly complex and very stable in the healthy human. Control is maintained by interbacterial and host-bacterial interactions.

The stomach, duodenum, and jejunum are essentially sterile. Acid within the stomach maintains gastric sterility and also prevents migration of live organisms into the duodenum; thus sterility in the proximal small bowel is maintained.

Table 9-1 The Effect of Dietary Change on Bacteria in the Ileum

Dietary change	Effect
Increased dietary fiber	Increase in all organisms
Increased dietary protein	Increase in aerobic organisms
	No change in anaerobic organisms
Increased dietary fat	Increase in total anaerobes and *Bacteroides* organisms
	No effect on aerobic organisms

From Hill M. In: Losowsky MS and Heatley RV, eds. Gut defences in clinical practice. Edinburgh: Churchill Livingstone, 1986; 148.

Table 9-2 The Composition of the Fecal Bacterial Flora

Organisms	Mean number/g feces
Bacteroides spp	10^{11}
Gram-positive nonsporing rods	10^{11}
Bifidobacteria	
Propionibacteria	
Eubacteria	
Veillonella spp	10^{15}
Clostridium spp	10^{6}
Lactobacillus spp	10^{7}
Escherichia coli and other coliform bacteria	10^{7}
Streptococcus—total	10^{7}
—fecal	10^{5}
Bacillus spp	10^{3}
Yeasts and fungi	10^{3}

From: Hill M. In: Losowsky MS and Heatley RV, eds. Gut defences in clinical practice. Edinburgh: Churchill Livingstone, 1986; 149.
Abbreviations: *g*, gram; *spp*, species (Latin plural).

The ileum contains a large number of both aerobic and anaerobic bacteria. Aerobes in the ileum include *Escherichia coli*, *Streptococcus faecalis*, and *Lactobacillus* and *Staphylococcus* organisms, and anaerobes include *Bacteroides*, *Bifidobacterium*, *Clostridium*, and *Veillonella* organisms.[21,22] It is of interest to note that dietary intake is a major factor influencing the bacterial population in the ileum (Table 9-1).

The bacterial flora is prolific in the large bowel and consists of a number of species (Table 9-2). Flora count and type remain fairly constant, and fecal flora is essentially unaffected by dietary intake.[23]

A symbiotic relationship exists between the mucosa and the GI flora. In fact, the bacteria found in the gut are thought to be part of the GI system's key defenses against invasion by pathogens. The normal flora competes with pathogenic species for nutrients and attachment sites and also produces inhibitory substances. Any alteration in the normal flora in the colon may actually allow overgrowth of such pathogenic organisms as *Clostridium difficile*, *Staphylococcus aureus*, and *Candida albicans*.[23]

PATHOPHYSIOLOGY

In ischemic and inflammatory events, the GI tract is injured, and the response alters normal gut function and leads to pathophysiologic derangements. Fig. 9-7 depicts causes and effects of splanchnic ischemia. The primary events include a breakdown in the mucosal barrier, changes in the intramural pH, and alterations in normal gut flora. These events can occur as a result of the maldistribution of circulating volume and tissue perfusion deficits seen in MSOF. The gut becomes a victim or target organ in the process. However, MSOF can exist in the absence of an identifiable source of infection, with symptomatology mimicking intraabdominal sepsis. This phenomenon has led to the hypothesis that the gut may, in some instances, initiate the MSOF process.

Gut as a target organ in MSOF

Because the GI luminal mucosa is highly vascular, it is extremely sensitive to ischemic changes. In ischemic events, the extent of destruction occurs along a time-dependent continuum: the longer the period of ischemia, the greater the mucosal damage. The effects on the gastric and intestinal mucosa are somewhat different because of differences in their functional anatomy.

Mucosal ischemia. The stomach is a well-established target organ in septic states. Elevated acid production, along with increased permeability and mucosal ischemia, contributes to the development of stress ulceration. Gastric mucosal ischemia is seen in 80% of patients with MSOF and may be

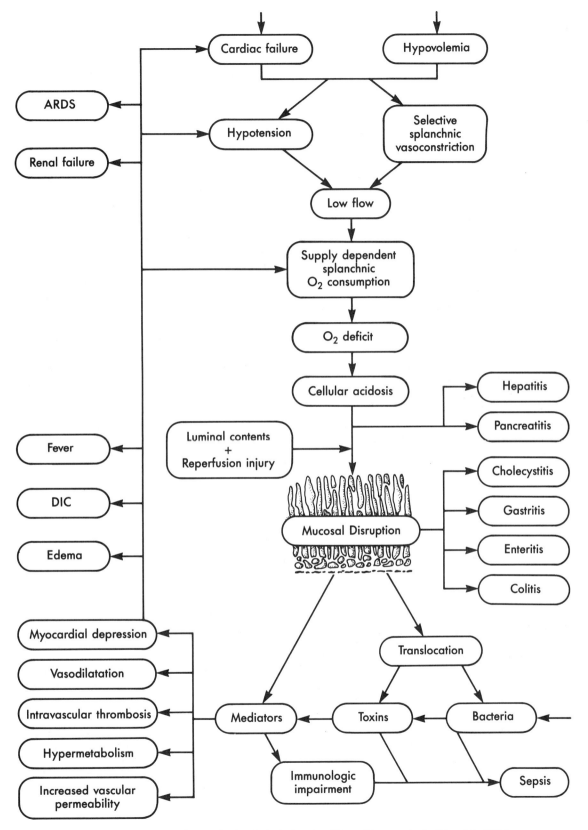

Fig. 9-7 Causes and effects of splanchnic ischemia. (From Marston A, Bulkley GB, Fiddian-Green RG, Haglund UH, eds. Splanchnic ischemia and multiple organ failure. London: Hodder and Stoughton Ltd., 1989; inside front page.)

one of the earliest manifestations of core tissue perfusion in the critically ill.[24] Use of antacids to prevent stress ulceration may lead to bacterial overgrowth in the stomach and proximal small bowel. This overgrowth occurs secondary to proliferation of the nosocomial organisms residing in the pharynx or from contaminated enteral feedings.[25]

The intestinal mucosa is also susceptible to ischemic injury. Within 5 minutes of superior mesenteric artery occlusion, ultrastructural changes are evident in the mucosal cells. In the small bowel, ischemia causes the basement membrane of the surface epithelium to detach. As the ischemic insult continues, subepithelial blebs develop. These blebs rupture, causing separation of the epithelium from the villus tips. The separation then causes an increase in capillary permeability and allows passage of plasma proteins, blood, and interstitial fluid into the intestinal lumen. Physical evidence of this includes diarrhea and guaiac-positive stools.[26,27]

If the ischemic event is gradual, collateral circulation may develop, and infarction rarely occurs. However, rapid ischemia causes mucosal infarction within 1 to 2 hours after initiation of the ischemia, and transmural infarction occurs within 8 to 10 hours.[24] Sloughing of intestinal mucosal cells, along with a decrease in mucus production and an increase in capillary permeability, has been demonstrated in dog models.[26]

Endogenous vasoconstrictors released as a consequence of sepsis and inflammation exacerbate the mucosal damage (see Chapter 3). Endogenous vasoconstrictors affecting the splanchnic circulation include angiotensin II, vasopressin, thyrotropin-releasing hormone (TRH), and prolactin. Of these, angiotensin II is a potent splanchnic vasoconstrictor, and these vasoconstrictive effects further destroy the luminal walls.

Impairment of motility. Motility is also adversely affected in critical illness. Ingested food is a strong stimulus for gut motility. Total parenteral nutrition may be initiated in the acute phase of critical illness when the patient is unable to tolerate enteral feedings. The initiation of total parenteral nutrition is associated with mucosal atrophy and decreased gut motility.

Motility functions to remove gut debris. The loss of motility (ileus), coupled with colonization of bacteria throughout the GI tract, may facilitate the migration of bacteria into areas that are normally sterile, such as the proximal GI tract.

Antibiotic administration. Antibiotic use is common in critically ill patients. However, antibiotic therapy can cause overgrowth of bacteria by altering the normally stable flora within the colon.[28] Exposure of the intestinal bacteria to systemic antibiotics causes the development of a population of organisms that are resistant to these antibiotics. These highly resistant and pathogenic organisms overgrow rapidly in the GI tract when the competing but nonresistant organisms are killed.

Reperfusion injury. During ischemic events, hypoxic metabolism generates cytotoxic substances through xanthine oxidase pathways (see Chapter 5). Degradation of adenine nucleotide compounds (ATP, ADP) produces hypoxanthine. Upon reperfusion of the ischemic tissue, the newly delivered oxygen reacts with the hypoxanthine and xanthine oxidase. By-products of this reaction include uric acid and oxygen-derived free radicals. Oxygen-derived free radicals mediate lipid peroxidation within the cell during reperfusion and cause cell injury. Recent evidence suggests that much of the injury to cells occurs within the first few moments of reperfusion and is the result of xanthine oxidase–mediated free radical production.[29]

Summary. With the breakdown of the mucosal barrier, translocation of viable organisms or endotoxin across the gut mucosal barrier represents a mechanism whereby gut organisms can produce systemic infection and shock by triggering the release of inflammatory mediators.[30] Substances from the GI tract move across the injured and dying gut and into the circulation. The entry of these metabolites into the circulation produces profound toxemia. Death is the end result.

These mechanisms (bacterial translocation and activation of the inflammatory response) demonstrate the effect of systemic alterations that occur in the MSOF syndrome on the gut. In addition, evidence exists which suggests that the phenomenon of translocation may occur before the onset of MSOF and in fact may initiate the MSOF process.

Etiologic role of the gut in MSOF

Some investigators hypothesize that MSOF initiation and/or progression may occur secondary to the effect of inflammatory mediators released into the bloodstream in response to translocated bacteria and/or endotoxin.[31,32] The actual mechanism for the migration of intestinal bacteria is unknown.

Bacterial translocation. Bacterial translocation involves the egress of bacteria and/or their toxins across the mucosal barrier and into the lymphatics or portal circulation. Evidence of translocation exists in both human and animal models.[15,30] Mechanisms associated with bacterial translocation include (1) compromised host defenses; (2) alteration in normal GI flora, especially proliferation secondary to bowel stasis; and (3) alteration in gut membrane permeability secondary to perfusion deficits, inflammatory mediators, and septic states.

Defense mechanisms. Host defenses, specifically the GALT, defend against invading pathogens and protect against extraluminal proliferation of bacteria. When these defenses are compromised, such as in immunosuppressed states, the GALT is no longer able to ward off invading pathogens. In fact, Wells et al have postulated that luminal bacteria are ingested by intestinal macrophages, transported to extraintestinal sites, and then released from the dead or dying macrophage.[30] Hence, the gut macrophage may actually facilitate translocation.

Kupffer cells (liver macrophages) play an important role in the maintenance of GI integrity and bacterial containment. Impaired Kupffer-cell function may facilitate translocation by allowing translocating bacteria or endotoxin to reach the systemic circulation.[33] The role of Kupffer cells is discussed in depth in Chapter 8.

Normal gut flora prevents overgrowth of more pathogenic bacteria in the gut. When gut flora is altered, as with antibiotic use, these pathogens proliferate and attach to the mucosa. This proliferation is a key factor in the translocation process.

Summary. Gut barrier integrity is maintained by an intact mucosa. This barrier protects the entire body by minimizing entry of pathogens into the GI system and preventing egress of normal gut flora into the systemic circulation. Unfortunately, impaired gut barrier function facilitates bacterial translocation (Fig. 9-8).

Intestinal Mucosal Layer

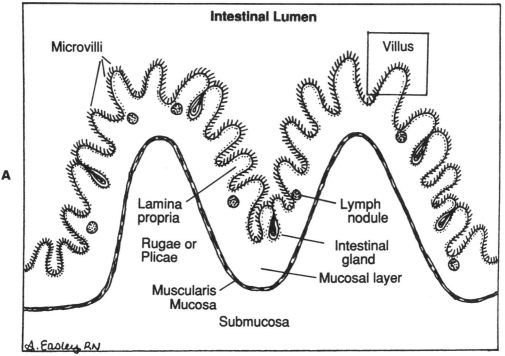

Fig. 9-8 Hypothesized mechanism of bacterial translocation from the gut. **A,** Longitudinal view of the morphologic layers of the small intestine. Note the villus, cross-sectioned and detailed in **B.** *Continued.*

Cross-section of Intestinal Villus

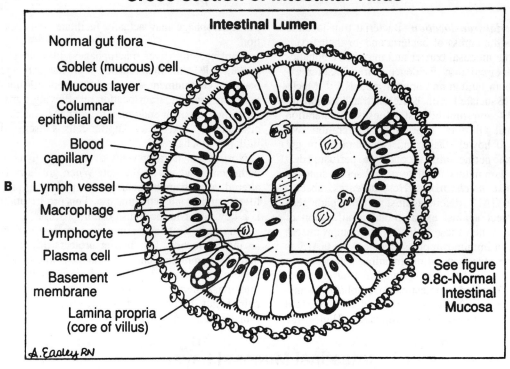

Intestinal Lumen

Normal gut flora

Goblet (mucous) cell

Mucous layer

Columnar epithelial cell

Blood capillary

B

Lymph vessel

Macrophage

Lymphocyte

Plasma cell

Basement membrane

Lamina propria (core of villus)

See figure 9.8c-Normal Intestinal Mucosa

A. Easley RN

Normal Intestinal Mucosa

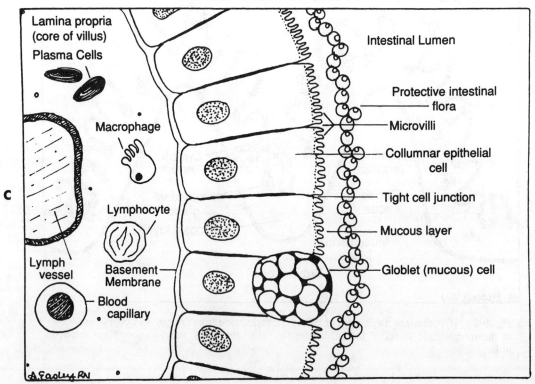

Lamina propria (core of villus)

Plasma Cells

Macrophage

C

Lymphocyte

Basement Membrane

Lymph vessel

Blood capillary

Intestinal Lumen

Protective intestinal flora

Microvilli

Collumnar epithelial cell

Tight cell junction

Mucous layer

Globlet (mucous) cell

A. Easley RN

Theory of Translocation

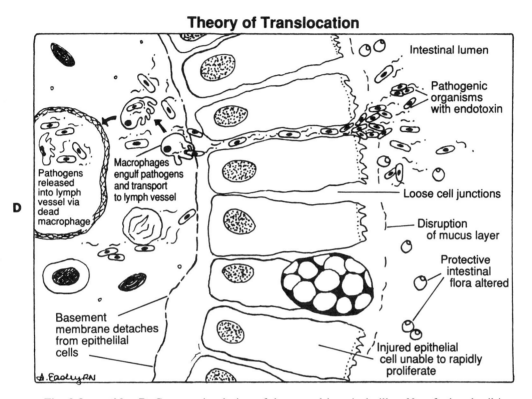

Intestinal lumen

Pathogenic organisms with endotoxin

Loose cell junctions

Disruption of mucus layer

Protective intestinal flora altered

Injured epithelial cell unable to rapidly proliferate

Macrophages engulf pathogens and transport to lymph vessel

D Pathogens released into lymph vessel via dead macrophage

Basement membrane detaches from epithelilal cells

A.Easley,RN

Fig. 9-8, cont'd **B,** Cross-sectional view of the normal intestinal villus. Note further detail in **C. C,** Detail of normal intestinal villus. The structural and functional components of the normal villus assist in maintaining overall gut integrity. Protective intestinal flora compete with pathogenic species for nutrients and attachment sites and produce inhibitory substances. Mucus production prevents adherence of pathogens to the luminal walls. Epithelial cells of the GI tract regenerate at a very rapid rate to ensure continued integrity of the mucous layer. Tight cell junctions are essentially impervious to large antigenic molecules and prevent paracellular transmission of microbes into the plasma compartment. A network of gut-associated lymphoid tissue, located in the lamina propria, protects the gut by preventing absorption or proliferation of anaerobes. **D,** Impaired intestinal villus. Dissolution of normal gut flora and alterations in mucus production allow pathogens to adhere to and colonize the luminal surface. Loose cell junctions and alterations in membrane integrity further compromise the mucous layer and allow transmission of bacteria and/or endotoxin into the lamina propria (core of the villus). Although the exact mechanism for translocation is unknown, it has been hypothesized that the intestinal bacteria are then ingested by gut macrophages. From here, they are transported to extraintestinal sites via the lymph system, and liberated upon lysis of the macrophages. (Courtesy Sheila Easley, R.N., Dallas, Tx.)

Translocation has been demonstrated in normal humans following ingestion of live *Candida albicans*.[34] The fact that translocation can occur in the absence of sepsis and shock supports the hypothesis that the gut plays a pivotal role in the initiation of the MSOF process.

CLINICAL PRESENTATION AND ASSESSMENT

Although the indicators of gut failure are not as immediately apparent as those associated with other organ systems, the extremely high mortality associated with MSOF warrants closer observation of all organ systems. This is especially true for the gut, which is a proven etiologic factor in the MSOF syndrome.

Ileus and GI bleeding

Development of an ileus and gastrointestinal bleeding are common responses of the gut to critical illness. However, these are often late manifestations of gut compromise that occur secondary to the breakdown of the mucous barrier and impairment of intestinal motility. Diarrhea and guaiac-positive stools may occur secondary to the breakdown of the gut barrier and result from the movement of plasma, interstitial fluid, and blood into the intestinal lumen. These are later, nonspecific signs that may result after mucosal damage has already occurred.

Overgrowth of pathogenic bacteria on stool culture

Antibiotic use, diarrhea, and alterations in GI motility can promote bacterial overgrowth in the small and large bowel. Normal anaerobes may decrease, with a subsequent increase in coliform bacteria (*Klebsiella, Proteus,* and *Enterobacter*). Alterations in bacterial counts on stool culture may be another indicator of gut compromise secondary to bacterial overgrowth.

Presence of enteric organisms on blood cultures

Enteric organisms on blood culture are often seen in critically ill patients. In fact, this clinical indicator led to the hypothesis that the gut might initiate the MSOF syndrome by releasing bacteria, yeast, and/or endotoxin from the GI tract into the portal and lymphatic systems. Enteric organisms on blood culture may be an early indicator that translocation of organisms is occurring.

Elevated gastric output

Gastric output can increase for a number of reasons including delayed emptying, increased production of gastric secretions, and reflux of material from the duodenum into the stomach. Although increased gastric output may be attributed to a number of factors, it can be an early indicator of gut compromise.

Endoscopic ulcerations/erosions

Shock states have been shown to produce stress ulcers in laboratory animals. Septic shock in dog models produces bleeding gastric erosions within 2 days, and hemorrhagic shock in rabbits causes gastric ulcers.[35,36] For this reason, ulcerative lesions seen on endoscopy can be a diagnostic indicator of mucosal compromise. Endoscopy will provide a definitive diagnosis for ulcerations in approximately 90% of the cases, and this can lead to early treatment measures (such as stress ulcer prophylaxis) designed to minimize mucosal injury and maintain gut integrity.

Abdominal distention

Abdominal distention can occur secondary to alterations in motility and excess gas production. The overgrowth of bacteria causes bacterial interactions that produce gas, and the alterations in gut function and motility prevent the gas from escaping the body. Distention may also be an early indicator of gut compromise.

In general, symptomatology of gut compromise is nonspecific. Definitive diagnosis of mucosal damage is at best difficult. Few diagnostic tools specific to GI function are available to assist the clinician. Direct measurement of mucosal pH may be one of the best and earliest indicators of gut compromise.

Mucosal pH

Gastric tonometry may allow for earlier detection of GI complications via indirect measurement of mucosal pH. A balloon-tipped catheter is inserted into the stomach or the sigmoid colon, and the intramural pH can be calculated. Fiddian-Green et al[37,38] have correlated low intramural pH values with a poor prognosis in critically ill patients. A normal pH indicates adequate perfusion, and an acidic pH is associated with tissue hypoxia.

Improved methods for monitoring visceral perfusion may be the hallmark for improved patient outcome. Treatment can then be initiated early and effectively, with increased survival and shortened hospital stays as the ultimate goal.

THERAPEUTIC MANAGEMENT
Surgical drainage

A common cause of MSOF is intraabdominal sepsis, which has an associated mortality rate of 60% to 90%.[39] Abdominal exploration should be considered for any patient who exhibits persistent evidence of mucosal ischemia, such as gastrointestinal bleeding, ulcerations, and low intramural pH values. The greater the period of ischemia, the higher the incidence of complete transmural infarction of the luminal wall, and the greater the mortality.

Although various studies show that early and repeated drainage of intraabdominal abscesses does not reverse MSOF in the majority of patients,[40] it is clearly a desirable therapuetic measure when compared with the alternative. In addition, there are studies which substantiate that intramucosal acidosis may be reversed by draining pus[41] and may therefore reduce mortality. However, the use of empiric laparotomy remains controversial.

Stress ulcer prophylaxis

Antacid therapy. Traditionally, antacids were thought to protect the stomach and duodenum from erosion by maintaining a neutral pH in the presence of mucosal breakdown and increased production of luminal acids. However, indiscriminant use of antacids can result in bacterial overgrowth in the stomach and the proximal small bowel. The GI tract may also become colonized by nosocomial organisms from the pharynx.[42] In addition, undesirable side effects such as diarrhea, hypermagnesemia, and/or alkalemia can result from antacid therapy.[43]

Histamine antagonists. Histamine antagonists (H_2 blockers) are an alternative or adjunct to antacid therapy. Since histamine is a stimulus to acid production, H_2 blockers antagonize acid secretion. In addition, intraluminal acids may impair hemostatic mechanisms[44]; therefore H_2 blockers have been used in treating significant gastric bleeding. However, histamine is not the only stimulus of acid

secretion, and use of H_2 blockers does not guarantee control of pH.[45] H_2 blockers may also contribute to bacterial colonization of the proximal GI tract.

Sucralfate. Sucralfate is an alternative to standard stress ulcer prophylaxis in the critically ill patient. Sucralfate is a nonabsorbable aluminum salt (sucrose octasulfate) with little or no effect on gastric acid secretion. Its therapeutic actions include antibacterial properties,[46] the exertion of trophic effects on the gastric mucosa, the ability to bind pepsin and bile acids, and the ability to coat existing ulcers with a protective layer.[47] Sucralfate may also prevent stress ulcers by stimulating bicarbonate, mucus, and prostaglandin release and by stimulating mucous cell renewal.[47]

The gastric acid barrier is very important in the pathogenesis and prevention of ventilator-associated pneumonia. In studies performed by Driks et al, nosocomial pneumonia was two times more frequent among ventilated patients receiving antacids and/or H_2 blockers than among ventilated patients receiving sucralfate.[25] Thus sucralfate is becoming an increasingly important agent in the prophylactic management of stress ulcers.

Selective decontamination

Considerable interest exists in using systemic, oral, and topical oropharyngeal antibiotics in the prophylactic treatment of bacterial translocation in critical illness. This treatment regimen is known as selective decontamination of the digestive tract (SDD). The goal of therapy is to decrease the number of aerobic and anaerobic organisms in the oropharynx and gut while maintaining adequate numbers of obligate anaerobes in the mucous membrane. It is based on the hypothesis that many infections in critically ill patients are caused by endogenous bacteria in the oropharynx and GI tract that are either aspirated into the lungs or translocate across the gut barrier and into the systemic circulation.

Several studies support the theory that SDD of the gut with oral nonabsorbable antibiotics reduces the incidence of translocation in immunosuppressed cancer patients and burn patients.[48,49] Other studies utilizing SDD have demonstrated a reduction in the colonization of the oropharynx, digestive tract, and respiratory tract by aerobic gram-negative organisms, which was accompanied by a reduction in lower respiratory tract, urinary tract, and intravenous line infections.[50,51]

Despite the evidence in favor of SDD, concerns exist about the risk of selecting out antibiotic-resistant bacterial strains. In addition, SDD can be a very costly regimen. Continued investigation of SDD is essential before employing it as standard clinical practice in the prophylactic treatment of bacterial translocation in MSOF.

Vasodilator agents

Splanchnic vasodilators, such as papaverine hydrochloride, have been employed in the clinical management of patients with nonocclusive mesenteric ischemia.[52] Studies on cat models have demonstrated that blood flow can be increased tenfold in the small and large intestine with infusions of vasodilators.[53] Other studies have demonstrated the return of normal pH in the gastric mucosa in response to low-dose dopamine.[52] This practice, however, remains controversial, and the risks may substantially outweigh the benefits.

Use of vasodilator agents is based on the theory that the therapy may override the effects of endogenous vasoconstrictors.[54] Opponents argue that many of the dilator drugs used exert a selective effect and may exert a "steal" syndrome, or may have opposing actions in different regions of the circulatory system. In addition, some may increase oxygen use, and the effects of individual vasodilators may be substantially different.

Although many questions remain unanswered concerning the efficacy of vasodilator therapy on gut failure, better monitoring techniques, such as tonometry (which measures the adequacy of perfusion to the gut), may substantiate its validity.

Enteral feedings

Recently, enteral feedings have been heralded as an important factor in the treatment of the gut in MSOF. Enteral feeding stimulates mucosal cell turnover. In fact, the presence of food in the gut has been cited as the most important stimulus for mucosal growth.[55] In addition, the feedings stimulate hormones that have trophic effects on the gut mucosa. They also assist in the sloughing of mucosal cells, thereby promoting new cell growth.[56,57] In essence, enteral feedings prevent intestinal mucosal atrophy. Adequate enteral feedings early in the treatment of MSOF appear to improve gut-

barrier function by maintaining and/or promoting mucosal integrity. For further information on enteral feedings and nutritional support, see Chapter 7.

Glutamine

Glutamine is an important nutrient that supports cell growth and replication. Although present in small quantities in enteral feedings, it is not routinely present in total parenteral nutrition. Glutamine is thought to play a major role in maintaining gut integrity. In studies where glutamine was substituted for other nonessential amino acids in total parenteral nutrition, mucosal thickness and protein content were significantly increased in the jejunum, ileum, and colon.[58,59] Thus glutamine-containing enteral/parenteral feedings have been associated with improved survival after gut mucosal injury. Studies on the addition of specific growth factors to the diet have demonstrated increased mucosal growth as well, and their interaction with glutamine may maximize mucosal healing.[55]

Antiendotoxin antibodies

Endotoxin is carried in the cell wall of gram-negative bacteria. Because of its detrimental effects following release from the bacterial cell wall, it has been studied extensively. At this time, much attention is focused on preventing intestinally caused endotoxemia. Antiendotoxin antibodies may limit the consequences of endotoxin activity.

Studies indicate that immunotherapy with antiendotoxin antibodies can improve survival in cases where endotoxemia is a key factor leading to morbidity. Although much of the research has been on animal models, a recent multicenter trial showed improved survival after infusion of a human monoclonal antibody against endotoxin[60] in patients with gram-negative septicemia.

Although more research is needed on the efficacy of treatment with antiendotoxin antibodies and other monoclonal therapy, there is a growing body of support for using immunotherapy to lessen the effects of intestinal endotoxemia.

Preventing reperfusion injury

Reperfusion injury is an important factor in the pathogenesis of GI mucosal injury. The longer the period of mucosal ischemia, the more significant a role reperfusion plays in cell injury and death.

Table 9-3   Summary of Gut Responses in MSOF

Gut defense	Evidence of failure	Treatment options
Barrier	Guaiac-positive stools	Surgical drainage
Mucus	Acid pH on tonometry	Vasodilator drugs
Epithelium	Ulcerations/erosions on endoscopy	Allopurinol/SOD may prevent reperfusion injury
Junctions	Enteric organisms on blood culture	Enteral feeds
		Glutamine
Motility	Ileus	Enteral feeds
	Distention	Glutamine
	High gastric output	
Gut immunity	Nonspecific	Support of all gut defenses
Gastric acid	Ulcerations/erosions on endoscopy	Stress ulcer prophylaxis:
	GI bleeding	Histamine antagonists
		Antacids
		Sucralfate
Gut flora	Bacterial overgrowth on stool culture	Selective decontamination
	Abdominal distention	
	Diarrhea	

Abbreviations: *SOD*, superoxide dismutase.

Evidence suggests that agents such as allopurinol and superoxide dismutase (SOD) limit mucosal damage by minimizing reperfusion injury.[61-63] Timely and aggressive intervention to prevent reperfusion injury may limit the extent of injury and improve survival in gut-associated complications of MSOF (see Chapters 3 and 5).

CONCLUSION

The gut plays a key role in the MSOF process. Table 9-3 summarizes gut defenses, clinical evidence of failure, and treatment modalities. As research continues, more information becomes available on the gut's interaction with other organ systems and how it is itself affected by the process. If it is an etiologic factor in MSOF development and progression as has been suggested, it is of the utmost importance to intervene and stop the cascade of events that culminates in MSOF. As a target organ, it extends the damage to the whole and exacerbates the MSOF syndrome. Improvement in monitoring and management will translate into decreased mortality and morbidity—the ultimate goal of therapy.

REFERENCES

1. Cannon WB. Traumatic Shock. New York: Appleton. 1923.
2. Fine J. Current status of the problem of traumatic shock. Surg Gynecol Obstet 1965;120:537-544.
3. Nagler AL, Zweifach BW. Pathogenesis of experimental shock. II. Absence of endotoxic activity in blood of rabbits subjected to graded hemorrhage. J Exp Med 1961;114:195-204.
4. Padykula HA. The digestive tract. In: Weiss L, Greep RO, eds. Histology. New York: McGraw-Hill. 1977:643-700.
5. Jacobsen ED. The gastrointestinal circulation. In: Johnson LR, ed. Gastrointestinal Physiology. St Louis: Mosby–Year Book. 1985:140-155.
6. Meyer JH et al. Sieving of solid food by the canine stomach and sieving after gastric surgery. Gastroenterology 1979;76:804-813.
7. Smith JN. Essentials of gastroenterology. St Louis: Mosby–Year Book. 1969.
8. Davenport HW. Intestinal secretion. In: Davenport HW, ed. Physiology of the digestive tract. 4th ed. St Louis: Mosby–Year Book. 1977:161-165.
9. O'Brien PE. Gastric acidity: The gastric microvasculature and mucosal disease. In: Marston A, Bulbley GB, Fiddian-Green RG, Haglung UH, eds. Splanchnic ischemia and multiple organ failure. London: Hodder and Stoughton, Ltd. 1989:145-157.
10. Silen W, Merher A, Simson JN. The pathophysiology of stress ulcer disease. World J Surg 1981;5:165-174.
11. Sarna S et al. Intrinsic nervous control of migrating myoelectric complexes. Am J Physiol 1981;4:G16-G23.
12. Lydyard P, Grossi C. The lymphoid system. In: Roitt I, Brostoff J, Male D, eds. Immunology. 2nd ed. London: Gower Medical Publishing. 1989:3.1-3.10.
13. Mayrhofer G. Physiology of the intestinal immune system. In: Newby TJ, Stokes CR, eds. Local Immune Responses of the Gut. Boca Raton: CRC Press. 1984:1-96.
14. Border JR et al. The gut origin septic states in blunt multiple trauma. Ann Surg 1987;206(4):427-448.
15. Berg RD. Translocation of indigenous bacteria from the intestinal tract. In: Hentges DJ, ed. Human Intestinal Microflora

in Health and Disease. Orlando: Academic Press. 1983;15:333-352.

16. Pounder RE et al. Effect of cimetidine on 24 hour intragastric acidity in normal subjects. Gut 1976;17:133-138.

17. McCloy RF, Baron JH. Intragastric pH and cimetidine, fasting and after food. Lancet 1981;1:609-610.

18. Ruddell WS et al. Gastric juice nitrite: A risk factor for cancer in the hypochlorhydric stomach. Lancet 1976;2:1037-1039.

19. Katz LA, Spiro HM. Gastrointestinal manifestations of diabetes. N Engl J Med 1966;275:1350-1361.

20. Reed PI et al. Gastric juice N-nitrosamines in health and gastroduodenal disease. Lancet 1981;2:550-552.

21. Hori S et al. The effect of dietary fibre on the bacterial flora of ileostomy fluid. J Med Microbiol 1983;16:VIII.

22. Fernandez F et al. Effect of changes in amount of dietary protein and fat on the composition of ileostomy bacterial flora. J Med Microbiol 1983;16:XV.

23. Hill M. Bacterial factors. In: Losowsky MS Heatley RV, eds. Gut defences in clinical practice. Edinburgh: Churchill Livingstone. 1986:147-154.

24. Fiddian-Green RG. Splanchnic ischaemia and multiple organ failure in the critically ill. Ann R Coll Surg Engl 1988; 70:128-134.

25. Driks MR et al. Nosocomial pneumonia in intubated patients given sucralfate as compared with antacids or histamine type two blockers. N Engl J Med 1987;317:1376-1382.

26. Bounous G et al. Biosynthesis of mucin in shock: Relation to tryptic hemorrhagic enteritis and permeability to curare. Ann Surg 1966;164:13-22.

27. Bounus G. Acute necrosis of intestinal mucosa. Gastroenterology 1982;82:1457-1467.

28. Marshall JC et al. The microbiology of multiple organ failure—the proximal gastrointestinal tract as an occult reservoir of pathogens. Arch Surg 1988;123:309-315.

29. Granger DN, Höllwarth ME, Parks DA. Ischemia-reperfusion injury: Role of oxygen-derived free radicals. Acta Physiol Scand 1986;(Suppl)548:47-63.

30. Wells CL et al. Intestinal bacterial translocate into experimental intraabdominal abscesses. Arch Surg 1986;121:102-107.

31. Fiddian-Green RG. Studies in splanchnic ischemia and multiple organ failure. In: Marston A, Bulbley GB, Fiddian-Green RG, Haglung UH, eds. Splanchnic ischemia and multiple organ failure. London: Hodder and Stoughton, Ltd., 1989:349-363.

32. Carrico CJ et al. Multiple organ failure syndrome. Arch Surg 1986;121:196-208.

33. Deitch EA. The role of intestinal barrier failure and bacterial translocation in the development of systemic infection and multiple organ failure. Arch Surg 1990;125:403-404.

34. Krause W, Matheis H, Wulf K. Fungaemia and funguria after oral administration of *Candida albicans*. Lancet 1969;2:598-599.

35. Menguy R, Masters YF. Mechanisms of stress ulcer. III. Effects of hemorrhagic shock on energy metabolism in the mucosa of the antrum, corpus, and fundus of the rabbit stomach. Gastroenterology 1974;66:1168-1176.

36. Odonkor P, Mowat C, Himal HS. Prevention of sepsis-induced gastric lesions in dogs by cimetidine via inhibition of gastric secretion and by prostaglandin via cytoprotection. Gastroenterology 1981;80:375-379.

37. Fiddian-Green RG, Amelin PM, Baker S. The predicted value of the pH in the wall of the stomach for complications after cardiac operations: A comparison with other forms of monitoring. Crit Care Med 1987;15:153-156.

38. Fiddian-Green RG, Gantz NM. Transient episodes of sigmoid ischemia and their relation to infection from intestinal organisms after abdominal aortic operations. Crit Care Med 1987;15:835-839.

39. Fry DE et al. Multiple system organ failure. Arch Surg 1980;115:136-140.

40. Norton LW. Does drainage of intraabdominal pus reverse multiple organ failure? Am J Surg 1985;149:347-350.

41. Fiddian-Green RG et al. Predictive value of intramural pH and other risk factors for massive bleeding from stress ulceration. Gastroenterology 1983;85:613-620.

42. Hillman KM et al. Colonization of gastric contents in critically ill patients. Crit Care Med 1982;10:444-447.

43. Derrida S et al. Occult gastrointestinal bleeding in high-risk intensive care unit patients receiving antacid prophylaxis: Frequency and significance. Crit Care Med 1989;17:122-125.

44. Green FW et al. Effect of acid and pepsin on blood coagulation and platelet aggregation. Gastroenterology 1978; 74:38-43.

45. Noseworthy TW et al. A randomized clinical trial comparing ranitidine and antacids in critically ill patients. Crit Care Med 1987;15:817-819.

46. Tryba M, Mantey-Stiers F. Antibacterial activity of sucralfate in human gastric juice. Am J Med 1987;83(suppl 3B):125-127.

47. Tarnawski A, Hollander D, Gergely H. The mechanism of protective, therapeutic, and prophylactic actions of sucralfate. Scand J Gastroenterol 1987;22(suppl 140):7-13.

48. Gurwith MS et al. A prospective controlled investigation of prophylactic trimethoprim/sulfamethoxazole in hospitalized granulocytopenic patients. Am J Med 1979;66:248-256.

49. Jarrett F et al. Clinical experience with prophylactic antibiotic bowel suppression in burn patients. Surgery 1978;83:523-527.

50. Ulrich C et al. Selective decontamination of the digestive tract with norfloxacin in the prevention of ICU-acquired infections: A prospective randomized study. Intensive Care Med 1989;15:424-431.

51. Hartenauer U et al. Effect of selective flora suppression on colonization, infection, and mortality in critically ill patients: A one-year prospective consecutive study. Crit Care Med 1991;19:463-473.

52. Boley SJ et al. Initial results from an aggressive roentgenologic and surgical approach to acute mesenteric ischemia. Surgery 1977;82:848-855.

53. Hulten L, Lindhagen J, Lundgren O. Sympathetic nervous control of intramural blood flow in feline and human intestines. Gastroenterology 1977;72:41-48.

54. Boley SJ, Brandt LJ. Selective mesenteric vasodilators: A future role for mesenteric ischemia? Gastroenterology 1986;91:247-249.

55. Wilmore DW et al. The gut: A central organ after surgical stress. Surgery 1988;104:917-923.

56. Johnson LR et al. Action of gastrin on gastrointestinal structure and function. Gastroenterology 1975;68:1184-1192.

57. Steiner M et al. Effect of starvation on the tissue composition of the intestine in the rat. Am J Physiol 1969;215:75-77.
58. Hwang TL et al. Preservation of the small bowel mucosa using glutamine enriched parenteral nutrition. Surg Forum 1986;37:56-58.
59. Jacobs DO et al. Trophic effects of glutamine-enriched parenteral nutrition on colonic mucosa. JPEN 1988;12, 1(suppl):6.
60. Ziegler EJ et al. Treatment of gram-negative bacteremia and septic shock with HA-1A human monoclonal antibody against endotoxin: A randomized double-blind, placebo-controlled trial. The HA-1A Sepsis Study Group. N Engl J Med 1991;324:429-436.
61. Smith SM et al. Gastric mucosal injury in the rat: Role of iron and xanthine oxidase. Gastroenterology 1987;92:950-956.
62. Sanfey H, Bulkley GB, Cameron JL. The role of oxygen-derived free radicals in the pathogenesis of acute pancreatitis. Ann Surg 1984;200:405-412.
63. Nordstrom G, Seeman T, Hasselgren PO. Beneficial effect of allopurinol in liver ischemia. Surgery 1985;97:679-683.

SUGGESTED READINGS

Alverdy JC, Aoys E, Moss GS. Total parenteral nutrition promotes bacterial translocation from the gut. Surgery 1988; 104:185-190.

Atherton ST, White DJ. Stomach as source of bacteria colonizing the respiratory tract during artificial ventilation. Lancet 1978;2(8097):968-969.

Baue AE. Gastrointestinal tract—an active metabolic organ that can fail. In: Multiple organ failure: Patient care and management. St Louis: Mosby—Year Book. 1990:364-373.

Border JR. Sepsis, multiple organ failure, and the macrophage (an editorial). Arch Surg 1988;123:285-286.

Bounous G. The intestinal factor in multiple organ failure and shock. Surgery 1989;107:118-119.

Carrico CJ et al. Multiple-organ-failure syndrome. Arch Surg 1986;121:196-208.

Collins AS. Gastrointestinal complications in shock. Crit Care Nurs Clin North Am 1990;2:269-277.

Deitch EA. Gut failure: Its role in the multiple organ failure syndrome. In: Multiple organ failure: Pathophysiology and basic concepts of theory. New York: Thieme Medical Publishers. 1990:40-59.

Dumoulin GC et al. Aspiration of gastric bacteria in antacid-treated patients: A frequent cause of postoperative colonization of the airway. Lancet 1982;1:242-245.

Fink MP. Why the GI tract is pivotal in trauma, sepsis, and MOF. J Crit Illness 1991;6(3):253-276.

Fry DE. Multiple system organ failure. Surg Clin North Am 1988;68:107-122.

Gallavan RH, Parks DA, Jacobsen ED. Pathophysiology of intestinal circulation. In: Schultz SG, Wood JD, Rauner BB, eds. The handbook of physiology—Section 6: The gastrointestinal system. Vol 1, Part 2. Bethesda: American Physiological Society, 1989:1713-1732.

Grendell JH, Ockner RK. Vascular diseases of the bowel. In: Sleisenger MH and Fordtran JS, eds: Gastrointestinal disease: Pathophysiology/Diagnosis/Management. 4th ed. vol 2. Philadelphia: WB Saunders, 1989: 1903-1932.

Gurd FN. Metabolic and functional changes in the intestine in shock. Am J Surg 1965;110:333-336.

Herndon DN et al. The effect of mucosal integrity and mesenteric blood flow on enteric translocation of microorganisms in cutaneous thermal injury. Prog Clin Biol Res: Second Vienna Shock Forum 1989; 308:377-382.

Herrerias-Gutierrez JM, Pardo L, Segu JL. Sucralfate versus ranitidine in the treatment of gastric ulcer. Am J Med 1989;86(suppl 6A):94-97.

Maddaus MA, Wells CL, Simmons RL. Role of cell-mediated immunity in preventing the translocation of intestinal bacteria. Surg Forum 1986;37:107-109.

Marston A et al, eds. Splanchnic ischemia and multiple organ failure. London: Hodder and Stoughton, Ltd., 1989.

Morris SE et al. Decreased mesenteric blood flow independently promotes bacterial translocation in chronically instrumented sheep. Surg Forum 1989;40:88-91.

Navaratnam RLN et al. Endotoxin (LPS) increases mesenteric vascular resistance and bacterial translocation. J Trauma 1990;30:1104-1115.

O'Dwyer ST et al. A single dose of endotoxin increases intestinal permeability in healthy humans. Arch Surg 1988; 123:1459-1464.

Runcie C, Ramsay G. Intraabdominal infection: Pulmonary failure. World J Surg 1990;14:196-203.

Saadia R et al. Gut barrier function and the surgeon. Br J Surg 1990;77:487-492.

Sarfeh IJ, Rypins EB. Physiology and pathophysiology of digestive organs in critical illness. Crit Care Clin 1987;3:395-404.

Spenney JG, Shoemaker RL, Sachs G. Microelectrode studies of fundic gastric mucosa: Cellular coupling and shunt conductance. J Membr Biol 1974;19:105-128.

Szabo S, Hollander D. Pathways of gastrointestinal protection and repair: Mechanisms of action of sucralfate. Am J Med 1989;86(suppl 6A):23-31.

Tasman-Jones C et al. Sucralfate interactions with gastric mucosa. Am J Med 1989;86(suppl 6A):5-9.

Tryba M. Side effects of stress bleeding prophylaxis. Am J Med 1989;86(suppl 6A):85-93.

Vantrappen G et al. The interdigestive motor complex of normal subjects and patients with bacterial overgrowth of the small intestine. J Clin Invest 1977;59:1158-1166.

Wells CL, Maddaus MA, Simmons RL. Role of the macrophage in the translocation of intestinal bacteria. Arch Surg 1987; 122:48-53.

10 Myocardial Dysfunction in Sepsis and Multisystem Organ Failure

Doris M. Gates

Cardiovascular and hemodynamic changes in sepsis and multisystem organ failure (MSOF) are of paramount concern for the critical care practitioner. Many advanced monitoring techniques and interventions are focused on supporting the myocardial and hemodynamic functions to meet the increased metabolic demands of the tissues. Failure to balance supply and demand at the tissue level ultimately leads to death. Thus the performance of the cardiovascular system is of central concern in the development of MSOF. Septic shock is the most common precursor to the development of MSOF, and much attention has been focused on myocardial performance in this disease state.

Myocardial dysfunction in the septic syndrome is the focus of this chapter. Many questions remain unanswered because research in this area is very difficult to conduct. Because of the severity of illness in patients, animal models have been used with varying degrees of congruence to human models in septic shock.[1] In addition, complex hemodynamic interactions between myocardial performance and changes in the peripheral vasculature hinder investigations exploring specific myocardial parameters.[2] Furthermore, methods of measuring myocardial function vary among studies, often resulting in conflicting conclusions.[3]

HISTORICAL PERSPECTIVE

The opinions concerning the pathogenesis and relative role of the myocardium in septic shock have evolved over the last 40 years. During the 1950s and early 1960s, the hyperdynamic and hypodynamic phases of septic shock were seen as two separate clinical syndromes. Many patients had symptoms of the hypodynamic phase. Invasive monitoring was minimal, and aggressive fluid therapy was avoided because of concern about inducing pulmonary edema. Thus hypovolemia was not recognized, and hypotension with a decreased cardiac output was viewed as acute cardiac failure. This acute failure was believed to be a major component in the pathogenesis of the septic syndrome.[1,4] With the advent of more sophisticated hemodynamic monitoring in the late 1960s and early 1970s, hypovolemia was recognized as the predominating cause for hypodynamic septic shock. Early fluid resuscitation became the standard, resulting in an initial hyperdynamic state often followed by hypotension with a decreased CO. Septic shock was now seen as a continuum of shock states.[1] Many hypothesized that myocardial failure was insignificant or absent in the hyperdynamic phase and instead was the mediating factor in progression to the hypodynamic phase and death. In addition, humoral myocardial depressant factors and mediators were implicated in contributing to the myocardial demise.[5] Furthermore, researchers began to recognize that survival was positively correlated with maintenance of the hyperdynamic state, adequate tissue perfusion, and oxygen delivery.[1,5,6]

Intensive research in myocardial dysfunction in sepsis has continued into the 1980s and 1990s. The definitive answer to the fundamental question of the role of the myocardium in sepsis and its progression to MSOF remains elusive. However, current research indicates the initial hyperdynamic cardiac state is the response to peripheral vasodilatation induced by alterations in tissue metabolism.[1,7] Significant and early myocardial depression occurs despite volume loading and increased cardiac index and hemodynamic parameters. In addition, biventricular failure is common, and myocardial systolic (contractility) and

178

diastolic (compliance) functions are unfavorably altered.[6,8-13] Multiple humoral mediators and altered cellular physiology are implicated in myocardial pump dysfunction, which may lead to the patient's ultimate demise.[1,7,14] Recent research has revealed significant differences between those who recover and those who die from sepsis, and patients who die 7 days or more after shock onset are usually victims of MSOF.[12] Thus, despite extensive research and advances in medical technology and knowledge, the mortality rate for sepsis and MSOF remains 40% to 60% and 90% to 100%, respectively.[15,16]

PATHOPHYSIOLOGY AND CLINICAL PRESENTATION
Overview

Cardiac performance in septic shock is intimately linked to the cardiovascular system's attempt to preserve oxygen delivery to the tissues. Normally, the tissue's oxygen supply and demand balance is maintained through peripheral vascular autoregulation and systemic compensatory mechanisms. In the septic syndrome, the peripheral autoregulatory mechanisms fail, leading to indiscriminate vasodilatation, maldistribution of flow, and decreased oxygen extraction. Consequently, the maintenance of tissue oxygenation is determined by the three major organ systems interacting to regulate systemic responses to oxygen requirements. The respiratory system oxygenates venous blood, the hematopoietic system contributes hemoglobin to carry oxygen, and the cardiovascular system strives to maintain tissue perfusion. The respiratory and hematopoietic systems may be limited in their ability to significantly affect tissue requirements; thus the cardiac system performs a pivotal role in preservation of oxygen supply in septic shock.[17]

Alterations occur in heart rate, preload, compliance, afterload, and contractility in an attempt to maintain cardiac function to meet the increased requirements of tissue metabolism. As various factors impinge on cardiac function and compensatory mechanisms are exhausted, oxygen transport becomes inadequate. Consequently, the combined effects of anaerobic cellular conditions, release of pathophysiologic mediators, and worsening cardiac failure may propel the patient with sepsis into MSOF. The inability to maintain hyperdynamic

tissue perfusion as a result of cardiac failure has been implicated in the pathogenesis of sepsis and MSOF. However, the exact mechanisms of this myocardial failure are unclear, and the myocardium may be a victim and not the originator of the sequence of events leading to the patient's ultimate demise.[17-21]

Septic shock is induced by a wide variety of organisms, all of which produce the typical clinical and cardiovascular picture of hypotension, severe peripheral vasodilatation, and enhanced cardiac output.[15] The severe decrease in systemic vascular resistance (SVR) is seen as the initiating event producing hypotension. Adequate volume loading to fill the expanded vascular space results in a compensatory increase in cardiac output. With appropriate fluid resuscitation, 90% of patients demonstrate the hyperdynamic response.[10,15]

Hyperdynamic vs. hypodynamic: misconceptions. It is a commonly held assumption that the hyperdynamic state is consistently followed by the hypodynamic state (hypotension, increased SVR, and decreased CO) as the patient's condition deteriorates. However, recent reports[10,15] demonstrate that only a small minority of patients die from a progressively deteriorating cardiac output. Unresponsive hypotension accounts for approximately 50% of deaths, because of either a severe and persistent decrease in SVR (40%) or a profoundly diminished cardiac output (10%). MSOF is responsible for the other 50% of deaths (Fig. 10-1). Patient mortality from unresponsive hypotension usually occurs within 7 days of disease onset, whereas deaths from MSOF occur more than 7 days after onset of shock symptoms.[10,13] Thus several as yet undetermined mechanisms appear to mediate the physiologic response and outcome of sepsis.

Whatever the etiology and progression of sepsis, myocardial dysfunction is evident early in the course of the disease.[12,13] Various factors adversely affect both right- and left-ventricular performance, leading to alterations in heart rate, preload, compliance, afterload, and contractility.[8,10,11]

Alterations in hemodynamic parameters

Systemic blood pressure and mean arterial pressure (MAP) are regulated through the inverse relationship between cardiac output (CO) and SVR. In the septic state, massive peripheral vasodilatation induces increases in cardiac output. Since car-

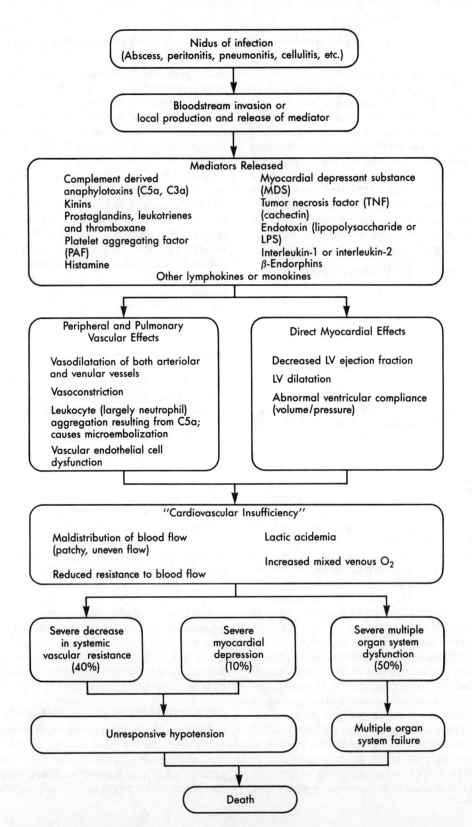

Fig. 10-1   The pathogenesis of human septic shock. (From Natanson C, Hoffman WD, Parrillo JE. Septic shock: The cardiovascular abnormality and therapy. J Cardiothor Anesth 1989:3:219.)

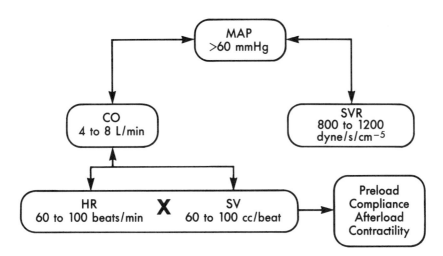

Fig. 10-2 Hemodynamic components and regulation. The hemodynamic components strive to maintain an MAP greater than 60 mm Hg. A negative change in any component of SV induces an increase in HR in order to maintain CO. If CO rises, SVR decreases. If CO falls, SVR increases. Conversely, changes in SVR induce changes in CO. If SVR falls, CO rises; if SVR rises, CO falls in order to maintain a constant MAP. Abbreviations: *MAP*, Mean arterial pressure; *CO*, cardiac output; *SVR*, systemic vascular resistance; *HR*, heart rate; *SV*, stroke volume; *L/min*, liters per minute; *dyne/sec/cm^{-5}*, dyne per second per cm^{-5}.

diac output is determined by heart rate and stroke volume (CO = HR × SV), these two parameters consequently are altered. Heart rate increases, and the myocardium attempts to maintain or increase stroke volume through alterations in the determinants of stroke volume: preload, compliance, afterload, and contractility (Fig. 10-2).

Ventricular preload

Physiologic role. Ventricular preload is defined as the volume of blood (end-diastolic volume, [EDV]) or the amount of myocardial tension at the end of diastole.[22] The end-diastolic volume determines the degree of myocardial fiber stretch and thus myocardial tension. According to the Frank-Starling law of the heart, the greater the myocardial

fiber length or tension, the more forceful the contraction. This relationship between preload and contractile force is termed stroke work and is measured as stroke work index (SWI). Assuming that the myocardium is healthy and will distend and stretch with added volume (compliance), increases in volume will increase SWI. Diseased myocardial fibers are stiff and resistant to lengthening (noncompliant) and do not demonstrate significant increases in SWI with added volume (Fig. 10-3). Factors affecting preload and thus SWI include fluid status, distribution of blood volume, venous return, ventricular compliance, atrial contraction (atrial kick), and valvular status.[22,23]

Impact of disease. In sepsis, fluid status, distribution of blood volume, and venous return are

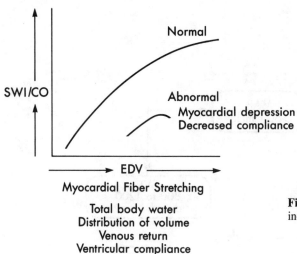

SWI/CO

Normal

Abnormal
Myocardial depression
Decreased compliance

EDV

Myocardial Fiber Stretching

Total body water
Distribution of volume
Venous return
Ventricular compliance
Atrial contraction
Valvular status

Fig. 10-3 Preload. Abbreviations: *SWI,* Stroke work index; *CO,* cardiac output; *EDV,* end-diastolic volume.

the significant determinants of preload. Vasodilatation, increased peripheral capillary permeability, and maldistribution of blood volume result in a relative and actual fluid deficit in the vascular space. The expanded vasculature requires a larger volume to "fill up the tank." Various inflammatory mediators enhance capillary permeability, leading to significant interstitial edema. Therapies such as positive pressure ventilation and PEEP reduce venous return and further displace volume into the periphery.[19] Thus preload volume and SWI are significantly depressed in the septic patient, and massive fluid resuscitation is necessary to maintain volume status and adequate myocardial stretch.

Ventricular compliance

Physiologic role. Compliance is an important factor in determining ventricular diastolic function. Ventricular compliance refers to the ability of the ventricle to stretch and dilate in response to volume and is demonstrated by the end-diastolic pressure to volume relationship. Increases in ventricular EDV result in increases in end-diastolic pressure (EDP), commonly measured as CVP or PCWP. However, this pressure-volume relationship is not linear: it is curvilinear. This relationship is illustrated in Fig. 10-4. In the normal ventricle, low volume exerts a low pressure. When a fluid bolus enters an empty ventricle, only small changes in

pressure occur because the ventricle is compliant and stretches, accommodating the increased volume and increasing the SWI (Fig. 10-4, point *A* to *B*). As the ventricle fills, a point is reached wherein a fluid bolus induces a larger increase in pressure (Fig. 10-4, point *C* to *D*). On the upward curve of the relationship, additional volume does not enhance ventricular performance and SWI but merely increases pressure without any benefit to hemodynamic status. Thus a normal ventricle becomes less compliant as it progressively fills.[15,23,24] As illustrated in Fig. 10-5, noncompliant ventricles demonstrate large pressure changes in response to volume infusions (the curve is shifted upward and to the left). Compliant, elastic ventricles exhibit smaller pressure changes in response to volume infusions (the curve is shifted downward and to the right).

The clinical significance of the pressure-volume relationship is that CVP and PCWP do not accurately reflect ventricular volume and SWI.[24] It is an erroneous assumption that any given CVP or PCWP reflects a certain ventricular EDV and amount of myocardial stretch (Fig. 10-5). Trends and changes in these pressure readings in response to fluid therapy are clinically important and significant, because they indicate the ventricular compliance at any given time and assist in directing therapy. For example, a fluid challenge of 250 cc

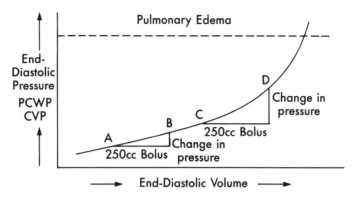

Fig. 10-4 Compliance. Abbreviations: *PCWP*, Pulmonary capillary wedge pressure; *CVP*, central venous pressure.

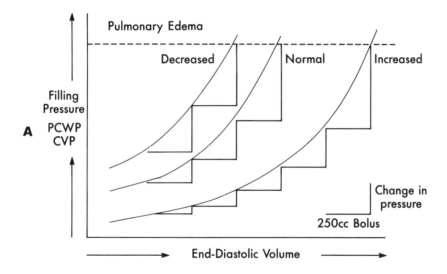

Decreased Compliance	Increased Compliance
Progressive ventricular filling Myocardial ischemia/infarction Inotropic agents Catecholamines PEEP Cardiac tamponade ARDS Hypertension Ventricular hypertrophy	Vasodilators Calcium-channel blockers Relief of myocardial ischemia Ventricular dilatation Dilated cardiomyopathy

Fig. 10-5 **A** and **B,** Compliance and volume loading. Abbreviations: *PCWP*, Pulmonary capillary wedge pressure; *CVP*, central venous pressure; *PEEP*, positive end expiratory pressure; *ARDS*, adult respiratory distress syndrome.

that induces a pressure change of greater than 5 mm Hg indicates a stiff ventricle—a large pressure change occurred in response to a small volume infusion. Administration of additional fluid would result in volume overload and greatly increase the filling pressure without increasing SWI and cardiac output. The abnormally elevated pressure would only predispose the patient to pulmonary edema. However, if several 250-cc fluid challenges are given before a 5-mm Hg change is detected, the ventricles are compliant—a larger volume was necessary to produce the same pressure change. Minimal pressure response to volume infusion indicates that the SWI and preload are not maximized, and the patient may be hypovolemic. Once volume status is optimized, other therapies are introduced as indicated by hemodynamic parameters.[15,22,24,25]

Impact of disease. The pressure-volume relationship is an important concept, especially in the septic patient. Changes in ventricular compliance occur early in the disease and affect the patient's ultimate outcome. Several studies demonstrate that alterations in compliance occur in both ventricles during sepsis.* Survivors demonstrate increased compliance with biventricular dilatation and increased end-diastolic volumes in order to maximize stroke work. The enhanced SWI maintains CI and tissue perfusion despite evidence of myocardial depression. Those who do not survive do not display this compensatory adaptation.[11,12]

Sepsis is often complicated by other factors that affect ventricular compliance. ARDS can have a significant impact on both left- and right-ventricular compliance. In ARDS characterized by mean PAPs of less than 30 mm Hg, the right ventricle dilates to maximize SWI and is therefore able to maintain forward flow to the left ventricle. However, in ARDS with mean PAPs of greater than 30 mm Hg, the right ventricle dilates, but resistance to outward flow is too great, and left-ventricle contractility diminishes.[20,26] Thus forward flow to the left ventricle is compromised, and left-ventricle preload diminishes. In addition, the extreme dilatation of the right ventricle impinges upon the left ventricle with interseptal shifts and crowding within the pericardium, further decreasing left ventricle compliance and preload. Furthermore, the

*References 8, 11, 12, 20, and 26.

use of positive pressure mechanical ventilation and PEEP exerts pressure against the pericardium, resulting in limited ventricular expansion. Other processes or therapies used in the septic state that may decrease ventricular compliance are myocardial edema, altered calcium metabolism, sympathetic stimulation, and vasopressor drugs (through direct cardiotonic actions or increases in afterload). Ventricular compliance is augmented through the use of vasodilators and calcium-channel blockers.[22-24,27,28] Thus it becomes evident that volume is but one determinant of ventricular pressure. Compliance plays a significant role, especially in disease states.

Ventricular afterload

Physiologic role. Ventricular afterload refers to the force or tension created in the myocardial muscle that ejects blood against a resistant vasculature. SVR, a clinical approximation of afterload, greatly influences the quantity of blood ejected from the ventricle. High afterloads (increased resistance) obstruct the outflow of blood while low afterloads (low resistance) facilitate forward flow and output. Ventricular afterload varies in response to local tissue metabolic needs, sympathetic autonomic function and stimulation, and vasoactive mediators. Right ventricular afterload is also affected by the presence of pulmonary hypertension and ARDS.[22,25] All of these factors contribute to the alterations in afterload associated with septic shock (Fig. 10-6).

Impact of disease. Massive peripheral vasodilatation in response to increased tissue metabolic demands is the clinical hallmark of septic shock and requires massive fluid resuscitation to fill the expanded vascular space. The reduction in left ventricular afterload facilitates ventricular ejection, resulting in an increased CO. However, severe and persistent vasodilatation increases venous pooling and diminishes venous return. This may result in a decreased preload and cardiac output. Perpetuation of the severe vasodilatation compounded by a failing myocardium leads to prolonged hypotension, cellular damage, and ultimately death.[11,12] Physiologic mechanisms that normally enhance vasoconstriction may be nonfunctional or ineffective. These mechanisms may include nonresponsive peripheral alpha-receptors and inhibition of endogenous norepinephrine release.[19] In addition, multiple

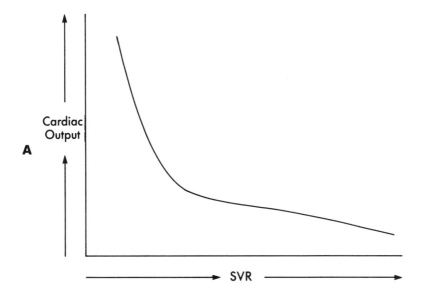

Decreased SVR	Increased SVR
Vasodilator agents	Vasopressor agents
Inflammatory mediators	Alpha stimulators
Increased cardiac output	Decreased cardiac output
Hypermetabolic tissue needs	ARDS (PVR, right ventricle)
	Atherosclerosis

Fig. 10-6 **A** and **B,** Afterload. Abbreviations: *SVR,* Systemic vascular resistance; *ARDS,* adult respiratory distress syndrome; *PVR,* pulmonary vascular resistance.

vasoactive mediators actively enhance vasodilatation. These may involve endotoxin, tumor necrosis factor, interleukin-1, interleukin-2, complement, prostaglandins, and beta-endorphins.[15] Therapeutic interventions in this setting include maximum volume administration, followed by the addition of vasopressor agents to increase SVR.

In a small number of cases, sepsis is complicated by such a severe myocardial depression that a compensatory increase in SVR mimics cardiogenic shock.[13,15] In this setting, vasodilator therapy, along with inotropic support, is appropriate to reduce afterload, facilitate forward flow, and enhance tissue perfusion.[15]

A special consideration for right-ventricular afterload is the presence and severity of ARDS. Unlike the muscular left ventricle, the thin-walled right ventricle has minimal ability to increase contractility in response to an acutely elevated resistance or myocardial depression. Instead, the right ventricle relies on its ability to accommodate large volumes in order to maintain stroke volume. Thus changes in right ventricle preload and compliance are of primary importance in maintaining forward flow to the left ventricle in disease states (ARDS) that result in increased right ventricular afterload.[17]

Studies have described the impact of ARDS on right ventricle function.[20,26] Sibbald et al[26] demonstrated an increasing trend in right ventricular end-diastolic volumes as mean PAPs increased. Significant right ventricle dilatation was seen with mean PAPs of greater than 30 mm Hg. In addition, right ventricular ejection fraction (RVEF) fell as volume increased. However, stroke volume was maintained through the Frank-Starling mechanism. Forward flow to the left ventricle was maintained; and left ventricle preload, left ventricular ejection fraction (LVEF), and contractility were unaltered in patients with ARDS without sepsis. In spite of ʼdequate left ventricle function, left ventricular nd-diastolic pressures (PCWP) were significantly igher as mean PAPs increased. This was seen as econdary to overdistention of the right ventricle, ight-to-left septal shifts, and crowding within the ʼericardium, which consequently decreased left ʼventricle compliance (small volumes exerting large ʼressures in a stiff, nonexpanding left ventricle). ʼOther studies have found similar results in septic patients, supporting the concept that right ventricle dilatation is an important compensatory mechanism in preserving right ventricular myocardial function in sepsis and MSOF complicated by ARDS with an increased afterload.[8,11,20]

Ventricular contractility

Physiologic role. Ventricular contractility is defined as the ability of the myocardial fibers to shorten and effectively propel blood from the ventricular chambers independent of variations in preload or afterload.[23] Alterations in contractility are offset by changes in preload and afterload under normal conditions. Experimentally, contractility is assessed in isolated myocardial fibers by determining velocity and strength of fiber shortening. Clinically, however, the objective determination of contractility is difficult because of the interdependence of hemodynamic components and effects of external factors such as circulating catecholamine levels, therapeutic measures, and intrinsic and extrinsic myocardial depressant factors (Fig. 10-7). Various derived measures of flow, volume, and pressure are used to infer contractile force.* These include cardiac output, cardiac index, ejection fraction,

stroke work index, and end-systolic volume (Table 10-1).

Cardiac output and cardiac index are measures of the flow of blood from the heart to the periphery. As a measure of flow only, CI does not take into account the work generated by the myocardium to produce the flow. CI is very dependent upon multiple variables, such as preload, afterload, heart rate, and contractility, that change substantially during the course of disease. As in the case of sepsis, a depressed myocardium that is stimulated by endogenous or exogenous catecholamines, has an increased EDV, and faces a low resistance to flow will usually exhibit a normal or increased CI. Thus, clinically, CI is a reliable indicator of the delivery of blood to the tissues but not the contractile force necessary to sustain that delivery of flow.[2,15]

Ejection fraction (EF) is the percentage of the end-diastolic volume ejected from the ventricle. EF is a better indicator than CI of baseline ventricular function; however, it is also affected by preload, afterload, and compliance.[1] In general, EF falls as the myocardial contractile force is insufficient to propel blood from the ventricles. The heart attempts to maintain stroke volume and flow through the use of preload reserve (ventricular dilatation). If the compensatory increase in compliance with larger preload volumes is inadequate to maintain forward flow, afterload increases, further restricting EF. In sepsis, an initially low EF is paradoxically associated with increased survival.[12] This phenomenon is explained by compensatory ventricular dilatation in response to myocardial depression that results in larger end-diastolic volumes to maintain stroke volume. Ventricular size, preload, and EF return to normal as the septic syndrome and myocardial depression subside (Fig. 10-8). Conversely, the EF in patients who do not survive is usually normal throughout the duration of the disease until death. For unknown reasons, compensatory ventricular dilatation does not occur (perhaps due to decreased compliance), and the lower peripheral resistance in those who do not survive is seen as facilitating the maintenance of EF.[8,10-12] These changes in EF have been demonstrated in both the right and left ventricles. In addition, the changes vary together in the majority of cases, thus indicating a biventricular contractile dysfunction.[11]

Stroke work index (SWI) is a composite variable

---

*References 3, 4, 8, 10, and 15.

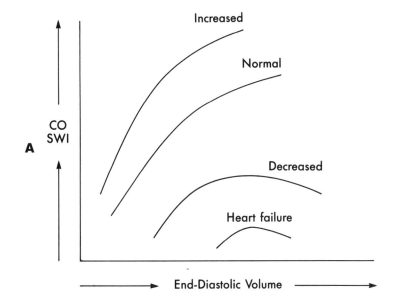

Increased contractility	Decreased Contractility
Catecholamines Inotropic agents Increased end-diastolic volume	Decreased sympathetic stimulation Decreased compliance Decreased end-diastolic volume Myocardial edema Loss of myocardial tissue Hypoxia Acidosis Inflammatory mediators Depressant factors Beta blockers Calcium-channel blockers

Fig. 10-7   **A** and **B,** Contractility. Abbreviations: *CO*, Cardiac output; *SWI*, stroke work index.

Table 10-1 Calculated Hemodynamic Variables

Parameter	Calculation	Normal range
Flow		
MAP	$\dfrac{S - D}{3} + D$	60-105 mm Hg
CI	$\dfrac{CO}{BSA}$	2.5-4.0 L/min
CO	$HR \times SV$	4.0-8.0 L/min
Volume		
SV	$\dfrac{CO \times 1000}{HR}$	60-100 mL/beat
SVI	$\dfrac{CI}{HR}$	33-47 mL/beat/m^2
PCWP		8-12 mm Hg
CVP	$cm\ H_2O = mm\ Hg \times 1.34$	2-6 mm Hg
Resistance		
SVR	$\dfrac{MAP - CVP}{CO} \times 80$	800-1200 dyne/s/cm^{-5}
SVRI	$\dfrac{MAP - CVP}{CI} \times 80$	1760-2600 dyne/s/cm^{-5}/m^2
PVR	$\dfrac{mPAP - PCWP}{CO} \times 80$	37-250 dyne/s/cm^{-5}
PVRI	$\dfrac{mPAP - PCWP}{CI} \times 80$	45-225 dyne/s/cm^{-5}/m^2
Contractility		
LVSWI	$SVI\ (MAP - PCWP) \times 0.0136$	38-85 g/m^2/beat
RVSWI	$SVI\ (mPAP - PAD) \times 0.0136$	7-12 g/m^2/beat

Abbreviations: *MAP*, mean arterial pressure; *S*, systolic; *D*, diastolic; *CI*, cardiac index; *CO*, cardiac output; *BSA*, body surface area; *L/min*, liters per minute; *HR*, heart rate; *SV*, stroke volume; *SVI*, stroke volume index; *PCWP*, pulmonary capillary wedge pressure; *CVP*, central venous pressure; *SVR*, systemic vascular resistance; *SVRI*, systemic vascular resistance index; *PVR*, pulmonary vascular resistance; *PVRI*, pulmonary vascular resistance index; *LVSWI*, left ventricular stroke work index; *RVSWI*, right ventricular stroke work index; *PAD*, pulmonary artery diastolic pressure; *mPAP*, mean pulmonary artery pressure.

used to assess ventricular contractility. It is a measure of the relationship between myocardial fiber tension (contractile force) and preload volume (i.e., Frank-Starling law of the heart). Given a set volume infusion, normal myocardial tissues exhibit greater increases in contractile force (SWI) than depressed myocardial tissues (Fig. 10-3). In other words, larger volumes and greater stretch are necessary to maintain contractile force and output in the depressed myocardium. Biventricular myocardial depression, indicated by low SWI, has been consistently demonstrated in survivors and non-survivors of sepsis. Decreases in SWI are noted early in the septic syndrome, and one study[10] indicated that depression of LVSWI frequently preceded falls in LVEF. Survivors demonstrate a return to normal SWI, while the SWI of patients who die continues to decline.[10,11]

End-systolic volume (ESV) is another useful measure in evaluating contractility. As contractile ability declines, less blood is propelled from the heart (falling EF) resulting in more blood remaining at the end of systole (ESV). In addition, alterations in afterload affect ESV. Increased resistance impedes outflow, resulting in an increased ESV; conversely, decreased resistance facilitates ventricular ejection, leading to smaller ESV. In sepsis, studies have demonstrated increased LVESV despite lower resistance, signifying a decrease in left ventricle contractility.[4,12] RVESV has also been

Acute Phase of Septic Shock

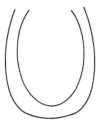

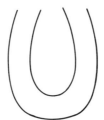

Stroke volume = 50 mL

$$\text{Ejection fraction} = \frac{200 \text{ mL} - 150 \text{ mL}}{200 \text{ mL}} = 25\%$$

Left-ventricular
end-diastolic
volume = 200 mL

Left-ventricular
end-systolic
volume = 150 mL

Recovery Phase of Septic Shock

Stroke volume = 50 mL

$$\text{Ejection fraction} = \frac{100 \text{ mL} - 50 \text{ mL}}{100 \text{ mL}} = 50\%$$

Left-ventricular
end-diastolic
volume = 100 mL

Left-ventricular
end-systolic
volume = 50 mL

Fig. 10-8 Ventricular changes in septic shock. A schematic representation of the reversible myocardial depression seen in the survivors of septic shock. (From Parker MM et al. Profound but reversible myocardial depression in patients with septic shock. Ann Intern Med 1984:100:488.)

shown to rise regardless of the presence of an elevated afterload (ARDS), thus leading researchers to conclude that right ventricular myocardial depression is also apparent during the septic syndrome.[1,8,11,26]

Impact of disease. In summary, biventricular diastolic and systolic dysfunction is evident in early sepsis. In response to myocardial depressant stimuli, diastolic components (preload and compliance) are altered to compensate for declining systolic function (contractility).[17] In addition, as illustrated in Table 10-2 and Table 10-3, these changes follow distinct patterns in survivors and nonsurvivors of septic shock. Regardless of the final outcome, most patients' (more than 90%) symptoms include an elevated CI, low SVRI, and hypotension. By 2 to 5 days after the onset of hypotension, survivors show evidence of significant myocardial depres-

sion. Despite a normal or elevated CI, these patients display a dilated left ventricle, increased LVEDV, low LVEF, a low LVSWI, and a normal or low SVRI. They tolerate large volumes of fluid before maximum filling pressure is reached (PCWP at 12 to 15 mm Hg) and may require only transient inotropic and vasopressor support, since hemodynamic parameters typically return to normal within 7 to 10 days. Symptoms of right ventricular dysfunction closely parallel those described in left ventricular dysfunction, indicating a severe but reversible biventricular abnormality.[4,10-12]

Conversely, nonsurvivors do not demonstrate adequate compensatory changes in diastolic function to offset systolic abnormalities. Significant increases in left ventricular dilatation and LVEDV do not occur in response to myocardial depression.

Table 10-2   Initial to Final Hemodynamic Changes in Survivors and Nonsurvivors of Septic Shock

Parameters	Survivors (n = 22)			Nonsurvivors (n = 17)		
	Initial	Final	p*	Initial	Final	p
Heart rate, beats/min	105	95	NS†	111	129	0.006
Mean arterial pressure, mm Hg	77	85	0.017	74	74	NS
Pulmonary artery wedge pressure, mm Hg	13.7	9.6	0.047	14	13.4	NS
Central venous pressure, mm Hg	9.5	4.4	0.016	9.8	10.7	NS
Cardiac index, L/min/m²	4.1	4.1	NS	4.9	4.8	NS
Stroke volume index, mL/m²	39.9	42	NS	45.5	38.6	NS
Systemic vascular resistance index, dynes·s·cm⁻⁵·m²	1470	1691	NS	1262	1176	NS
Pulmonary artery mean pressure, mm Hg	22	17	0.036	22	24	NS
Pulmonary vascular resistance index, dynes·s·cm⁻⁵·m²	204	150	NS	144	193	NS
Left ventricular stroke work index, g·m/m²	34	41	NS	37	34	NS
Right ventricular stroke work index, g·m/m²	5.4	7.3	.03	7.2	6.3	NS

*Paired sample *t* test.
†NS indicates not statistically significant.
From Parker MM et al. Right ventricular dysfunction and dilatation, similar to left ventricular changes, characterize the cardiac depression of septic shock in humans. Chest 1990:97:126-131. Abbreviations: *L/min/m²*, liters per minute per meter²; *mL/m²*, milliliters per meter²; *dynes·s·cm⁻⁵·m²*, dynes per second per centimeter⁻⁵ per meter²; *g·m/m²*, grams·meter per meter².

Table 10-3   Initial to Final Ejection Fraction and End Diastolic Volume Index in Survivors and Nonsurvivors of Septic Shock

Parameters	Survivors (n = 22)			Nonsurvivors (n = 17)		
	Initial	Final	p*	Initial	Final	p
Left ventricular ejection fraction	.31	.47	.001	.40	.43	NS†
Left ventricular end diastolic volume index, mL/m²	145	106	.012	124	102	NS
Right ventricular ejection fraction	.35	.51	.001	.41	.39	NS
Right ventricular end diastolic volume index, mL/m²	124	88	.03	120	114	NS

*Paired sample *t* test.
†NS indicates not statistically significant.
From Parker MM et al. Right ventricular dysfunction and dilatation, similar to left ventricular changes, characterize the cardiac depression of septic shock in humans. Chest 1990:97:126-131. Abbreviation: *mL/m²*, milliliters per meter².

Their stiff ventricles render them intolerant to massive fluid resuscitation, and other therapies (inotropes, vasopressors) are necessary to support hemodynamics. Despite persistent hypotension, nonsurvivors typically maintain a hyperdynamic profile with a normal or elevated ejection fraction, stroke volume, and CI until death. They exhibit a more severe vasodilatory response to sepsis than survivors, which perhaps enables the depressed myocardium to continue to propel blood through the tissues. In addition, the higher heart rate of nonsurvivors aids in maintaining CI in the event SVI falls (CO = HR × SV). Considerable cardiac reserve is necessary to support such abnormal demands, and eventually irreversible failure ensues. Thus the ability of the ventricles to dilate and use preload reserve in response to myocardial depression is positively correlated with survival. Stiff, noncompliant ventricles are associated with higher mortality rates.[4,10-12]

ETIOLOGY OF MYOCARDIAL DYSFUNCTION

Although most authors and researchers agree that myocardial depression is evident early in the course of sepsis, the pathogenesis of this altered performance is ill defined and controversial. However, several factors and multiple mediators have been implicated in the development of myocardial dysfunction in sepsis and overwhelming inflammation.

Coronary blood flow

Global perfusion. Reduction in coronary blood flow producing global myocardial ischemia has been postulated as a precursor to myocardial failure in septic shock, and early animal studies suggested its possibility.[29] However, several other studies demonstrate significant increases in coronary blood flow without parallel increases in myocardial demands.[30-32] Under physiologic conditions, coronary perfusion is directly determined by myocardial metabolic demands. The myocardium maintains an almost complete (70% to 75%) extraction of arterial oxygen.[30] Increases in oxygen demand that cannot be met by enhanced extraction are met by changes in coronary blood flow. Through autoregulatory mechanisms, the coronary vasculature precisely maintains perfusion to match myocardial requirements. Even over a wide range of perfusion pressures (60 to 140 mm Hg), abrupt changes do not disturb this delicate balance.[30,31,33]

Loss of autoregulation. In sepsis, this autoregulatory ability is lost. Although myocardial requirements do not increase in sepsis, excessive vasodilatation, high coronary blood flow, and reduced oxygen extraction are apparent. Net lactate production is not increased, indicating the absence of global myocardial hypoxia and ischemia.[30-32] Global measure of myocardial metabolism, however, may not detect local ischemia resulting from possible maldistribution of flow within the myocardium. Several authors have described microcirculatory disturbances and scattered necrosis in the septic heart, but the role of these symptoms in the pathogenesis of myocardial failure has not been resolved.[2,19,21,34]

Maldistribution of coronary blood flow. The changes in coronary circulation are similar to the alterations of high cardiac output, low SVR, and reduced oxygen extraction described in the systemic circulation. Factors precipitating myocardial circulatory changes are unclear but may result from the release of vasoactive mediators such as epinephrine, histamine, kinins, and prostacyclin.[31] The vasodilatation may also be a compensatory mechanism to counteract the negative effects of decreased oxygen extraction.[30] In addition, alterations in myocardial energy metabolism may contribute to coronary vasodilatation and myocardial dysfunction. Dhainaut et al[31] described alterations in myocardial substrate extraction that were associated with poor cardiac performance in patients with sepsis. Patients with sepsis relied primarily on lactate and endogenous cardiac reserves for metabolism and did not appropriately use exogenous glucose, fatty acids, and ketone bodies for energy production. The decrease in exogenous substrate use was more pronounced in patients who did not survive, indicating a greater metabolic derangement. The precise relationship between altered myocardial circulation, energy metabolism, and myocardial depression remains to be defined through further research.[30-32]

Calcium metabolism, coronary artery disease, and myocardial edema. Altered calcium metabolism[2] and the presence of preexisting coronary artery disease[35] has been shown to decrease ventricular compliance and thus reduce the available preload reserve necessary to compensate for decreased intrinsic contractility. In addition, myocardial edema has been implicated in contributing to both systolic and diastolic myocardial dysfunction. Edematous myocardial tissues do not contract or relax adequately; thus contractile force and compliance are diminished. Myocardial edema may be more pronounced in nonsurvivors,[8,25] contributing to the inability of the myocardium to dilate in response to acute contractile depression. Furthermore, edema may interfere with myocardial microperfusion by compression of the coronary circulation and increasing diffusion distance.[36] Thus the presence of myocardial edema may be a critical determinant of early cardiac dysfunction.[2]

Sympathetic nervous system responsiveness

Alterations in sympathetic nervous system responsiveness may contribute to diminished ventricular performance in septic shock. Contractility and cardiac output are enhanced through sympathetic stimulation of myocardial beta receptors. In shock states, such sympathetic stimulation is a vital compensatory mechanism that maintains ventricular performance, and may, in fact, obscure any underlying primary cardiac dysfunction.[9,36] Increased circulating catecholamine levels and enhanced beta-adrenergic stimulation have been demonstrated in early sepsis (preshock).[37,38] In addition, administration of beta-blockers, such as propranolol, have indeed resulted in reduced contractility and hemodynamic deterioration indicative of early underlying myocardial dysfunction.[18,36] However, following the initial compensatory period and as the septic syndrome progresses, the myocardium becomes less sensitive to circulating catecholamines and contractility declines.[2] Contractile reserves are reduced through this down-regulation of beta-adrenergic receptors, contributing to biventricular depression that is increasingly refractory to elevated plasma levels of epinephrine and norepinephrine.[2,9,19,21]

Mediator activity

Myocardial depressant factor. Circulating cardiodepressant and vasoactive mediators have been described in the pathogenesis of sepsis. The existence of myocardial depressant factor (MDF) and its potential role in myocardial dysfunction in shock states have been intensely researched and debated for nearly 20 years, and general consensus has yet to be achieved.[36] However, recent animal and human studies have demonstrated a direct effect of MDF, or other humoral factors, on myocardial function. MDF has been shown to decrease contractility in animals by as much as 54% within 1 hour of administration and ultimately induce shock.[36] In humans, Parrillo et al[39] demonstrated that serum from patients with sepsis exhibiting acute myocardial dysfunction (low LVEF) produced a 25% to 34% decrease in contractility of rat myocytes. As the patients with sepsis recovered and LVEF returned to normal, their sera no longer contained MDF nor affected the rat myocyte contractility. In addition, the degree of LVEF reduction in patients paralleled the extent of rat myocyte depression. Furthermore, increased levels of MDF were associated with substantially elevated LV filling pressures, ventricular dilatation, and mean peak lactate concentrations. Serum from normal volunteers, critically ill patients without sepsis, and patients with structural heart disease demonstrated no depression of the rat myocardial cells.

Strong evidence exists that supports the presence of a circulating myocardial depressant factor in septic shock; however, this factor has yet to be isolated and its precise mechanism of action determined. In addition, conflicting evidence exists as to its site of origin. It is hypothesized that the pancreas, stimulated by hypoperfusion and ischemia, produces MDF through a series of cellular autolytic reactions. MDF is then released into the bloodstream,

where it is transported to the heart. However, removal of the pancreas does not necessarily prevent myocardial depression in septic animals. Therefore the presence, actions, and relative importance of humoral depressant factors require further research.[36]

Endotoxin. The cardiodepressant effect of endotoxin is controversial. Studies in dogs have shown a direct depressant effect, while recent studies in rat myoctyes demonstrated no change in contractility when exposed to endotoxin.[40,41] In humans, detectable serum levels of endotoxin were found in only 43% of patients with septic shock, and its presence was intermittent during the 24-hour study period. However, the presence of endotoxin was associated with a higher mortality, myocardial depression, renal failure, ARDS, and MSOF.[29,42] In another human study, endotoxin administered to healthy volunteers resulted in the classic septic hemodynamic response of high cardiac output, left ventricle dilatation, decreased LVEF, and systemic vasodilatation.[41] Although these studies suggest that endotoxin plays a role in the cardiovascular changes and myocardial depression in septic shock, the mechanism for its action is not clear. The effects may be the result of direct myocardial depression, or endotoxin may stimulate the release of other humoral mediators that reduce cardiac contractility.[29,42,43]

Tumor necrosis factor. After exposure to endotoxin, tumor necrosis factor (TNF) has been found in the plasma of healthy human volunteers. Peak levels of TNF coincided with the onset of the hyperdynamic cardiovascular state. As the septic event progressed to the stage of myocardial depression and ventricular dilatation, TNF was no longer detectable in the serum of the subjects.[41] In animal models, TNF demonstrated no direct contractile depression on cardiac cells.[40] Thus TNF may be generated in response to endotoxin and either have a delayed effect on myocardial contractility or itself generate other cardiac depressants and mediators.[41]

Other mediators. Various other mediators have been studied in relation to the hemodynamic changes exhibited in septic shock. Interleukin-2 produced heart failure and hemodynamic changes consistent with septic shock when administered intravenously to cancer patients as immunotherapy.[44] Complement has been associated with severe vasodilatation and hypotension in human septic shock.[45] Thromboxane A_2 may act as an intermediary by generating plasma myocardial depressant substances.[46] Prostaglandin F_2 demonstrated direct dose-dependent depression on rat myocardial cells, and prostaglandin E_2, leukotrienes B_4, C_4, and D_4,[40] and prostacyclin[46] exhibited no cardiac depression. Platelet activating factor has also been shown to depress the contractility of animal and human heart tissue.[47] Therefore many endogenous mediators may be involved directly or indirectly in the production of cardiac dysfunction.

In conclusion, myocardial depression is the result of numerous physiologic derangements and humoral mediators. The precise interaction and roles of these factors and mediators are unknown. Research continues in this area to identify and clarify the mechanisms producing the abnormal cardiovascular sequelae described in the septic syndrome.

ROLE OF MONITORING

Patients in septic shock typically present with hypotension, warm and flushed skin, bounding pulses, and alterations in mental status. Other associated clinical symptoms include fever, positive blood cultures, evidence of end-organ insufficiency (i.e., elevated creatinine, jaundice, hyperbilirubinemia, elevated lactate), and occasionally cold and clammy skin with weak pulses.[25,48] Once the diagnosis of septic shock is made, patients must be admitted to the critical care unit. Analysis of survival rates in sepsis has demonstrated a decrease in mortality rates for patients admitted to critical care units staffed by full-time critical care physicians and nurses with knowledge and capabilities for hemodynamic monitoring and support.[49]

Arterial access

Invasive monitoring in the intensive care unit begins with an arterial line. An arterial line is essential for continuous monitoring of blood pressure because cuff pressures are often inaccurate in shock states. An adequate systolic pressure (> 90 mm Hg) is often indicative of flow; however, when coupled with a very low diastolic pressure as often seen in septic shock, perfusion to some vascular beds may be impaired. Thus mean arterial pressure (MAP) is the best indicator of perfusion since it takes into account both systolic and diastolic values. An MAP greater than 60 mm Hg is necessary to maintain perfusion to the vital organs. In addition to blood pressure monitoring, arterial lines allow frequent blood sampling for various parameters such as arterial blood gases, electrolytes, lactate, and metabolites that can change rapidly during the course of the disease.[4,15,48] Common metabolic derangements in sepsis such as acidosis, hypoxia, hypophosphatemia, and hypocalcemia are known cardiac depressants and must be avoided to optimize cardiac output.[50]

Pulmonary artery catheter

A pulmonary artery catheter allows for the initial differential diagnosis of the cause of shock (Table 10-4). Ongoing cardiac status and fluid balance are

Table 10-4 Hemodynamic Parameters in Shock States

Shock state	MAP	CO	SVR	PCWP	CVP	Treatments
Distributive Septic Neurogenic Anaphylactic	↓	↑	↓	↓	↓	Fluid Vasopressors Inotropes
Cardiogenic	↓	↓	↑	↑	↑	Fluid Inotropes Vasodilators
Hypovolemic	↓	↓	↑	↓	↓	Fluid/blood
Obstructive Cardiac tamponade	↓	↓	↑	↑	↑	Pericardiocentesis Reentry sternotomy

Abbreviations: *MAP*, mean arterial pressure; *CO*, cardiac output; *SVR*, systemic vascular resistance; *PCWP*, pulmonary capillary wedge pressure; *CVP*, central venous pressure.

evaluated through serial analysis of cardiac filling pressures (PCWP and CVP), cardiac flow (CO, CI), cardiac contractility (SV, SVI, SWI), and afterload (SVR). Mixed venous blood gases and pulmonary artery oxygen saturations allow for calculations of total body oxygen consumption. Correct assessment and interpretation of these parameters is important in choosing the appropriate treatments, determining the response to interventions, and monitoring the patient's progress.[4,48,50]

Venous access

A central line (single or multiple infusion) and two or more peripheral lines are often required to allow for simultaneous administration of resuscitation fluids, antibiotics, vasoactive infusions, and blood products. In addition, continuous cardiac monitoring is necessary. Atrial arrhythmias (atrial fibrillation, atrial flutter, or supraventricular tachycardia) are more common than ventricular arrhythmias in patients with sepsis. Atrial arrhythmias can significantly diminish cardiac output and exacerbate the hypotension and abnormal organ flow. Conversion to normal sinus rhythm can be accomplished with medications or synchronized cardioversion. The use of cardioversion may necessitate concurrent administration of sedatives and analgesics that can further lower blood pressure. Therefore the use of such agents must be considered on an individual basis. Pharmacologic agents such as verapamil, procainamide, or quinidine may also be useful in slowing tachyarrhythmias or holding a conversion rhythm. Again, side effects of hypotension and direct myocardial depression must be weighed in light of the patient's overall condition.[48] The guiding principle when using these therapies is to begin at the lowest dose or watt-seconds and titrate up until the desired effect is achieved.

THERAPEUTIC MANAGEMENT

The septic syndrome and MSOF are complex disease states that require prompt and knowledgeable interventions in order to maximize the patient's probability of survival. The high mortality rate associated with these disease states reflects our inability to reverse the underlying pathologic process that results in persistent hypotension, maldistribution of flow, and eventual end-organ demise. The use of antimediator therapy is promising but requires further investigation before it can be ap-

plied effectively. Thus maintenance of cardiac and end-organ function is the cornerstone of therapy while the injurious processes run their course and the infection is treated.[15,48]

In treating septic shock, it is important to distinguish between high output (hyperdynamic) and low output (hypodynamic) states. Almost all patients (90%) present in the hyperdynamic state following volume infusion. The majority of patients maintain the hyperdynamic state until they begin to recover or death occurs. These patients require volume infusion, inotropes, and vasoconstricting drugs. A small minority of patients progresses to the hypodynamic state, and their treatment includes volume infusion, inotropes, and vasodilating drugs.

Volume infusion

Goal. Increasing preload through volume infusion is the best initial hemodynamic therapy to treat hypotension. Initially, preload and cardiac filling pressures (CVP and PCWP) are significantly reduced as a result of vasodilatation. Ongoing preload reduction results from increased capillary leakage, displacement of volume, and maldistribution of blood flow. Fluid infusion increases ventricular volume, maximizes myocardial stretch (Frank-Starling mechanism), and maintains cardiac output.[51] Although CO is often elevated in septic shock, MAP and SVR are reduced. The goal of fluid resuscitation is to increase CO to supranormal levels and keep MAP greater than 60 mm Hg to preserve adequate perfusion and oxygen transport to the hypermetabolic organs.[4,48]

Response. Response to volume infusion is determined through serial measures of filling pressures (PCWP), ventricular performance parameters (CO, CI, SVR, SVI, SWI), and end-organ function. Trends and magnitude of changes in PCWP during volume infusion are interpreted, since isolated PCWP values do not accurately reflect end-diastolic volume (preload) and are influenced by ventricular compliance. Fluid challenges of 250 to 500 cc are administered when the PCWP is less than 10 to 12 mm Hg. If the PCWP increases 3 to 5 mm Hg, the ventricle is compliant and can accommodate more fluid to maximize stretch. Fluid challenge continues as long as the PCWP changes no more than 3 to 5 mm Hg with subsequent boluses. However, when the PCWP increases by more than 5 to 7 mm Hg in response to a fluid bolus, maximal preload volume and stretch have been achieved, and further fluid administration will only increase filling pressure and put the patient at risk for developing pulmonary edema (Fig. 10-5).[22,25] Measures of ventricular performance are assessed along with PCWP to give the total picture of response to fluid therapy. Stroke volume, stroke work index (a measure that considers both ventricular volume and pressure), and cardiac output should increase as preload is augmented. As optimal fluid status is achieved, further increases in these ventricular function measures will be absent or minimal with additional volume infusion. If maximum volume infusion fails to alleviate hypotension, vasopressor therapy is added.[52]

In general, PCWP is maintained between 12 and 15 mm Hg in patients with sepsis. However, decreases in ventricular compliance as a result of either instrinsic changes in myocardial muscle fibers (myocardial edema) or extrinsic causes (ARDS, PEEP) may require pressures between 15 and 18 mm Hg to maintain stroke volume. Patients with a PCWP of greater than 20 mm Hg often develop pulmonary edema.[4]

Crystalloids vs. colloids. Because of myocardial and peripheral vascular abnormalities, large quantities of fluid are necessary to maintain blood pressure and organ perfusion. The use of colloids or crystalloids continues to be debated, but neither has proven to be superior over the other in terms of cardiovascular performance or ultimate mortality.[53] Crystalloids (normal saline and lactated Ringer's solutions) are inexpensive and have relatively few if any side effects. Colloids (albumin, protein solutions, and blood products) and synthetic colloids (hetastarch and dextran) are more expensive and have increased side effects, but they remain in the vascular space longer. However, opponents of colloidal use argue that the colloids leak into the interstitial space in the presence of increased vascular permeability and exacerbate vascular fluid loss and peripheral edema.[4,53] Assessment of the individual patient's needs is the best guide to fluid therapy. If the patient is anemic (hematocrit <30%), blood should be administered to maintain not only volume status but also oxygen-carrying capacity of the blood. If the patient is hypoalbuminemic (< 2 g/dL), albumin solutions (50 to 100 g given as a 25% solution) are appropriate. Given an acceptable hematocrit and albumin level, crystalloid solutions are indicated.[48]

Survivors vs. nonsurvivors. Recent studies demonstrate that preload requirements change as the septic syndrome evolves and are different in survivors and nonsurvivors.[4,10-12] Survivors demonstrate acute ventricular dilatation (more fluid must be infused before maximum PCWP and ventricular performance are attained), decreased ejection fraction, high cardiac output, tachycardia, and low systemic vascular resistance that return to normal within 7 to 10 days. Thus fluid requirements decrease as the patient progresses toward recovery. Patients who do not survive typically maintain an elevated CO, severe vasodilatation, tachycardia, and hypotension without ventricular dilatation and decreased ejection fraction. Decreased ventricular compliance renders patients less tolerant to fluid resuscitation measures, and they exhibit higher filling pressures with less volume. If the patient develops ARDS, further decreases in left ventricular compliance and size occur as a result of right ventricle dilatation, interventricular shifts, and PEEP therapy and are reflected in even higher filling pressures. These higher filling pressures (15 to 18 mm Hg) are necessary to maintain stroke volume, and the persistence of the peripheral vascular abnormalities and capillary leakage require continued fluid support.[4,10-12,48,54]

Vasopressor therapy

Goal. Vasopressive agents are indicated if maximum volume infusion (up to a PCWP of 15 to 18 mm Hg) does not normalize blood pressure and organ perfusion as judged by an MAP > 60 mm Hg, decreased lactate levels, adequate urine output, and normal organ function studies. Persistent hypotension is usually secondary to profound vasodilatation and not a reduced cardiac output. Vasopressors are necessary at this point to either induce vasoconstriction, increase cardiac output, or both. Vasopressors vary in their influence on the heart and peripheral vasculature (Table 10-5).[50] In addition, their prolonged use in profound sepsis and MSOF may require increasingly larger doses to maintain hemodynamic stability. This phenomenon may be due to the decreased responsiveness of the alpha- and beta-receptors, circulating mediators, and continued losses of intravascular volume through capillary leakage and maldistribution

Table 10-5 Commonly Used Vasopressor Agents: Relative Potency*

Agent	Dose	Cardiac		Peripheral vasculature		
		Heart rate	Contrac- tility	Vasocon- striction	Vasodila- tation	Dopami- nergic
Dopamine	1–10 μg/kg/min	2+	2+	0	2+	4+
	>10 μg/kg/min	2+	2+	2–3+	0	0
Levarterenol (norepinephrine)	2–8 μg/min	2+	2+	4+	0	0
Dobutamine	1–10 μg/kg/min	1+	4+	1+	2+	0
Isoproterenol	1–4 μg/min	4+	4+	0	4+	0
Epinephrine	1–8 μg/min	4+	4+	4+	3+	0
Phenylephrine	20–200 μg/min	0	0	4+	0	0

From Parrillo JE. Septic shock: Clinical manifestations, pathogenesis, hemodynamics, and management in a critical care unit. In: Parrillo JE, Ayres SM. Major issues in critical care medicine. Baltimore: Williams & Wilkins Co, 1984:111-125.
Abbreviation: *μg/kg/min,* micrograms per kilogram per minute.
*The 1 to 4+ scoring system represents an arbitrary quantitative scoring system to allow a judgment of comparative potency among these vasopressor agents.

of flow (sympathomimetics are ineffective in the presence of hypovolemia) seen in the septic syndrome.[51,54-56] As the resistance builds to the vasopressive drugs, it may become more difficult to maintain vascular tone and blood pressure than cardiac output.[54]

Dopamine. Low-dose dopamine (1 to 5 μg/kg/min) is the initial inotrope of choice because of its ability to improve cardiac function and blood pressure while preserving renal function and improving flow to the liver and gut. Dopamine in the range of 1 to 5 μg/kg/min (and up to 10 μg/kg/min in some patients due to considerable interpatient variability) stimulates cardiac and peripheral beta-receptors to produce moderate inotropic, chronotropic, and peripheral vasodilatory effects that increase stroke volume, heart rate, cardiac output, and blood pressure. This dose also stimulates the renal and splanchnic vasculature dopaminergic receptors, resulting in renal vasodilatation that protects the kidneys from the detrimental effects of shock and improved flow to the gut. If hypotension persists within the low-dose range, dopamine can be titrated up to a maximum of 20 μg/kg/min to keep the MAP > 60 mm Hg and optimize hemodynamic and organ function parameters. At dosage ranges of 10 to 20 μg/kg/min, dopamine continues to have positive inotropic and chronotropic effects; however, renal and splanchnic vasodilatation is lost, and peripheral vasoconstriction occurs in all vascular beds as a result of alpha-adrenergic stimulation. At dosages greater than 20 μg/kg/min,

dopamine is an unreliable vasoconstrictor and adverse effects (extreme tachycardia, atrial dysrhythmia, ventricular dysrhythmia) are more common.[4,48,50] Some patients exhibit tachycardias at even low doses of dopamine. In these patients, the use of dopamine may not be beneficial.[48]

Levarterenol. If the dopamine dose exceeds 20 μg/kg/min and hypotension continues, another vasopressor is required. Levarterenol (Levophed) is a potent vasoconstrictor and is one of a few vasopressors that can produce an adequate blood pressure in the septic shock patient if volume infusion and high-dose dopamine fail. Levarterenol is infused at 2 to 10 μg/min until the MAP is greater than 60 mm Hg. Elevating the MAP is necessary to maintain tissue perfusion and preserve life. However, excessive levarterenol-induced vasoconstriction could potentially worsen the shock syndrome by vasoconstricting vascular beds and aggravating flow abnormalities. This excessive vasoconstriction results in organ tissue damage. In addition, if vasoconstriction produces too high an afterload, myocardial contractility and cardiac output are reduced. Therefore the minimal effective dose of levarterenol is administered to guard against its powerful vasoconstrictive side effects.[48,52,57]

The kidneys are particularly sensitive to the vasoconstrictive effects of levarterenol. A recent study has demonstrated that the simultaneous administration of low-dose dopamine (1 to 4 μg/kg/min) increases renal flow during levarterenol therapy.[58] Thus once maximum dopamine dosage has been achieved, levarterenol is begun and the dopamine titrated down to 1 to 4 µg/kg/min. By following serial hemodynamic and renal function studies, the combination therapy can be adjusted to maximize the patient's status.[52,58]

Other agents. If the patient remains hypotensive despite high-dose levarterenol and renal-dose dopamine therapy, the patient's prognosis is poor.[15] Other sympathomimetics may be administered to the patient with sepsis, but they often demonstrate more adverse reactions. Phenylephrine (Neo-Synephrine) is a pure alpha-agonist. As such, it produces powerful vasoconstriction without direct cardiac effects. If the patient requires intense vasoconstriction or adversely responds to dopamine or levarterenol with arrhythmias, phenylephrine can be used effectively.[48] Epinephrine is an alpha- and beta-agonist that has effects similar to those of levarterenol. In patients who are hypotensive because of profound myocardial depression (cardiogenic shock superimposed on septic shock) and are refractory to high-dose levarterenol, high-dose epinephrine administration may result in their stabilization and survival.[1,4] The major disadvantage of epinephrine use is its tendency to produce arrhythmias and tachycardias and increase myocardial oxygen needs.[48]

Dobutamine (Dobutrex) is a synthetic beta-agonist that produces a significant increase in myocardial contractility and peripheral vasodilatation. It decreases SVR, increases contractility, and results in no appreciable change in MAP. It may be useful in combination with dopamine in the minority of patients with sepsis with profound cardiac depression and vasoconstriction,[59] but its vasodilatory effects render it ineffective in maintaining blood pressure in the majority of patients with sepsis.[48] Isoproterenol (Isuprel) is a pure beta-agonist that has similar effects to those of dobutamine. However, it has limited clinical usefulness because of its profound effects of lowering SVR and MAP, increasing myocardial oxygen requirements, and producing arrhythmias.[48,50] Amrinone (Inocor), a phosphodiesterase inhibitor, increases cardiac contractility and produces potent vasodilatation. Thus its usage is also limited in hyperdynamic sepsis. However, patients in hypodynamic sepsis with serious heart failure and vasoconstriction may benefit from its cardiac and peripheral effects.[59]

Vasodilator therapy

Goal. Patients who maintain a high cardiac output and low systemic resistance during the course of their disease do not require vasodilating therapy; in fact, such therapy would only compound the hypotension and provide no clinical benefit. However, sepsis and MSOF can progress to a hypodynamic state in which the patient demonstrates profound cardiac failure characterized by a low cardiac output and stroke volume, high left ventricular filling pressure, and increased systemic vascular resistance.[7,17,48] The intense vasoconstriction is deleterious to cardiac function and must be treated. This cardiogenic shock picture results from severe biventricular myocardial depression, and perhaps is more pronounced in patients with overt or occult cardiac disease.[7,35] The status of this patient population is also often complicated by the presence of ARDS and MSOF. The goal of vasodilator therapy in this setting is to reduce the obstruction to flow (afterload), enhance ventricular performance (contractility), decrease filling pressures, increase cardiac output, and sustain tissue perfusion and oxygen delivery.

Nitroprusside. Sodium nitroprusside (Nipride) is usually the vasodilator of choice because of its balanced effect on arterial resistance and venous capacitance. Nitroprusside simultaneously reduces SVR and venous return (preload) and is especially useful in the presence of pulmonary edema. Its afterload reducing effects enhance contractility and allow a higher ejection of blood. The decreased venous return coupled with enhanced ejection reduces myocardial and pulmonary congestion, and filling pressures (CVP and PCWP) are reduced.[15,51] Nitroprusside infusion is begun at 0.5 µg/kg/min and is increased in small increments every 5 to 10 minutes until MAP falls 5 to 10 mm Hg below previous levels but systolic pressure remains above 95 to 90 mm Hg. The normal therapeutic range of nitroprusside administration is 0.5 to 8.0 µg/kg/min. Hemodynamic, oxygenation, and organ function parameters are repeated and assessed for improvement in the patient's status, and therapy is adjusted appropriately.[51]

Nitroglycerin. Nitroglycerin is predominantly a venous dilator; thus its effect on arterial resistance and SVR is minimal. However, one study demonstrated that nitroglycerin ointment was successful in reducing SVR and increasing CO in patients with hypodynamic sepsis.[51] If nitroglycerin is the vasodilator of choice, infusions are begun at 400 µg/hr and titrated up every 5 to 10 minutes until the desired PCWP is attained and the MAP falls no more than 5 to 10 mm Hg. Reassessment of the patient's status determines further needs for manipulation of the infusion.[51]

Other agents. Phentolamine (Regitine) is primarily an arterial vasodilator and has significant effects on SVR but minimal influence on PCWP. However, tachycardia is a major side effect. Hydralazine and isosorbide dinitrate have also been used experimentally in patients with sepsis; however, these drugs are not commonly used in the clinical setting for treatment of septic shock.[51] Prostacyclin and PGE₁ have been researched in relation to decreasing pulmonary vascular resistance and right ventricular afterload in patients with ARDS. Although initial hemodynamic and oxygenation parameters improved, long-term survival and development of MSOF were not affected.[60-62]

Combination therapy. Combination therapy with an inotrope and vasodilator is the most common form of unloading therapy used in the treatment of sepsis-induced cardiogenic shock. The inotrope, usually dopamine, maintains MAP and enhances contractility while the vasodilator, usually nitroprusside, reduces afterload and PWCP. The combined effects result in a greater increase in cardiac output than either medication alone.[51] As noted earlier, if maximum dopamine infusion fails to enhance cardiac performance, other inotropes such as dobutamine, epinephrine, and amrinone may be effective. However, patients who require such massive hemodynamic support have a poor prognosis.[15]

Mechanical support

Other therapies for cardiac augmentation are the mechanical support devices: the intraaortic balloon pump (IABP) and ventricular assist devices (VAD). Both devices have been effective when used in the population of patients with primary cardiac disease. Their use in the patient with septic MSOF is not supported by the literature.[48,63-67]

Intraaortic balloon pump. The IABP is the most commonly used support device (Fig. 10-9). The balloon is usually inserted percutaneously through the femoral artery into the aorta and lies just distal to the left subclavian artery. Balloon inflation occurs during diastole. This inflation drives blood into the aortic root, increasing aortic root diastolic

pressure and thereby increasing coronary artery perfusion. Balloon deflation occurs immediately before systole. The deflation of the balloon leaves a dead space that acts as a vacuum and "pulls" blood from the heart and functionally reduces afterload.[66]

Current studies indicate that the coronary arteries are hyperperfused during septic shock.[30-32] In addition, reduced afterload with a high cardiac output is the usual sequela in sepsis. For those patients who exhibit cardiogenic shock–like symptoms superimposed on sepsis, the IABP does not reverse or improve the pathologic mechanisms ongoing at the cellular level such as vasoconstriction, arteriovenous shunting, microembolization, alterations in oxygen use, and end-organ dysfunction. Thus the successful use of the IAPB in septic MSOF is rare.[48]

Ventricular assist devices. The right and left ventricular assist devices (RVAD and LVAD) serve to temporarily replace the patient's ventricle with a mechanical device while the heart recovers from a potentially reversible injury. Support can be either univentricular or biventricular. For left ventricular support (Fig. 10-10), blood exits the body through the left atrial cannula, is pumped through the LVAD, and is returned to the systemic circulation through the aortic cannula. For right ventricular support (Fig. 10-11), blood exits through the right atrial cannula, is pumped through the RVAD, and is returned to the pulmonary system through the pulmonary artery cannula. Biventricular support would include simultaneous placement and usage of the RVAD and LVAD for complete cardiac support (Fig. 10-12).[63,65,67]

Selection criteria for VAD use include failure to wean from cardiopulmonary support following cardiac surgery, cardiogenic shock following acute myocardial infarction, acute cardiac deterioration while awaiting cardiac transplantation, and drug-induced cardiac failure.[63,65,67] Patients who are not potential candidates for cardiac transplantation should not be placed on VADs.[63] Thus, like the IABP, current indications for the use of the VAD do not include the patient with septic MSOF, and use does not reverse the pathophysiologic conditions at the cellular level.

CONCLUSION

Myocardial dysfunction in septic shock is a complex phenomenon that results from numerous phys-

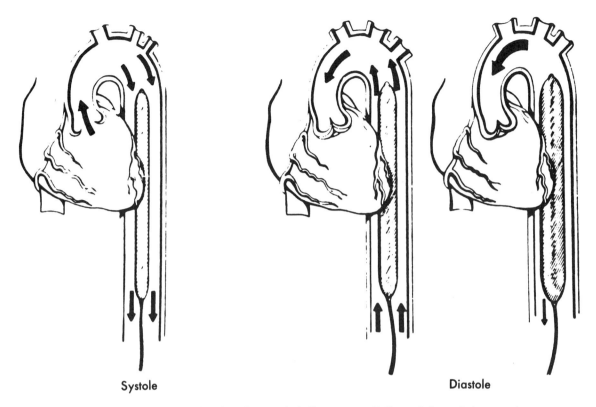

Systole   Diastole

Fig. 10-9 Mechanisms of action: intraaortic balloon pump. Balloon deflates during systole, unloading ventricle; balloon inflates during diastole, increasing coronary perfusion pressure and myocardial oxygen supply. (From Reemtsma K, Bregman D, Cohen SS, Kaskel P. Mechanical circulatory support: Advances in intraaortic balloon pumping. In: Shoemaker WC, Ayres S, Grenvik A, Holbrook PR, and Thompson WL, ed. Textbook of critical care. Philadelphia: WB Saunders Company, 1989:420.)

iologic derangements and humoral mediators. The biventricular systolic and diastolic alterations lead to critical changes in hemodynamic parameters that vary significantly between survivors and nonsurvivors. The ability of the ventricles to dilate and use preload reserve in response to the declining pump function appears to be a key determinant in survival. In addition, early and aggressive interventions by a knowledgeable health-care team are essential. The goal of therapy is to increase and maintain perfusion, often at supranormal levels, in order to meet the demands of the hypermetabolic organs. Initial treatment includes volume resuscitation to achieve an MAP greater than 60 mm Hg, a PCWP of 12 to 15 mm Hg, and end-organ perfusion. In the event volume resuscitation is inef-

fective, inotropes and vasopressor agents are added to the treatment regimen. Systemic vasodilators are indicated only in the minority of patients who demonstrate a clinical picture that is consistent with cardiogenic shock (elevated SVR). Mechanical support is sometimes attempted in patients with severe myocardial depression, but such support rarely improves the final outcome.

Despite advances in critical care technology and science, the mortality of patients with septic shock remains at 40% to 60%; MSOF mortality remains at 60% to 100%. However, research in this area continues in order to identify, clarify, and inhibit the mechanisms producing the abnormal cardiovascular sequelae characteristic of sepsis and the MSOF syndrome.

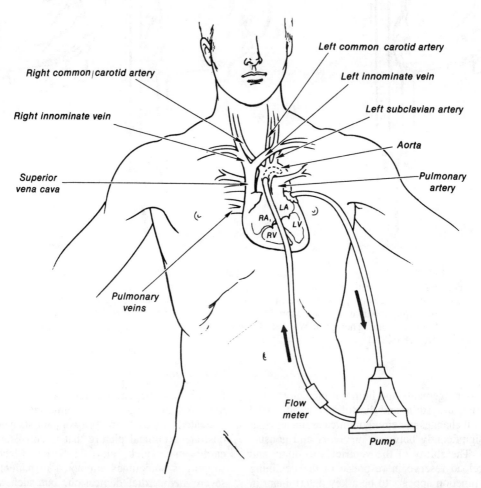

Fig. 10-10 Left ventricular assist device. (From Mulford E. Nursing perspectives for the patient receiving postoperative ventricular assistance in the critical care unit. Heart Lung 1987:16:247.)

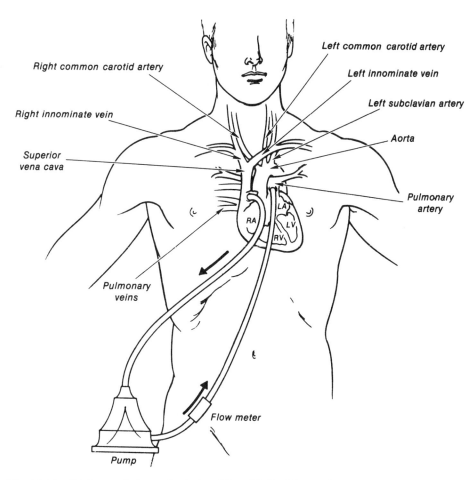

Fig. 10-11 Right ventricular assist device. (From Mulford E. Nursing perspectives for the patient receiving postoperative ventricular assistance in the critical care unit. Heart Lung 1987:16:248.)

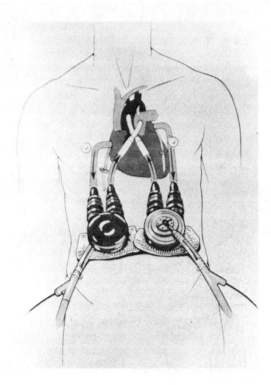

Fig. 10-12 Biventricular mechanical assistance. (From Ruzevish SH, Swartz MT, Pennington DG. Nursing care of the patient with a pneumatic ventricular assist device. Heart Lung 1988:17:401.)

REFERENCES

1. Cunnion RE, Parrillo JE. Myocardial dysfunction in sepsis. Crit Care Clin 1989:5:99-118.
2. Archer LT. Myocardial dysfunction in endotoxin- and *E coli*-induced shock: Pathophysiological mechanisms. Circ Shock 1985:15:261-280.
3. Goldfarb RD. Cardiac mechanical performance in circulatory shock: A critical review of methods and results. Circ Shock 1982:9:633-653.
4. Natanson C, Hoffman WD, Parrillo JE. Septic shock: The cardiovascular abnormality and therapy. J Cardiothor Anesth 1989:3:215-227.
5. Hess ML, Hastillo A, Greenfield LJ. Spectrum of cardiovascular function during gram-negative sepsis. Prog Cardiovasc Dis 1981:23:279-298.
6. Rackow EC et al. Hemodynamic response to fluid repletion in patients with septic shock: Evidence of early depression of cardiac performance. Circ Shock 1987:22:11-22.
7. Siegel JH. Cardiorespiratory manifestations of metabolic failure in sepsis and the multiple organ failure syndrome. Surg Clin North Am 1983:63:379-399.
8. Dhainaut JF et al. Right ventricular dysfunction in patients with septic shock. Intensive Care Med 1988:14:488-491.
9. McDonough KH, Lang CH, Spitzer JJ. The effect of hyperdynamic sepsis on myocardial performance. Circ Shock 1985:15:247-259.
10. Ognibene FP et al. Depressed left ventricular performance: Response to volume infusion in patients with sepsis and septic shock. Chest 1988:93:903-910.
11. Parker MM et al. Right ventricular dysfunction and dilatation, similar to left ventricular changes, characterize the cardiac depression of septic shock in humans. Chest 1990:97:126-131.
12. Parker MM et al. Profound but reversible myocardial depression in patients with septic shock. Ann Intern Med 1984:100:483-490.
13. Parrillo JE. Cardiovascular dysfunction in human septic shock. Prog Clin Biol Res 1989:308:191-199.
14. Fry DE. Multiple system organ failure. Surg Clin North Am 1988:68:107-122.
15. Parrillo JE. Septic shock in humans: Clinical evaluation, pathogenesis, and therapeutic approach. In: Shoemaker WC, Ayres S, Grenvik A, Holbrook PR, Thompson WL, eds. Textbook of critical care. Philadelphia: WB Saunders, 1989:1006-1024.
16. Knaus WA, Wagner DP. Multiple systems organ failure: Epidemiology and prognosis. Crit Care Clin 1989:5:221-232.
17. Sibbald WJ. Myocardial function in the critically ill: Factors influencing left and right ventricular performance in patients with sepsis and trauma. Surg Clin North Am 1985:65:867-1003.
18. Adams HR, Parker JL, Laughlin MH. Intrinsic myocardial dysfunction during endotoxemia: Dependent or independent of myocardial ischemia? Circ Shock 1990:30:63-76.
19. Bersten MB, Sibbald WJ. Circulatory disturbances in multiple systems organ failure. Crit Care Clin 1989:5:233-254.
20. Russell JA et al. Oxygen delivery and consumption and ventricular preload are greater in survivors than in nonsurvivors of the adult respiratory distress syndrome. Am Rev Respir Dis 1990:141:659-665.
21. Sibbald WJ. Circulatory responses to the sepsis syndrome. Prog Clin Biol Res 1989:308:1075-1085.
22. Calvin JE, Sibbald WJ. Applied cardiovascular physiology in the critically ill with special reference to diastole and ventricular interaction. In: Shoemaker WC, Ayres S, Grenvik A, Holbrook PR, Thompson WL, ed. Textbook of critical care. Philadelphia: WB Saunders, 1989:312-326.
23. Braunwald E, Sonnenblick EH, Ross J. Mechanisms of cardiac contraction and relaxation. In: Braunwald E, ed. Heart disease: A textbook of cardiovascular medicine, Volume 1. Philadelphia: WB Saunders, 1988:383-414.
24. Raper R, Sibbald WJ. Misled by the wedge? The Swan-Ganz catheter and left ventricular preload. Chest 1986:89:427-434.
25. Weil MH, von Planta M, Rackow EC. Acute circulatory failure (shock). In: Braunwald E, ed. Heart disease: A textbook of cardiovascular medicine, Volume 1. Philadelphia: WB Saunders, 1988:561-578.
26. Sibbald WJ et al. Biventricular function in the adult respiratory distress syndrome: Hemodynamic and radionuclide assessment, with special emphasis on right ventricular function. Chest 1983:84:126-134.
27. Glantz SA, Parmley WW. Factors which affect the diastolic pressure-volume curve. Circ Res 1978:42:171-180.

28. Lewis BS, Gotsman MS. Current concepts of left ventricular relaxation and compliance. Am Heart J 1980:99:101-112.

29. Parrillo JE. The cardiovascular pathophysiology of sepsis. Annu Rev Med 1985:40:469-485.

30. Cunnion RE et al. The coronary circulation in human septic shock. Circulation 1986:73:637-644.

31. Dhainaut JF et al. Coronary hemodynamics and myocardial metabolism of lactate, free fatty acids, glucose, and ketones in patients with septic shock. Circulation 1987:75:533-541.

32. Shapiro R et al. Sepsis induced coronary vasodilatation (Abstract). Circ Shock 1985:16:79-80.

33. Braunwald E, Sobel BE. Coronary blood flow and myocardial ischemia. In: Braunwald E, ed. Heart disease: A textbook of cardiovascular medicine, Volume 2. Philadephia: WB Saunders, 1988:1191-1203.

34. Hersch M et al. Histopathological evidence of tissue ischemia in a hyperdynamic and nonhypotensive septic animal model (Abstract). Crit Care Med 1988:16:421.

35. Raper RF, Sibbald WJ. The effects of coronary artery disease on cardiac function in nonhypotensive sepsis. Chest 1988:94:507-511.

36. Parker JL, Jones CE. The heart in shock. In: Hardaway RM. Shock: The reversible stage of dying. Littleton: PSG Publishing Company, 1988:348-363.

37. Raymond RM. When does the heart fail during shock? Circ Shock 1990:30:27-41.

38. Smith LW, McDonough KH. Inotropic sensitivity to beta-adrenergic stimulation in early sepsis. Am J Physiol 1988:255:H699-H703.

39. Parrillo JE et al. A circulating myocardial depressant substance in humans with septic shock: Septic shock patients with a reduced ejection fraction have a circulating factor that depresses *in vitro* myocardial cell performance. J Clin Invest 1985:76:1539-1553.

40. Brenner M et al. Determination of direct myocardial contractile effects of eicosanoids, endotoxin, tumor necrosis factor and other mediators using a newly designed quantitative cellular contractility assay (Abstract). Clin Res 1987:35:785A.

41. Suffredini AF et al. The cardiovascular response of normal humans to the administration of endotoxin. N Engl J Med 1989:321:280-287.

42. Danner RL. Mediators and endotoxin inhibitors, 235-237. In: Parrillo JE, moderator. Septic shock in humans: Advances in the understanding of pathogenesis, cardiovascular dysfunction, and therapy. Ann Intern Med 1990:113:227-242.

43. Beutler B, Cerami A. Cachectin: More than a tumor necrosis factor. N Engl J Med 1987:316:379-385.

44. Ognibene FP et al. Interleukin-2 administration causes reversible hemodynamic changes and left ventricular dysfunction similar to those seen in septic shock. Chest 1988:94:750-754.

45. Ognibene FP et al. Neutrophil aggregation activity and septic shock in humans: Neutrophil aggregation by a C5a-like material occurs more frequently than complement component depletion and correlates with depression of systemic vascular resistance. J Crit Care 1988:3:103-111.

46. Hechtman HB et al. Prostaglandin and thromboxane mediation of cardiopulmonary failure. Surg Clin North Am 1983:63:263-283.

47. Lefer AM. Induction of tissue injury and altered cardiovascular performance by platelet-activating factor: Relevance to multiple systems organ failure. Crit Care Clin 1989:5:331-352.

48. Parker MM, Parrillo, JE. Septic shock and other forms of distributive shock. In: Parrillo JE, ed. Current therapy in critical care medicine. Philadelphia: BC Decker, 1987:44-55.

49. Li TCM et al. The impact of tertiary physicians on a community hospital intensive care unit. JAMA 1984:252:2023.

50. Parrillo JE. Septic shock: Clinical manifestations, pathogenesis, hemodynamics, and management in a critical care unit. In: Parrillo JE, Ayres SM, ed. Major issues in critical care medicine. Baltimore: Williams & Wilkins, 1984:111-125.

51. Sibbald WJ et al. Concepts in the pharmacologic and non-pharmacologic support of cardiovascular function in critically ill surgical patients. Surg Clin North Am 1983:63:455-482.

52. Ognibene FP. Management of septic shock, 239-240. In: Parrillo JE, moderator. Septic shock in humans: Advances in the understanding of pathogenesis, cardiovascular dysfunction, and therapy. Ann Intern Med 1990:113:227-242.

53. Luce JM. Pathogenesis and management of septic shock. Chest 1987:91:883-888.

54. Thijs LG, Teule GJJ, Bronsveld W. Problems in the treatment of septic shock. Resuscitation 1984:11:147-155.

55. Chernow B, Roth BL. Pharmacologic manipulation of the peripheral vasculature in shock: Clinical and experimental approaches. Circ Shock 1986:18:141-155.

56. Fajfer LI, Goldberg LI. Sympathomimetic amines in the treatment of shock. In: Shoemaker WC, Ayres S, Grenvik A, Holbrook PR, Thompson WL, eds. Textbook of Critical Care. Philadelphia: WB Saunders, 1989:438-440.

57. Meadows D et al. Reversal of intractable septic shock with norepinephrine therapy. Crit Care Med 1988;16:663-666.

58. Schaer GL, Fink MP, Parrillo JE. Norepinephrine alone versus norepinephrine plus low-dose dopamine: Enhanced renal blood flow with combination pressor therapy. Crit Care Med 1985:13:492-496.

59. Schremmer B, Dhainaut JF. Heart failure in septic shock: Effects of inotropic support. Crit Care Med 1990:18:S49-S55.

60. Bone RC et al. Randomized double-blind, multicenter study of prostaglandin E_1 in patients with the adult respiratory distress syndrome. Chest 1989:96:114-119.

61. Russell JA, Ronco JJ, Dodek PM. Physiologic effects and side effects of prostaglandin E_1 in the adult respiratory distress syndrome. Chest 1990:97:684-692.

62. Shoemaker WC, Appel PL. Effects of prostaglandin E_1 in adult respiratory distress syndrome. Surgery 1986:99:275-282.

63. Kormos RL, Griffith BP. Ventricular assist devices. In: Shoemaker WC, Ayres S, Grenvik A, Holbrook PR, Thompson WL, eds. Textbook of critical care. Philadelphia: WB Saunders, 1989:428-438.

64. Mulford E. Nursing perspectives for the patient receiving postoperative ventricular assistance in the critical care unit. Heart Lung 1987:16:246-255.

65. Minsinski M. Role of conventional management and alternative therapies in limiting infarct size in acute myocardial infarction. Heart Lung 1987:16:746-755.

66. Reemtsma K et al. Mechanical circulatory support: Advances in intraaortic balloon pumping. In: Shoemaker WC, Ayres S, Grenvik A, Holbrook PR, Thompson WL, eds. Textbook of critical care. Philadelphia: WB Saunders, 1989:420-428.

67. Ruzevish SH, Swartz MT, Pennington DG. Nursing care of the patient with a pneumatic ventricular assist device. Heart Lung 1988:17:399-405.

11 Adult Respiratory Distress Syndrome

Margaret T. Morris

Adult respiratory distress syndrome (ARDS) is responsible for respiratory failure in approximately 150,000 to 250,000 patients a year, having an overall mortality rate of 40% to 60%.[1] The exact cause of death in patients with ARDS is difficult to determine because various underlying pathologic conditions are often present: sepsis, disseminated intravascular coagulation (DIC), and multisystem organ failure (MSOF). Furthermore, death may not be due to failure of gas exchange alone, but rather the multiple organ failure often associated with ARDS.

Adult respiratory distress syndrome can occur in isolation, but it occurs more frequently in the setting of MSOF. ARDS can incite the development of MSOF, or it may develop secondary to the pathophysiologic derangements accompanying the MSOF syndrome. Whether culprit or victim, ARDS contributes to the self-perpetuating nature of MSOF syndrome by exacerbating tissue hypoxia and activating mediators of the inflammatory cascade. ARDS is a complex syndrome manifested by increased capillary permeability, atelectasis, and intraalveolar and interstitial noncardiogenic pulmonary edema, all of which cause a derangement in gas exchange and refractory hypoxemia.

Acute lung injury, noncardiogenic pulmonary edema, and shock lung are terms used to describe the scenario of respiratory failure in the setting of sepsis, MSOF, and critical illness. The most common term, ARDS, will be used in this chapter.

Since the ARDS syndrome was first described by Ashbaugh et al[2] more than 20 years ago, the understanding of the mechanisms of lung injury and clinical manifestations has evolved considerably. It is now clear that a cascade of inflammatory/immune reactions, including activation of the coagulation system, greatly contributes to lung injury. The exact role of each mechanism has not been fully defined.

A variety of clinical conditions are responsible for initiating the cascade of events that cause lung injury, ARDS, and MSOF. Causes can be differentiated as direct (pulmonary) and indirect (systemic) (see box below).[3] Overt signs and symptoms can be evident immediately or as late as 48 to 72 hours after the initial insult. Clinical features of ARDS include refractory hypoxemia, decreased

---

ETIOLOGY OF ARDS

Direct causes

Inhalation of toxins
Aspiration of gastric contents
Pulmonary contusion
Thoracic trauma
Bacterial/viral pneumonia
Oxygen toxicity
Fat emboli
Near drowning

Indirect causes

Septic shock
Other shock states
Multiple trauma
Disseminated intravascular coagulation
Pancreatitis
Thermal injuries
Anaphylaxis
Multiple blood transfusions

From Vaughan P, Brooks C. Adult respiratory distress syndrome: A complication of shock. Crit Care Nurs Clin North Am 1990;2:236.

pulmonary compliance, radiographic evidence of noncardiogenic pulmonary edema, and normal pulmonary capillary wedge pressures (PCWP).[4] For the critically ill patient, it is sometimes difficult to determine when the initial injury precipitating the development of ARDS occurred. Distinguishing ARDS from other causes of respiratory failure in these patients is also difficult, especially in the presence of underlying chronic disease and other host-related factors such as age, immunosuppression, and previous infection.

LUNG INJURY SCORE

Chest roentgenogram score

No alveolar consolidation	0
Alveolar consolidation in 1 quadrant	1
Alveolar consolidation in 2 quadrants	2
Alveolar consolidation in 3 quadrants	3
Alveolar consolidation in all 4 quadrants	4

Hypoxemia score

$Pao_2/Fio_2 \geq 300$	0
Pao_2/Fio_2 225-299	1
Pao_2/Fio_2 175-224	2
Pao_2/Fio_2 100-174	3
$Pao_2/Fio_2 <100$	4

Respiratory system compliance score (when ventilated) (mL/cm H_2O)

≥ 80	0
60-79	1
40-59	2
20-39	3
≤ 19	4

Positive end-expiratory pressure (PEEP) score (when ventilated)(cm H_2O)

≤ 5	0
6-8	1
9-11	2
12-14	3
≥ 15	4

The final value is obtained by dividing the aggregate sum by the number of components that were used.

Score

No injury	0
Mild to moderate injury	0.1-2.5
Severe injury (ARDS)	>2.5

From Murray JF et al. An expanded definition of the adult respiratory distress syndrome. Am Rev Respir Dis 1988;138:721.

The purposes of this chapter are to review the definition and diagnosis of ARDS; discuss principles of ventilation, perfusion, and gas transport; describe the pathophysiology of ARDS; discuss the clinical presentation; and outline therapeutic strategies used in the management of ARDS.

DEFINITION AND DIAGNOSIS

Defining and diagnosing ARDS involves three components.[1,5,6] First, an acute lung injury score is determined. Second, the clinical disorder associated with the development of ARDS is identified. Third, nonpulmonary organ involvement is determined. This systemic approach allows for a more accurate estimate of the actual incidence and prognosis of ARDS.[1] By providing an expanded definition of ARDS, this system shifts the focus of management from the treatment of an isolated severe lung injury to treating the severe lung injury, underlying systemic process, and multisystem organ involvement.

Acute lung injury score

The acute lung injury scoring system provides an objective measure for diagnosing and determining the severity of ARDS.[1] Four component scores are included in the scoring system: chest roentgenogram, hypoxemia, respiratory system compliance, and positive end-expiratory pressure (PEEP) (see box at the left).

Clinical disorders

Sepsis and gastric aspiration are the leading causes of ARDS; however, many factors are associated with the development of ARDS (see box on p. 204). It is not uncommon for a patient to have several direct and indirect pulmonary insults. One may actually potentiate another. For example, the lung with ARDS is more at risk for bacterial colonization and pneumonia.[7]

Nonpulmonary organ failure

Nonpulmonary organ failure is common in ARDS and must be identified early to minimize morbidity and mortality. The combination of ARDS with another organ failure carries a much greater mortality rate than either occurring in isolation. For example, hepatic failure with ARDS has almost a 100% mortality rate.[8] The box

---

EXPANDED DEFINITION OF ARDS

Severity of acute lung injury

Arterial oxygenation (Pao_2/Fio_2)
Chest radiograph
Static lung compliance
PEEP level

Associated clinical disorder(s)

Sepsis (microbiology, anatomic site)
Aspiration (type)
Major trauma
Drug overdose
Cardiopulmonary bypass
Others (bone marrow transplant)

Systemic organ function

Acid/base status
Renal function
Hematologic abnormalities
Hepatic function
Central nervous system function
Cardiovascular function

From Matthay MA. The adult respiratory distress syndrome: New insights into diagnosis, pathophysiology and treatment. West J Med 1989;150:190.

above summarizes the criteria for the expanded definition of ARDS.

PULMONARY PHYSIOLOGY

Through the process of gas exchange, the respiratory system provides oxygen for transport to the tissues. Oxygen moves from the atmosphere into the blood, and carbon dioxide moves from the blood out to the atmosphere. The respiratory process can be divided into three different phases: (1) ventilation, (2) diffusion/perfusion, and (3) gas transport. Disorders of the respiratory system can include abnormalities of one or all of these phases. An understanding of normal pulmonary physiology is an integral step in the appreciation of ARDS pathophysiology.

Ventilation

Ventilation involves air movement from the atmosphere through all branches of the airway to the terminal alveoli. The involuntary process of ventilation involves active motion of the thorax during inspiration and passive elastic recoil of the lungs and thoracic cage during expiration.

Muscles of ventilation. The diaphragm and the external intercostal muscles perform most of the work of normal, quiet ventilation. The diaphragm, a domed-shaped muscle located between the thorax and the abdomen, is innervated by the phrenic nerve of the autonomic nervous system.[9,10] When the diaphragm contracts, the lower portions of the lungs are pulled downward, increasing the vertical dimension of the chest. Contraction of the external intercostal muscles during inspiration increases the anteroposterior diameter of the thorax. Both of these muscular activities increase lung volume, thereby decreasing the intrathoracic and intraalveolar pressure. Slightly negative intraalveolar pressure with respect to atmospheric pressure causes air to flow inward from the mouth through the lungs.

Exhalation occurs passively through elastic recoil of the lungs and thorax. The lungs return to the resting volume, intraalveolar pressure increases above atmospheric, and air rushes out of the lungs.

Ventilatory control. Ventilation is regulated by neuronal control and chemical control. Other factors that contribute to the control of ventilation are changes in body temperature, pressoreceptors responding to changes in the blood pressure, stretch receptors located in the lungs, and pharmacologic agents.

Neuronal control. Spontaneous involuntary ventilation occurs through innervation of the respiratory muscles. The respiratory center is located in the medulla oblongata and the pons, and impulses travel down the phrenic nerve to stimulate contraction of the diaphragm.

Chemical control. Central chemoreceptors, located in the medulla, and peripheral chemoreceptors, located in the carotid bodies and aortic bodies, are the two main components of chemical control for respiration. In chemical regulation, changes in respiratory neuronal activity occur in response to the concentration of carbon dioxide (CO_2), hydrogen ions (H^+), and oxygen (O_2) in the body fluids.[9,10]

Distribution of ventilation. In the healthy lungs of a person standing or sitting, the alveoli in the apices remain more distended than those in the bases. The alveoli at the bases are slightly compressed by the weight of the tissue in the upper portions of the lung. Because the apical alveoli are more distended, they expand less during inspiration compared to the alveoli located in the bases.[10,11]

In the supine position, the alveoli in the apices and bases are ventilated equally, with the dependent portions of the lungs most affected by gravity and the weight of the tissue. Ventilation and perfusion are more equally matched in the supine position[10] (Fig. 11-1).

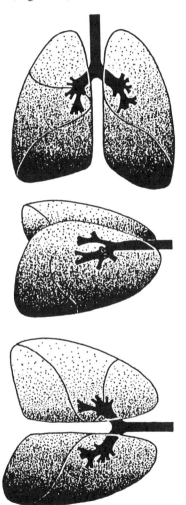

Fig. 11-1 The effects of position on pulmonary blood flow and gas exchange. (From Shapiro BA, Harrison RA, Walton JR. The physiology of external respiration. In: Shapiro BA, Harrison RA, Walton JR, eds. Clinical application of blood gases. 3rd ed. St Louis: Mosby–Year Book, 1982;56.)

Dead-space ventilation. Anatomic dead space refers to that portion of ventilation in the tracheobronchial tree that is not involved in gas exchange. Alveolar dead space refers to alveoli that are ventilated but not perfused.[9,10] The combination of anatomic dead space and alveolar dead space is termed physiologic dead space.[9,10] Increased dead space contributes to ventilation-perfusion (V/Q) mismatching and impaired gas exchange. The addition of ventilator tubing and artificial airways increases the calculated dead space.

Lung mechanics

Compliance. Lung compliance refers to the distensibility of the lungs. The pressure required to achieve a change in the lung volume is the lung compliance, and it is opposed by the elastic recoil of the lung.[9-11] The greater the elastic recoil or stiffness of the lung secondary to pathologic changes, the lower the compliance.

The compliance of the entire respiratory system is influenced by the lung compliance and chest-wall compliance. Chest-wall compliance decreases with age (the chest wall becomes stiff), obesity, and chest deformities such as kyphoscoliosis.[11]

Surface tension. Forces between molecules of a liquid are very strong (stronger than gas-liquid interface), so the liquid surface area becomes as small as possible. Pulmonary surfactant, a surface layer phospholipid produced by type II alveolar epithelial cells, decreases the surface tension of the alveolar sac.[11] By decreasing surface tension, surfactant stabilizes patent alveoli and increases lung compliance.

Airway resistance. Four major factors determine airway resistance: cross-sectional area of the airways, velocity of gas flow, the density of gas, and the total lung volume.[11] Airway resistance increases secondary to pathologic obstruction to airflow resulting from secretions, inflammation, edema, airway collapse or constriction, or mass lesions in the airways. Normally, most of the energy expended for ventilation is used to overcome the elasticity and airway resistance of the respiratory system.[12] However, if an underlying pathologic condition is present, energy is expended to overcome this frictional resistance to airflow as well. The pathologic conditions causing respiratory failure can affect both airway resistance and lung compliance. Artificial airways (endotracheal tube) and mechanical ventilation also increase airway resistance and the work of breathing.

The work of breathing for a normal individual at rest consumes approximately 5% of the body's total oxygen uptake.[13] Voluntary exercise may increase this value 25% to 30%.[13] When there is significant pulmonary disease, the oxygen consumption of the work of breathing may exceed 30% of the total body consumption.[13]

Lung perfusion

Gas exchange occurs at the level of the pulmonary capillary bed. The capillary bed is a low pressure system that contains approximately 50 to 60 mL of flowing blood. The pulmonary capillary endothelium is one cell thick and has very little support from surrounding structures; therefore the capillaries may collapse or expand depending on internal or external pressures. Only 25% to 35% of the pulmonary capillaries are open under normal resting conditions.[10] This percentage can increase dramatically through the process of recruitment (opening of capillaries not previously opened) and dilatation (expansion of currently opened capillaries) to accommodate changes in the cardiac output.[10] These mechanisms are responsible for decreased pulmonary vascular resistance as blood flow through the lungs increases. Conversely, vasoconstriction or collapse of capillaries resulting from increased surrounding pressures will cause increased pulmonary vascular resistance.

Patient positioning affects blood flow to lung regions in the same way that it affects ventilation (Fig. 11-1). The blood flow is greater in the dependent portions of the lung, which may not match the areas that have the greatest number of ventilated alveoli (see Ventilation/Perfusion Matching). Blood flow may also be affected by positive-pressure ventilation, PEEP, exercise, or a change in cardiac output.[10]

Diffusion

Diffusion is a passive process involving gas transfer across the alveolocapillary membrane in the presence of a concentration gradient. Factors that affect diffusion include (1) pressure difference between the concentration of alveolar gas and the gas in the capillary blood, (2) surface area of alveolocapillary membrane, (3) membrane thickness and integrity, (4) the diffusion coefficient of the gas, and (5) amount of hemoglobin in the blood.[9]

The alveolocapillary membrane includes the (1) surfactant lining, (2) alveolar epithelium and its basement membrane, (3) tissue in the intercalated interstitial space, and (4) capillary endothelium and its basement membrane.[14] The alveolar epithelium is composed of two important cell types: alveolar type I cells have large, thin surfaces with very little cytoplasm and provide the major structural anatomy of the alveolus. They are vulnerable to injury from direct or indirect causes. Alveolar type II cells produce surfactant and are also damaged easily. Another important cell type abundant in the lung is the alveolar macrophage, which constitutes the most important mechanism for fighting pulmonary infection. Macrophages release several mediators as part of the inflammatory process. Both a deficiency in function and the inability to down regulate can facilitate injury and infection in the lung. This injury and infection can alter both diffusion and V/Q matching.

Ventilation/perfusion matching

Ventilated alveoli must come into contact with perfused capillaries for gas exchange to occur. Total lung perfusion slightly exceeds ventilation because normally there is some perfusion of nonventilated alveoli; therefore the normal ventilation-to-perfusion ratio (V/Q) is approximately 0.8 rather than 1.0 (a 1.0 ratio would indicate exact match between ventilation and perfusion).[9,15]

The V/Q ratio differs in various zones of the lungs. Intravascular hydrostatic pressures change in different areas of the pulmonary capillary bed in relation to the vertical distance from a particular capillary to the heart. The intraalveolar pressure also differs at any particular point in relation to gravity. As described by West,[16] in zone I, intravascular pressure is lower than the intraalveolar pressure, and the capillary is totally collapsed because of pressure from surrounding alveoli. In zone II, the intravascular inflow (arterial) pressure exceeds intraalveolar pressure, but alveolar pressures are higher than intravascular outflow (venous) pressures. The result is a narrowed capillary and intermittent flow regulated, in part, by the cardiac cycle. In zone III, greater intravascular inflow and outflow pressures are unaffected by alveolar pressures, and the capillary remains fully dilated throughout the respiratory and cardiac cycle[16] (Fig. 11-2). High levels of PEEP decrease the number of perfused capillary beds and increase the area of

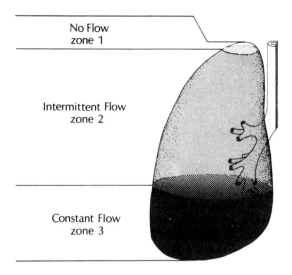

Fig. 11-2 The three-zone model illustrating the effects of gravity and pulmonary perfusion. (From Shapiro BA, Harrison RA, Walton JR. The physiology of external respiration. In: Shapiro BA, Harrison RA, Walton JR, eds. Clinical application of blood gases. 3rd ed. St Louis: Mosby–Year Book, 1982;57.)

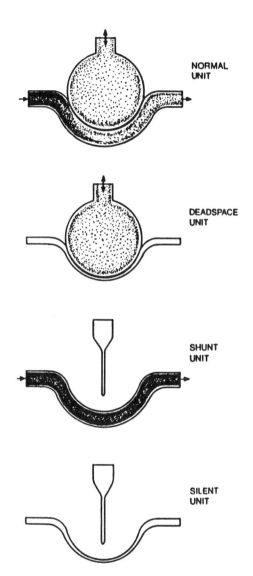

Fig. 11-3 The respiratory unit: Abnormalities of ventilation/perfusion matching. (From Shapiro BA, Harrison RA, Walton JR. The physiology of external respiration. In: Shapiro BA, Harrison RA, Walton JR, eds. Clinical application of blood gases. 3rd ed. St Louis: Mosby–Year Book, 1982;65.)

zones I and II as the increased intraalveolar and intrathoracic pressure compresses the poorly supported capillaries.

Alterations in ventilation, perfusion, or their matching impair gas exchange (Fig. 11-3). For example, if ventilation is decreased because of conditions such as pulmonary edema, mucous plugging, atelectasis, or pneumonia, the V/Q ratio is less than 0.8 and may produce hypoxemia.[17] If perfusion becomes impaired as in pulmonary emboli, vasoconstriction secondary to hypoxia, low cardiac output, and loss of capillary flow, the V/Q ratio will be greater than 0.8, also potentiating hypoxemia.

Intrapulmonary shunt. A pulmonary shunt is the component of pulmonary blood flow that is perfusing unventilated alveoli, and therefore not participating in gas exchange.[9] Pulmonary shunting is a severe form of V/Q mismatch. Normally, a shunt of 3% to 5% exists secondary to the venous drainage of the bronchial, pleural, and thebesian veins mixing with oxygenated blood in the pulmonary veins and left atrium. Also, perfusion slightly exceeds ventilation.[9]

In ARDS, intrapulmonary shunts may exceed 15% to 20%, since perfusion of collapsed and poorly functioning alveolar units does not contribute to gas exchange.[11] The shunt percentage can be estimated by dividing the fraction of inspired oxygen (FiO_2) by the arterial oxygen tension (PaO_2). Normal PaO_2/FiO_2 ratio is more than 300 to 400.[15] A lower value usually indicates the presence of a shunt (see box on p. 205). Large shunt fractions indicate that a large percentage of the cardiac output is returning to the left side of the heart unoxygenated. Poor oxygen content and tissue oxygen delivery are the ultimate results.

Gas transport

Approximately 98% of oxygen transported in the blood is bound to hemoglobin, with the remaining 2% dissolved in the plasma.[9] The amount dissolved in the plasma (measured by PaO_2) determines the saturation of hemoglobin. Oxygen combined with hemoglobin is referred to as oxyhemoglobin, and the percent saturation (SaO_2) refers to the amount of oxygen actually carried by the hemoglobin in relation to the hemoglobin's total oxygen-carrying capacity. Oxygen saturation and the partial pressure of oxygen have a curvilinear relationship. On the steep portion of the curve (PaO_2 less than 50 to 60 mm Hg), saturation of hemoglobin dramatically decreases with small changes in PaO_2. Factors that affect the oxyhemoglobin dissociation curve and thus SaO_2 are pH, temperature, 2,3-diphosphoglycerate (2,3-DPG), and $PaCO_2$ levels (see Chapter 6).[9]

Carbon dioxide (CO_2) is the end-product of cellular metabolism. It is transported in the blood in three forms: (1) a dissolved state measured as $PaCO_2$ (5% to 10%), (2) as carbamino compounds (10% to 20%), and (3) as bicarbonate (70% to 90%). In the lungs, the bicarbonate combines with H^+ to form carbonic acid (H_2CO_3), which dissociates into CO_2 and water.[10] The CO_2 diffuses out of the plasma and red blood cells into the alveoli under the influence of a pressure gradient. Carbon dioxide diffuses 20 times more readily than oxygen does and is the most accurate indicator of minute ventilation (respiratory rate × tidal volume)[15]; therefore alterations in ventilation cause abnormal CO_2 levels.

There is an intricate relationship between PaO_2 and $PaCO_2$ loading and unloading both in the peripheral tissues and in the lung. At the tissue level, increased $PaCO_2$ levels shift the oxyhemoglobin dissociation curve to the right, which facilitates oxygen unloading by the hemoglobin.[9] At the lung level, CO_2 and H^+ levels decrease rapidly as CO_2 diffuses into alveoli; pH increases, and the curve shifts to the left. The affinity for oxygen and hemoglobin increases, thus facilitating the uptake of oxygen at the lung.

Adequate tissue oxygenation involves ventilation, diffusion, and oxygen transport. ARDS primarily affects ventilation and diffusion. Refractory hypoxemia causing inadequate tissue oxygenation at the cellular level is the severe consequence of ARDS.

PATHOPHYSIOLOGY

The cascade of events responsible for the acute lung injury seen in ARDS and other organ dysfunction represents the host response to injury. Both cellular and humoral activity contributes to microvascular permeability, pulmonary hypertension, cellular necrosis, epithelial hyperplasia, inflammation, and fibrosis. The exact sequence of mediator activation and release is unknown. Investigators postulate that the initial event precipitating ARDS may determine the progression of mediator responses.[4] It is important to remember that various inflammatory/immune processes contributing to lung injury are initially activated to maintain host defense homeostasis; however, persistent activation (or absence of down regulation) and multiple inflammatory systems combine to cause damage to healthy tissue (such as the endothelium) as well as the targeted injured tissue or foreign substances.[3]

Endothelial damage results in increased capillary permeability, which allows protein-rich fluid to move into the interstitial and alveolar space. Pulmonary hypertension and microvascular obstruction contribute to the fluid shifts, overwhelming the lymphatic vessels. Pulmonary edema and alveolar flooding occur, further disrupting gas exchange.[18-20] The damaged endothelium releases mediators, such as eicosanoids, complement-split products, and tissue factor. Endothelial cell–white blood cell interaction is often accompanied by further mediator release. The following paragraphs summarize the mediators responsible for these changes and their mechanism of action. For an in-depth discussion of the inflammatory mediators, refer to Chapter 3.

Neutrophils

The neutrophils are thought to play a key role in the pathogenesis of ARDS. Following major systemic insults, large numbers of neutrophils are sequestered in the pulmonary vasculature, where they marginate along the endothelial lining.

Activated neutrophils phagocytize injured tissue and foreign debris. This process requires an increased oxygen consumption and is referred to as the "respiratory burst." Oxygen-derived free radicals (ODFRs) are produced as metabolites. In large amounts, ODFRs damage the pulmonary endothelium, contributing to the increased capillary permeability and coagulation abnormalities. Neutrophil aggregation also can cause direct damage to the pulmonary vasculature through vascular obstruction or endothelial damage; tissue ischemia and inflammation result.[3,21] Although it has been shown that ARDS can occur in the neutropenic patient, the majority of research demonstrates a strong correlation between increased neutrophil activity and pulmonary damage.[22]

Alveolar macrophages

Macrophages located in the alveoli and pulmonary vasculature are stimulated by bacteria, foreign substances in the alveoli, activated neutrophils, and endotoxin. Once stimulated, macrophages produce two potent monokines, tumor necrosis factor (TNF) and interleukin-1 (IL-1).[23] Macrophages also produce lysozymes, ODFRs, and arachidonic acid metabolites.[23,24] The macrophages' role in the pathology of ARDS is directly related to the production of these substances and their mechanism of action.

Tumor necrosis factor

TNF is believed to play a major role in the development of ARDS. Direct adverse effects include enhanced release of ODFRs by neutrophils, indirect endothelial damage, decreased vascular responsiveness to catecholamines, and increased capillary permeability.[25-27] The importance of TNF stems not only from its direct toxic effects but also from its ability to promote the elaboration of many secondary mediators of inflammation.

Interleukin-1

Interleukin-1 is primarily produced by macrophages but also by fibroblasts, natural killer cells, and damaged endothelium.[28] Its major contribution to ARDS is related to its synergistic activity with TNF. Both TNF and IL-1 are believed to contribute to increased vascular permeability and the development of microthrombosis.[3] TNF and IL-1 may also indirectly contribute to vascular or tissue damage by causing increased neutrophil aggregation and adhesion to the endothelium.[28]

Arachidonic acid metabolites (eicosanoids)

Arachidonic acid (eicosatetraenoic acid) is present in most cell membranes. When stimulated by tissue injury, endotoxin, and other substances, arachidonic acid is released and metabolized through one of two pathways. Prostaglandins (PG) and thromboxanes (TX) are produced through the cyclooxygenase pathway, and leukotrienes (LT) are produced through the lipoxygenase pathway.[29,30] Many different eicosanoids are produced within these three major classes. In the lung, prostacyclin (PGI_2) causes vasodilatation and decreased platelet aggregation. It acts in opposition to thromboxane A_2 (TXA_2), which causes pulmonary vasoconstriction, platelet aggregation, and bronchoconstriction.[31] Leukotrienes cause vasoconstriction and bronchoconstriction and facilitate increased pulmonary capillary permeability. In ARDS, the ratio of PGI_2 and TXA_2 may shift in the favor of increased TXA_2 production.[29,32]

Proteolytic enzymes

Activated neutrophils and macrophages are responsible for the elaboration of proteolytic enzymes at the site of injury. Elastase is abundant in acute lung injury. Normally, antiproteases inactivate the elastase. In ARDS, there is an imbalance in the protease-antiprotease ratio, resulting in high levels of protease activity.[33] The proteases cause direct injury to the vasculature as well as to lung parenchyma. ODFRs have been implicated in damaging or inhibiting antiprotease activity, thus perpetuating the damage done by the proteases.[34]

Platelet activating factor

Platelet activating factor (PAF) is present in cell membranes and is released by neutrophils, alveolar macrophages, mast cells, platelets, and damaged endothelium.[4] PAF stimulates platelet activation and aggregation, and it also enhances neutrophil adhesion and respiratory burst activity.[35,36] Excessive PAF activity incites increased endothelial damage, increased clot formation, bronchoconstriction, increased pulmonary artery pressures, and further exacerbation of coagulopathies.[36]

Platelets

Activated platelets release eicosanoids, serotonin, PAF, and platelet-derived growth factor.[36] These substances attract and activate neutrophils and cause vasoconstriction and bronchoconstriction. Platelet activation is thought to contribute to pulmonary vascular damage and pulmonary hypertension.

Complement

The complement cascade operates through enzymatic reactions involving more than 20 different plasma proteins. The complement system initiates, facilitates, and enhances the inflammatory/immune response[37] and becomes activated in response to tissue injury, antigen/antibody complexes, endotoxin, and bacteria. Complement contributes to the development of ARDS by increasing neutrophil activity, increasing microvascular permeability, and directly lysing target cells.[38,39] The C5a component of complement has been isolated in the plasma and bronchial alveolar lavage of patients with ARDS.[39]

Other vasoactive substances

The kallikrein/kinin system produces a metabolite, bradykinin, which is a potent vasodilator and increases capillary permeability. The kinins have also been demonstrated to stimulate neutrophil chemotaxis, phagocytosis, and respiratory burst activity.[40]

Histamine, a vasoactive amine, is released by mast cells during the inflammatory/immune response. A potent bronchoconstrictor, histamine, also increases vasodilatation and capillary permeability.

Summary

Regardless of the precipitating event, the combined effects of numerous inflammatory mediators are ultimately responsible for the vascular and lung tissue changes that result in the development of ARDS. Pulmonary hypertension occurs early in ARDS secondary to pulmonary vascular occlusion and uncontrolled vasoconstriction. Bronchocon-

striction also occurs in response to various eicosanoids and humoral substances.

Increased capillary permeability, the hallmark of ARDS, allows protein-rich fluid to leave the intravascular space and fill the surrounding interstitial area. The lymphatic system of the lung is overwhelmed and may be unable to reabsorb fluid adequately. This interstitial fluid increases interstitial pressure, facilitating the movement of fluid through the enlarged epithelial junctions of the alveoli. The protein-rich fluid creates an osmotic gradient in lung tissue, which further enhances fluid movement out of the vasculature. Atelectasis occurs as a result of interstitial edema compressing alveoli and decreased surfactant production. Without surfactant, surface tension increases and alveoli collapse. Reexpanding collapsed alveoli becomes even more difficult.

Lung parenchymal damage results from direct injury by macrophages and various mediators, in addition to cellular necrosis from hypoxia. Eventually, fibrotic tissue replaces the altered lung tissue, and compliance decreases further.[41] Hyaline membranes may form as the body attempts to digest this extracellular protein and cellular debris.[41] Fig. 11-4 diagrams the pathophysiologic cascade of ARDS.

The pathology described above is the result of an exaggerated inflammatory/immune response to some initial event. As endothelial damage continues, more mediators are released, which contribute to further endothelial damage. Current management focuses on supportive care and the prevention of secondary injury related to treatment methods. The future direction of management involves therapies that block or modulate the response of the uncontrolled mediators described above.

CLINICAL PRESENTATION AND ASSESSMENT

Patients may present in various stages of ARDS. Their signs and symptoms indicate respiratory failure, but a definitive diagnosis of ARDS and injury severity score may not be possible until the lung injury progresses and oxygenation worsens.

Signs and symptoms

In general, the patient in early phases of acute respiratory failure will experience dyspnea, tachypnea, tachycardia, and restlessness.[42] An increased

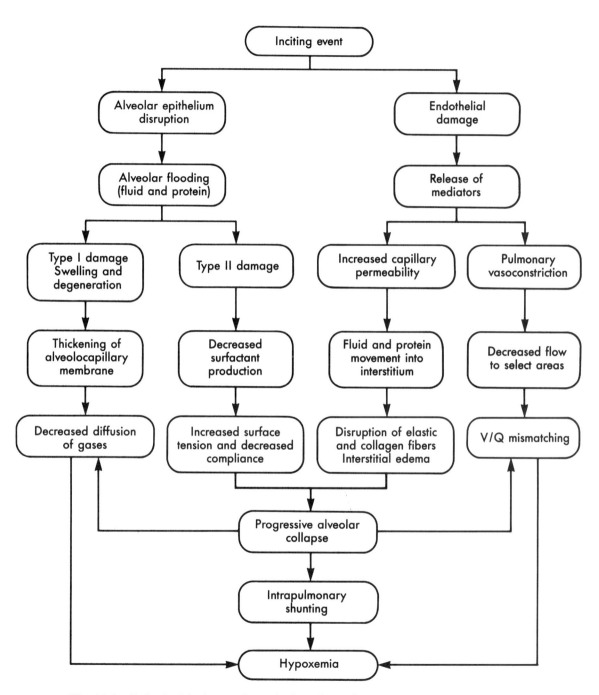

Fig. 11-4 Pathophysiologic cascade mechanism of ARDS. (From Huddleston VB. Pulmonary problems. Crit Care Nurs Clin North Am 1990;2:531.)

Table 11-1 Assessment of Tissue Hypoxia

CNS	Cardiovascular	Pulmonary	Renal	Gastrointestinal/hepatic	Musculoskeletal
Restlessness	Tachycardia	↑ Respiratory rate	↓ Urine output	↓ Bowel sounds	Muscle tremors
Agitation	↑ BP	↑ Tidal volume	Edema	Abdominal distention	Muscle fatigue
Confusion	Widened pulse pressure	Dyspnea	↑ BP	Vomiting	Muscle aches
Irritability	Dysrhythmias	Use of accessory muscles	↑ BUN	Jaundice	Generalized fatigue
Headache	ST- and T-wave changes	Cyanosis (late)	↑ Creatinine	Lactic acidosis	
↓ LOC	↑ CO	↑ PAP	Hyperkalemia	Anorexia	
Impaired judgment and memory	Bounding pulse	Respiratory alkalosis (early)	Metabolic acidosis	Nausea	
Altered sleep patterns	Diaphoresis	Respiratory acidosis (late)		Constipation	
Lethargy	Angina	↓ PaO₂		Abdominal pain	
Drowsiness		↓ SaO₂		Liver tenderness	
Coma					
Seizures					

Modified from Rice V. Clinical hypoxia. Crit Care Nurs 1980;1(1):21-29.
Abbreviations: *LOC*, level of consciousness; *BP*, blood pressure; *CO*, cardiac output; *PAP*, pulmonary artery pressures; *Hgb*, hemoglobin; *Hct*, hematocrit; *BUN*, blood urea nitrogen.

use of accessory muscles and a discoordinated respiratory pattern (abdominal muscle movement in opposition to chest wall expansion) may be seen. Lung sounds will vary from clear, isolated or generalized crackles to wheezes. Overall, physical signs and symptoms are specific to hypoxemia and decreased pulmonary compliance (Table 11-1). The following paragraphs discuss specific diagnostic findings.

Radiographic findings

Patients with impending or acute respiratory failure typically are too ill to undergo upright posterior/anterior (PA) and lateral chest roentgenograms (CXR). Usually, only portable CXRs are available for review. Early in the course of ARDS, CXR findings are nonspecific. Virtually clear lung fields, scant infiltrates, unilateral lobar consolidations, and diffuse lung involvement have all been noted.[43] Large pleural effusions are typically absent, but diffuse alveolar consolidation appears later in the course of ARDS.[43] Low lung volumes may also be present.[42]

Laboratory findings

Laboratory values in ARDS are often nonspecific, especially in the early stages. White blood cell counts may be high or low. Early arterial blood gas analysis reveals a normal or slightly alkalotic pH and low to normal carbon dioxide tensions with hypoxemia. As the lung injury progresses and respiratory failure worsens, the carbon dioxide tension increases, hypoxemia becomes refractory, and respiratory and metabolic acidosis are both present.[13] Circulating inflammatory mediators such as complement split products and TNF are also present.[39]

Alterations in lung mechanics

Patients with ARDS have increased extravascular lung water (EVLW). This pathologic process decreases the lung compliance: thus more pressure is required to ventilate the lungs. Normal dynamic lung compliance is approximately 100 mL/cm H_2O, and static effective compliance (SEC) is greater than 50 mL/cm H_2O.[15] Patients with ARDS have a reduced SEC of 20 to 30 mL/cm H_2O or lower.[15] Decreased lung compliance contributes to the difficulty in ventilating the lungs. Each tidal volume delivered by the ventilator requires a higher pressure as compared to the same tidal volume delivered to healthy lungs. Atelectasis and secretions contribute to poor lung compliance and decrease the amount of alveolar surface area available for gas exchange.[15] Decreased lung compliance contributes to an increased work of breathing.

Respiratory failure occurs when a patient's work of breathing becomes excessive and the patient becomes too fatigued to sustain the necessary effort to maintain oxygenation and ventilation. The percentage of oxygen consumption by the respiratory muscles in a resting normal adult is approximately 5% of total body consumption. In patients with ARDS, the percentage of oxygen consumption in the respiratory muscles alone may exceed 30% of total body consumption.[13]

Ventilation/perfusion mismatching

Ventilation/perfusion matching is a heterogeneous process throughout the lung fields in both normal and abnormal conditions. V/Q mismatching occurs secondary to venous admixture, shunting, and increased alveolar dead space and is the source of hypoxemia in the ARDS patient[44] (Fig. 11-3).

Venous admixture. Venous admixture occurs when partially ventilated alveoli receive blood flow.[44] Alveolar compression and secretions impair oxygen diffusion; therefore the blood leaving the dysfunctional alveoli has a lower oxygen tension. It mixes with oxygenated blood draining from other areas of the lung, and the overall SaO_2 decreases. In venous admixture, increasing the FiO_2 will improve the defect.[15]

Intrapulmonary shunt. In the region of a true shunt, unventilated alveoli are still receiving blood flow.[44] Distinguishing a true shunt from venous admixture is helpful for two reasons: determining severity and deciding on treatment. The presence of a large shunt indicates severe lung injury. In the partially ventilated alveoli, some gas exchange still occurs. In areas that have a true shunt, no gas exchange occurs. Therefore, if a large shunt is present, high oxygen concentrations will not increase the PaO_2. This is referred to as refractory hypoxemia, and other methods of ventilator management, such as PEEP, are more beneficial in this situation (see Therapeutic Management).

Alveolar dead space. When alveoli continue to inflate in regions of poor or absent perfusion, increased alveolar dead space occurs. Mediators such as serotonin and thromboxane A_2 contribute to increased pulmonary vasoconstriction and platelet aggregation. Other inflammatory mediators incite neutrophil adhesion and aggregation, endothelial damage, and microvascular permeability. The combination of mechanical obstruction, edematous tissue compression of vessels, and vascular constriction along with low flow states of shock and decreased cardiac output contributes to poor perfusion through the lung fields and thus alveolar dead space. The result is hypoxemia. Increasing the FiO_2 may do very little to improve this condition.

Hemodynamic parameters

Pulmonary hypertension is usually present early in the development of ARDS. Numerous mediators such as TXA_2 and serotonin as well as decreased levels of PGI_2 contribute to pulmonary vasoconstriction. Pulmonary systolic and diastolic pressures elevate, but the pulmonary capillary wedge pressure will usually be normal unless there is abnormal cardiac function present or underlying chronic pulmonary disease.[45] A third heart sound indicates the possibility of heart failure as a cause for the respiratory failure.

THERAPEUTIC MANAGEMENT

The goals of management for ARDS with or without MSOF are to maintain adequate gas exchange, prevent nonpulmonary organ failure, and prevent further lung injury while the lungs heal. Achieving these goals involves a management strategy that includes a balance of ventilatory techniques, pharmacologic intervention, hemodynamic support, and nutritional support.

Mechanical ventilation in ARDS

Goals. Different philosophies abound concerning the use of mechanical ventilation in the patient with ARDS. The controversy focuses on the balance between using components of mechanical ventilation that cause the least additional injury to the lungs while attempting to maintain adequate gas exchange. Regardless of the ventilation mode employed, management falls into two categories: full and partial support. Full support is recommended during the acute phase and partial support during the recovery and weaning phase of ARDS.[46]

The two goals of mechanical ventilation are maintaining gas exchange and avoiding secondary injury associated with mechanical ventilation, specifically barotrauma, oxygen toxicity, and structural damage to the airways.[46] Table 11-2 compares the various modes of ventilation.[46,47]

Complications

Barotrauma. Barotrauma refers to damage caused by excessive airway and/or alveolar pressures. Alveolar ruptures producing a tension pneumothorax, pneumomediastinum, subcutaneous air, and air emboli are common results of barotrauma, but pulmonary edema may also occur secondary to excessive intrathoracic pressures.[13] In ARDS, some lung regions are stiff and noncompliant, but other areas may be relatively unaffected. The high pressures required to ventilate the injured lung tissue and recruit alveoli are also transmitted to unaffected compliant areas as well, causing further damage. The literature suggests that both high peak inspiratory pressures and high mean airway pressures are responsible for causing barotrauma to the lungs.[48]

Oxygen toxicity. High fractions of inspired oxygen (FiO_2) are believed to increase oxygen radical formation, decrease surfactant production, contribute to reabsorptive atelectasis, contribute to the formation of hyaline membranes, and facilitate pulmonary fibrotic changes.[49] Although increased FiO_2 is often necessary, the use of PEEP can enhance arterial oxygenation and allow reduction of FiO_2.

Structural damage. Structural damage to the airway can occur secondary to the insertion and presence of artificial airways. Long-term use of endotracheal tubes and mechanical ventilation has been shown to cause permanent changes in the upper airway.[50,51]

Depressed myocardial function. Myocardial function in the ARDS patient can be adversely affected either as a direct result of the underlying pathologic conditions of the lung or as a result of mechanical ventilation. Positive pressure ventilation with or without high airway pressures, pressure support, PEEP, or inverse ratio ventilation increases the intrathoracic pressure. Impaired venous return, decreased filling pressures on the right side of the heart, and decreased cardiac output can result.[45,52] Since decreased cardiac output can contribute to decreased delivery of oxygen to the tissues, this adverse effect of positive pressure ven-

Table 11-2 Ventilator Strategies

	Assist control (AC)	Synchronized intermittent mandatory ventilation (SIMV)	Positive end-expiratory pressure (PEEP)	Pressure support ventilation (PSV)	Pressure control ventilation (PCV)	Inverse ratio ventilation (IRV)	High-frequency ventilation (HFV)
Respiratory rate	Machine set plus patient-triggered breaths	Machine set in synchrony with patient triggered breaths	May be used with any mode and all settings	Patient determined	Patient determined	Patient determined or machine set	Machine set 30-600 BPM
Apnea protection				Depends on model	Depends on model	Depends on mode and model	Continuous ventilation
Tidal volume	Machine set for both preset and patient's breaths	Machine set for machine breaths only		Patient determined	Patient determined	Patient determined or machine set	Machine set (very small)
Peak flow	Machine set	Machine set		Patient determined	Patient determined	Patient determined	Machine set
Inspiratory time	Machine set	Machine set		Patient determined	Patient determined	Machine set	Machine set
Peak airway pressure	High	High	High	Lower	Lower	Lower	Very low
Advantages	Full and partial support	Full and partial support	Full and partial, keeps alveoli open, redistributes intraalveolar fluid	Allows spontaneous breathing, full and partial support, low pressures	Allows spontaneous breathing, full and partial support, low pressures	Full and partial support, gas trapping keeps alveoli open	Full support
Spontaneous breathing	Present	Present with patient own rate and TV	May or may not be present			Present	Not present
Complications	Can facilitate respiratory alkalosis and ↑WOB	↑WOB	Barotrauma, ↓CO, ↑ICP, overdistention of alveoli compressing capillaries	Used with severe ARDS as partial support causes ↑WOB. PSV + PEEP = ↓CO	Same as for PSV and IRV	I:E ratios of 2:1 and 3:1 allow gas trapping causing "auto-PEEP" and ↓CO	No major complications. Controversial as to benefit.

Abbreviations: *BPM*, Breaths per minute; *TV*, tidal volume; *WOB*, work of breathing; *CO*, cardiac output; *ICP*, intracranial pressure.

tilation is an important concept to consider when creating a strategy for ventilation.

Considerations for the patient treated with mechanical ventilation

Airway management on mechanical ventilation. Specific patient care issues for the ARDS patient treated with mechanical ventilation are similar for all patients in respiratory failure. A pulmonary toilet regimen consisting of irrigation and suctioning airways as needed, in-line bronchodilatation treatments, and frequent repositioning is important.[15] Frequently, patients with ARDS are "PEEP-dependent," and they do not tolerate suctioning while off of PEEP. Several suctioning systems and ventilator circuits are available that maintain PEEP during suctioning. The rigid suction catheter and high suction pressures used can traumatize the airways[13] and increase the likelihood of bacterial contamination; therefore suctioning is performed only when indicated.

Repositioning. Repositioning the patient frequently facilitates blood flow to all lung regions, which may contribute to intermittent periods of decreased shunt (more blood flow to ventilated areas of lung). Recent evidence demonstrates positive effects of the prone position on oxygenation in patients.[53] The primary mechanism for the success of this position is believed to be related to a decreased shunt. Despite the practical difficulties of caring for patients in a prone position, this may be an important component of "ventilation strategies" used to improve oxygenation in the future. Since ARDS affects the lungs heterogeneously, it is impossible to know which areas of the lung contribute the most to gas exchange. Unlike the patient with a unilateral lung injury where placing the "good lung" down facilitates gas exchange, the ARDS patient may benefit most from frequent repositioning. Monitoring oxygen saturations of a patient while repositioning gives the practitioner information about the best position to facilitate gas exchange.

Work of breathing. Management theories related to the problem of "increased work of breathing" have changed throughout the years. The goal is to prevent the work of breathing from increasing respiratory muscle oxygen consumption. The balance between that concept and the theory that maintaining active use of respiratory muscles prevents atro-

phy is difficult to maintain.[12] Stoller and Kacmarek[46] promote the use of full ventilatory support to decrease the work of breathing in early ARDS.

Falling oxygen saturations may reflect excessive work of breathing. If the patient increases respiratory effort or becomes restless for other reasons and the oxygen saturation decreases, a change in the ventilatory strategy or sedation should be considered. Another tool recently employed in critical care areas is the continuous end-tidal CO_2 monitor (etCO_2). As with any form of respiratory failure, monitoring indicators of effective ventilation (PaCO_2 values and minute ventilation) can provide information about increased work of breathing and worsening respiratory failure.[15] The etCO_2 monitor provides an in-line estimate of the patient's PaCO_2 (carbon dioxide tension in the *alveolus*). In the absence of chest trauma, fistulas, and other anomalies, the etCO_2 values are considered to be an accurate reflection of the patient's PaCO_2.[54,55] Changes in the patient's ventilation process, as a result of either ventilator changes or the patient's condition, can be identified immediately.

Pharmacologic support

Currently, most of the pharmacologic agents used in patients with ARDS are considered supportive therapy. Several drugs that block or inhibit various mediators are under investigation in vitro, in vivo, and in clinical studies.

Specific supportive drug therapy includes antibiotics, bronchodilators, and paralytic agents. Antibiotics are used to treat specific infections. Bronchodilators can be used to reverse airway obstruction secondary to inflammation and mediator-induced bronchoconstriction.

Paralytic agents and sedatives can be used to relieve discomfort, decrease anxiety, and decrease oxygen consumption. The use of paralytic agents is usually restricted to patients with severe ARDS and subsequent problems with oxygen delivery and oxygen consumption. Disadvantages of paralytic therapy include development of respiratory muscle atrophy and lethal consequences of ventilator equipment malfunction.

Cardiovascular support

One of the more difficult aspects of ARDS management is maintenance of cardiovascular function.

Maximizing cardiac output and oxygen delivery with the appropriate combination of fluids, adequate hemoglobin levels, and inotropic support is critical. Fluid therapy should provide optimal filling pressures yet prevent further pulmonary edema as much as possible. A great deal of controversy remains concerning the use of crystalloids or colloids in fluid therapy (see Chapter 5). Crystalloids third-space more easily but may be used more frequently because of the theory that leaky pulmonary capillaries will also leak plasma albumin and other colloids. The increased oncotic pressure secondary to colloid movement into the interstitium would facilitate further fluid accumulation in the interstitial and intraalveolar space. It should also be noted that the cost of colloids far exceeds the cost of crystalloids; however, patient needs and responses to therapy should dictate the type of fluid used. A combination of vasoactive and inotropic agents is also used to treat the derangements of cardiac output, systemic vascular resistance, and pulmonary vascular resistance.

Hemodynamic monitoring plays a critical role in the practitioner's ability to accurately assess and treat variations in cardiac function. Mixed venous oxygen saturation monitoring will also assist the practitioner in diagnosing problems with oxygen transport and use, unless the patient demonstrates a pathologic oxygen supply dependency (see Chapter 6). This tool is helpful in assessing the effect of various nursing care procedures on patient status.[42]

Nutritional support

Early, aggressive nutritional support should be implemented. Patients with ARDS generally need 35 to 45 kcal/kg/day, and that value will increase if an additional systemic injury or illness is present.[56] The distribution of calories will vary depending on the presence of nonpulmonary organ failure; however, high levels of the appropriate type of protein should be included. These patients remain in a catabolic state that contributes to further metabolic and infectious complications.[42,57] Large feedings of high-carbohydrate solutions may contribute to fluid overload and increased CO_2 production. A multidisciplinary approach is needed to accurately assess patient need and response to therapy[58] (see Chapter 7).

INVESTIGATIONAL THERAPIES

Experimental studies of newer therapies used to provide prophylactic immunotherapy, block inflammatory effects, provide antibody protection against endotoxin, and inhibit effects of various activated mediators are ongoing. Laboratory animal studies and clinical trials using these investigational agents are currently underway, but it may be several years before substantial findings demonstrate significant decreases in mortality in the ARDS patient related to the administration of these drugs.[59]

Prostaglandin E_1

Prostaglandin E_1 inhibits platelet aggregation, neutrophil chemotaxis, and macrophage activity.[60] It also causes vasodilatation and may actually increase V/Q mismatching. Studies report conflicting results in ARDS patients receiving PGE_1. Improvement in overall oxygen delivery has been noted, but it may be at the expense of further V/Q mismatching.[59,61,62] Investigation continues to further define the role of vasodilatory prostaglandins in the pathogenesis and management of ARDS.

Exogenous Surfactant

Surfactant is a naturally occurring phospholipid that reduces surface tension in the alveoli. The use of exogenous surfactant (Exosurf) in neonates with premature hyaline membrane disease has been studied for several years. Some studies report significant positive effects, and others report no change in mortality rates. However, the use of surfactant is increasing in neonatal intensive care units. The benefits of surfactant in adult ARDS patients have not been demonstrated, but research is ongoing.[60]

Monoclonal antibody to WBC adhesion molecules

Autopsied lungs from ARDS patients show large numbers of white blood cells in both the parenchyma and pulmonary vasculature. Various efforts have been made to prevent adherence of white blood cells to the pulmonary endothelium by way of their adhesion molecules. Investigators have developed monoclonal antibodies against the adhesion molecules on the WBC,[63] and these monoclonal antibodies have decreased the incidence of tissue injury and inflammation in several animal studies.[64,65]

Extracorporeal membrane oxygenation

Extracorporeal membrane oxygenation (ECMO) is a form of extracorporeal bypass used to oxygenate the blood of critically ill patients. It was previously investigated in adult patients with ARDS with disappointing results,[66] although it had positive results in neonates. The studies demonstrated no significant difference in mortality rates and greater associated complications with the ECMO. Recent technology has allowed the development of more sophisticated techniques in ECMO administration, and ECMO is once again being investigated in the adult.[67]

CONCLUSION

Adult respiratory distress syndrome represents a major insult to the host, either as an isolated event or as a piece of the overall MSOF picture. Refractory hypoxemia and further stimulation of the inflammatory cascade exacerbate maldistribution of circulating volume, imbalance of oxygen supply and demand, and alterations in metabolism. Whether ARDS is the source of remote organ damage or the victim of the existing MSOF process, acute lung injury greatly contributes to the increased morbidity and mortality seen in this patient population. Prevention, early identification of respiratory deterioration, and prompt, aggressive intervention are key factors in minimizing the morbidity and mortality of ARDS in the critically ill.

REFERENCES

1. Murray JF, Matthay MA, Luce J. An expanded definition of the adult respiratory distress syndrome. Am Rev Respir Dis 1988;138:720-723.
2. Ashbaugh DG et al. Acute respiratory distress in adults. Lancet 1967;2:319-323.
3. Bersten A, Sibbald WJ. Acute lung injury in septic shock. Crit Care Clin 1989;5:49-79.
4. Vaughan P, Brooks C. Adult respiratory distress syndrome: A complication of shock. Crit Care Nurs Clin North Am 1990;2:235-253.
5. Petty TL. Adult respiratory distress syndrome: Refinement of concept and redefinition. Am Rev Respir Dis 1988;138:724-742.
6. Matthay MA. The adult respiratory distress syndrome: New insights into diagnosis, pathophysiology and treatment. West J Med 1989;150:187-194.

7. Niederman MS, Fein AM. Sepsis syndrome, the adult respiratory distress syndrome, and nosocomial pneumonia. Clin Chest Med 1990;6:635-661.
8. Dorinsky PM, Gadek JE. Multiple organ failure. Clin Chest Med 1990;11:581-591.
9. Guyton AC. Pulmonary ventilation: Textbook of medical physiology. Philadelphia: WB Saunders, 1986:466-525.
10. Brooks-Brunn J. Respiration. Critical care nursing: A physiologic approach. St Louis: Mosby–Year Book, 1986:168-251.
11. Murray JF. Ventilation: The normal lung. St Louis: Mosby–Year Book, 1986:83-107.
12. Marini JJ. Strategies to minimize breathing effort during mechanical ventilation. Crit Care Clin 1990;6:635-661.
13. Marini JJ. Lung mechanics. Respiratory medicine and intensive care. Baltimore: Williams & Wilkins, 1985:1-10.
14. Crapo JD, Barry BE, Gehr P, Bachofen M, Weibel ER. Cell number and cell characteristics of the normal lung. Am Rev Respir Dis 1982;125:740-745.
15. Marini JJ, Wheeler AP. Respiratory failure. Critical care medicine: The essentials. Baltimore: Williams & Wilkins, 1989:175-184.
16. West JB, Dollery CT, Naimark A. Distribution of blood in isolated lung: Relation to vascular and alveolar pressures. J Appl Physiol 1964;19:713-724.
17. Murray JF. Circulation: The normal lung. Philadelphia: WB Saunders, 1986:139-150.
18. Freudenberg N. Reaction of the vascular intima to endotoxin in shock. Prog Clin Biol Res: Second Vienna Shock Forum 1989;308:77-89.
19. Del Vecchio PJ, Malik AB. Thrombin-induced neutrophil adhesion. Prog Clin Biol Res: Second Vienna Shock Forum 1989;308:101-112.
20. Muller-Berghaus G. Septicemia and the vessel wall. In: Verstraete M, Vermylen J, Lijnen R, Arnout J, eds. Thrombosis and Haemostasis. Belgium: Leuven University Press, 1987:619-671.
21. Brigham KL, Meyrick B. Interactions of granulocytes with lungs. Circ Res 1984;54:623-635.
22. Ognibene FP et al. Adult respiratory distress syndrome in patients with severe neutropenia. N Engl J Med 1986;315:547-551.
23. Ford HR et al. Characterization of wound cytokines in the sponge matrix model. Arch Surg 1989;124:1422-1428.
24. Lazarou SA et al. The wound is a possible source of post-traumatic immunosuppression. Arch Surg 1989;124:1429-1431.
25. Beutler B. Cachectin in tissue injury, shock, and related states. Crit Care Clin 1989;5:353-368.
26. Tracey KJ et al. Shock and tissue injury induced by recombinant human cachectin. Science 1986;234:470-474.
27. Debets JM et al. Plasma tumor necrosis factor and mortality in critically ill patients. Can J Surg 1988;31:172-176.
28. Dinarello CA. Biology of interleukin-1. FASEB J 1988;2:108-115.
29. Sprague RS et al. Proposed role for leukotrienes in the pathophysiology of multiple systems organ failure. Crit Care Clin 1989;5:315-330.
30. Petrak RA, Balk RA, Bone RC. Prostaglandins, cyclooxygenase inhibitors, and thromboxane synthetase inhibitors in the pathogenesis of multiple systems organ failure. Crit Care Clin 1989;5:302-314.

31. Yellin SA et al. Prostacyclin and thromboxane A2 in septic shock: Species differences. Circ Shock 1986;20:291-297.

32. Brigham KL, Sheller JR. Leukotrienes and adult respiratory distress syndrome. Intensive Care Med 1989;15:422-423.

33. Rinaldo JE, Christman JW. Mechanisms and mediators of the adult respiratory distress syndrome. Clin Chest Med 1990;11:621-632.

34. Weiss SJ. Tissue destruction by neutrophils. N Engl J Med 1989;320:365-376.

35. Lefer AM. Induction of tissue injury and altered cardiovascular performance by platelet-activating factor: Relevance to multiple systems organ failure. Crit Care Clin 1989;5:331-352.

36. Braquet P, Hosford D. The potential role of platelet-activating factor (PAF) in shock, sepsis and adult respiratory distress syndrome. Prog Clin Biol Res: Second Vienna Shock Forum 1989:425-439.

37. Walport M. Complement. In: Roitt I, Brostoff J, Male D, eds. Immunology 2nd ed. London: Gower Medical Publishing, 1989:13.1-13.16.

38. Bengtson A, Heideman M. Anaphylatoxin formation in sepsis. Arch Surg 1988;123:645-649.

39. Langlois RF et al. Accentuated complement activation in patient plasma during the adult respiratory distress syndrome: A potential mechanism for pulmonary inflammation. Heart Lung 1989;18:71-84.

40. Ichinose M, Barnes PJ. Bradykinin-induced airway microvascular leakage and bronchoconstriction are mediated via a bradykinin B2 receptor. Am Rev Respir Dis 1990;1104-1107.

41. Pratt PC. Pathology of the adult respiratory distress syndrome. In: Thurlbeck WM, Abell MR, eds. The lung: Structure, function and disease. Baltimore: Williams & Wilkins, 1978:44-57.

42. Mims BC. Adult respiratory distress syndrome. Lewisville, Tx: Barbara Clark Mims Associates, 1990.

43. Aberle DR, Brown K. Radiologic considerations in the adult respiratory distress syndrome. Clin Chest Med 1990;11:737-754.

44. Shapiro BA, Harrison RA, Walton JR. Clinical application of blood gases. 3rd ed. St Louis: Mosby–Year Book, 1982.

45. Biondi JW et al. Mechanical heart-lung interaction in the adult respiratory distress syndrome. Clin Chest Med 1990;11:691-714.

46. Stoller JK, Kacmarek RM. Ventilatory strategies in the management of the adult respiratory distress syndrome. Clin Chest Med 1990;11:755-772.

47. Sassoon LS, Mahutte CK, Light RW. Ventilatory modes: Old and new. Crit Care Clin 1990;6:605-634.

48. Pierson DJ. Complications associated with mechanical ventilation. Crit Care Clin 1990;6:711-724.

49. Lodato RF. Oxygen toxicity. Crit Care Clin 1990;6:749-765.

50. El-Naggar M et al. Factors influencing choice between tracheostomy and prolonged translaryngeal intubation in acute respiratory failure: A prospective study. Anesth Analg 1976;55:195-210.

51. Elliott CG, Rasmussen BY, Crapo RO. Upper airway obstruction following acute respiratory distress syndrome: An analysis of 30 survivors. Chest 1988;94:526.

52. Pinsky MR. Multiple systems organ failure: Malignant intravascular inflammation. Crit Care Clin 1989;5:195-198.

53. Langer M et al. The prone position in adult respiratory distress syndrome patients: A clinical study. Chest 1988;94:103-107.

54. Von Reuden KT. Noninvasive assessment of gas exchange in the critically ill patient. Clin Issues Crit Care Nurs 1990;6:679-709.

55. Tobin MJ. Respiratory monitoring during mechanics of ventilation. Crit Care Clin 1990;6:679-709.

56. Pingleton SK. Nutritional support in the mechanically ventilated patient. Clin Chest Med 1988;9:101-112.

57. Cerra FB. Hypermetabolism, organ failure and metabolic support. Surgery 1987;101:1-14.

58. Holtzman GM et al. Nutritional support of pulmonary patients: A multidisciplinary approach. Clin Issues Crit Care Nurs 1990;1:300-312.

59. Goldstein G, Luce JJ. Pharmacologic treatment of the adult respiratory distress syndrome. Clin Chest Med 1990;11:773-787.

60. Bone RC et al. Randomized double-blind multicenter study of prostaglandin E_1 in patients with the adult respiratory distress syndrome. Chest 1989;96:114-119.

61. Silverman HJ et al. Effects of prostaglandin E_1 on oxygen delivery and consumption in patients with the adult respiratory distress syndrome. Chest 1990;98:405-410.

62. Melot C et al. Prostaglandin E_1 in the adult respiratory distress syndrome: Benefit for pulmonary hypertension and cost of pulmonary gas exchange. Am Rev Respir Dis 1989;139:106-110.

63. Wegner CD et al. Intercellular adhesion molecule-1 (ICAM-1) in the pathogenesis of asthma. Science 1990;247:456-459.

64. Tuomanen EI et al. Reduction of inflammation, tissue damage, and mortality in bacterial meningitis in rabbits treated with monoclonal antibodies against adhesion-promoting receptors of leukocytes. J Exp Med 1989;170:959-968.

65. Mileski WJ et al. Inhibition of CD18-dependent neutrophil adherence reduces organ injury after hemorrhagic shock in primates. Surgery 1990;108:206-212.

66. Zapol WM et al. Extracorporeal membrane oxygenation in severe acute respiratory failure. JAMA 1979;242:2193-2196.

67. Villar G, Winston B, Slutsky AS. Nonconventional techniques of ventilatory support. Crit Care Clin 1990;6:579-603.

12 Acute Renal Failure*

Larry E. Lancaster

The kidneys and other organ systems, especially the cardiovascular system, possess an intricate, inextricable interrelationship. Each minute the kidneys receive a percentage of the cardiac output far in excess of that required to nourish the renal cells. Yet the kidneys depend on this large, uninterrupted blood supply to maintain adequate function. Thus any event that alters the vascular volume or the cardiac contractility and, consequently, the cardiac output, also invariably affects kidney function. Renal function is also affected by numerous vasoactive substances and exogenous and endogenous toxins. Multisystem organ failure (MSOF) is one of those conditions that, based on its underlying cause, can affect various aspects of cardiovascular and renal function. Therefore damage to the kidneys is common from both ischemic insult and direct vascular and tubular damage by inflammatory and vasoactive mediators. Hence the purposes of this chapter are to review some basic renal physiologic concepts, discuss acute tubular necrosis (ATN) as a participant in MSOF, describe the pathophysiology and stages of ATN, and outline assessment parameters and intervention principles during each stage of ATN.

BASIC PHYSIOLOGIC CONCEPTS

To understand alterations in renal function during MSOF, it is first essential to understand some basic renal anatomic and physiologic concepts. These basic concepts are explained below and serve as a foundation for the remainder of this chapter.

Nephron

The functional unit of the kidney is the nephron; therefore overall renal function may be explained

in terms of single nephron function. There are approximately 1,000,000 nephrons in each kidney for a total of 2,000,000 in both kidneys. Each nephron is composed of a vascular component and a tubular component (Fig. 12-1). Blood from the aorta flows into the renal arteries, which branch into smaller and smaller arteries and arterioles before finally terminating in the afferent arterioles. Each afferent arteriole then divides into a capillary tuft called the glomerulus. The glomerular capillaries rejoin to form the efferent arteriole, which continues to become the peritubular capillaries and vasa recta. The peritubular capillaries and vasa recta are in close juxtaposition to the renal tubules, allowing for constant movement back and forth (i.e., reabsorption and secretion) between the filtrate of the renal tubules and the plasma of the peritubular capillaries and vasa recta[1-3] (Fig. 12-1).

Glomerular filtration

The two kidneys receive approximately 25% of the cardiac output each minute for a total of 1200 mL/min. Because of its large blood supply, the glomerular capillary bed is a high pressure area. As a result of this high pressure, fluid continually filters from the glomerular capillary bed into Bowman's capsule at an average rate of 125 mL/min.[1-3] The glomerular filtration rate (GFR) normally remains quite constant even with wide variations in arterial blood pressure. For example, a change in arterial blood pressure from 70 mm Hg to 160 mm Hg has almost no effect on the GFR.[1] This ability of the kidneys to maintain a constant GFR is called autoregulation[1]; mechanisms responsible for autoregulation are explained below. Based on an average GFR of 125 mL/min, approximately 180 L is filtered from the glomerulus into Bowman's capsule every 24 hours. Under the influence of various hormones, 98% to 99% of this

*This chapter is modified from Lancaster LE. Renal response to shock. In: Rice V, ed. Shock. Crit Care Nurs Clin North Am 1990; 2:221-234.

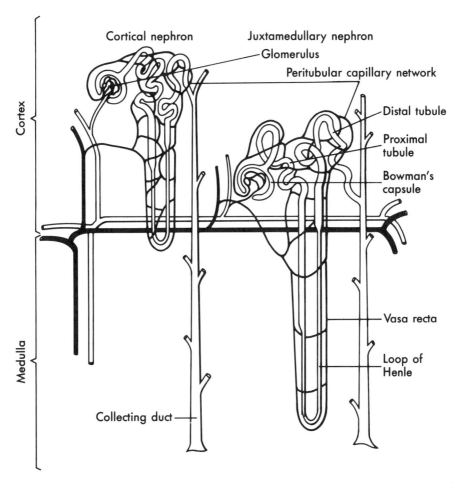

Fig. 12-1 Anatomy of cortical and juxtamedullary nephrons. Note relationship between vascular and tubular components. (From Lancaster LE. Renal response to shock. In: Rice V, ed. Shock. Crit Care Nurs Clin North Am 1990; 2:222).

filtrate is reabsorbed, leaving a urine output of about 1.5 to 2 L/day. However, the kidneys can make significant changes in the urine output, depending on the state of hydration. In conditions of fluid deficit, maximal amounts of tubular filtrate are reabsorbed, and a small amount of concentrated urine is excreted. Conversely, in conditions of fluid excess, tubular reabsorption decreases, and a large amount of dilute urine is excreted.[1,2]

Autoregulation and tubuloglomerular feedback

The process responsible for renal autoregulation is called tubuloglomerular feedback.[1] The two

mechanisms involved in tubuloglomerular feedback are afferent arteriolar vasodilator feedback and efferent arteriolar vasoconstrictor feedback.[1] The juxtaglomerular apparatus (JGA) controls most of the feedback mechanisms. The JGA consists of specialized cells located at the point at which the distal convoluted tubule of each nephron loops and comes into contact with the angle of the afferent and efferent arterioles of that nephron.[1,2] The cells of the distal tubule located at this junction are called the macula densa, which respond to ischemic changes; and the cells of the afferent and efferent arterioles at this point are called juxtaglomerular cells, which secrete renin. A decreased amount of glomerular filtrate decreases the sodium and chloride concentration in the area of the macula densa, which causes dilatation of the afferent arteriole.[1] As the afferent arteriole dilates, blood flow and hydrostatic pressure in the glomerular capillary bed increase, thus maintaining the glomerular capillary pressure and GFR.[1] Conversely, an increase in sodium and chloride at the macula densa causes afferent arteriole constriction, decreased glomerular blood flow, and decreased GFR.

The decrease in sodium and chloride at the macula densa also causes renin release from the juxtaglomerular cells. Through several physiologic reactions, renin is converted to angiotensin II, which causes efferent arteriole constriction. Efferent arteriole constriction also helps maintain the hydrostatic pressure in the glomerular capillary bed and helps the GFR remain normal.[1]

To summarize, autoregulation maintains renal blood flow and GFR within a narrow range despite wide fluctuations in arterial blood pressure. However, once the mean arterial pressure (MAP) falls below 50 to 70 mm Hg, the renal autoregulatory processes are no longer able to maintain adequate renal blood flow and GFR. As a result, in states of prolonged hypotension and renal hypoperfusion, drastic changes occur in renal function. MSOF is one of those conditions characterized by hypotension, renal hypoperfusion, and ischemia. Renal responses to hypoperfusion, ischemia, and toxic mediators of MSOF are discussed later in this chapter.

Renal function

To understand the effects of renal dysfunction, it is necessary to have a comprehension of normal renal function. An extensive discussion of normal renal physiology is beyond the scope of this chapter; however, to orient the reader a brief summary of essential renal functions is presented. The kidneys are responsible for:

1. Regulation of water balance through the processes of glomerular filtration and tubular reabsorption under the influence of aldosterone and antidiuretic hormone (ADH)[1,2]
2. Regulation of electrolyte balance by the processes of glomerular filtration and selective tubular reabsorption and secretion under the influence of various hormones, such as aldosterone and parathyroid hormone[1,2]
3. Along with the buffer and respiratory systems, regulation of acid-base balance through glomerular filtration of hydrogen ions and tubular reabsorption and secretion of hydrogen ions, bicarbonate regeneration, tubular ammonia synthesis and ammonium excretion, and secretion of other titratable acids[1,2]
4. Excretion of end products of metabolism (uremic toxins)[1,2]
5. Regulation of red blood cell production by erythropoietin production[1,2]
6. Metabolism of weak vitamin D precursors to the active, potent form (1,25-dihydroxycholecalciferol [1,25-DHCC])[1]
7. Blood pressure regulation through renin production by the juxtaglomerular apparatus
8. Synthesis of prostaglandins[4-6]

DEFINITION AND CLASSIFICATION OF ACUTE RENAL FAILURE

Acute renal failure (ARF) is a clinical syndrome with diverse causes characterized by sudden, rapid deterioration in renal function. There is usually an associated decrease in GFR and oliguria; however, some forms of ARF may be nonoliguric.[3,5,7] Concomitantly, there are increases in blood urea nitrogen (BUN) and plasma creatinine, fluid-electrolyte abnormalities, acid-base derangements, and altered renal hormonal functions. With appropriate, expeditious treatment return to normal or near-normal renal function is often possible.[3,5,7] Without appropriate treatment or adequate patient response to treatment, chronic renal failure or death from MSOF may be the outcome of an acute episode.

ARF falls into three categories depending on its cause: prerenal, postrenal, and renal parenchymal (also called intrinsic or primary acute failure). Acute prerenal failure occurs as the result of decreased blood flow to the kidneys. With decreased blood reaching the glomerular capillary bed, there is decreased GFR and a corresponding decrease in urinary output.[5,7] Causes of prerenal failure include any condition that alters the renal blood flow, including hypovolemia, increased intravascular capacity (sepsis, anaphylaxis, and neurogenic shock), abnormal myocardial contractility (myocardial infarction, dysrhythmias, and tamponade), alterations in the renal vasculature (stenosis, emboli, thrombi, trauma, and occlusion), and the hepatorenal syndrome.[3,5,7-10] Early in the course of prerenal problems, the nephrons remain functional.

The management of prerenal problems consists of rapidly and aggressively treating the underlying cause of the decreased renal blood flow. Once the underlying cause is alleviated, renal function usually returns rapidly to normal.

Acute postrenal failure refers to obstruction of urine outflow. The blockage may occur in the ureter (calculi and strictures), bladder (tumors and neurogenic bladder), or urethra (prostatic hypertrophy).[3,5,7] As in prerenal problems, early in the course of postrenal failure the nephrons remain functional. The management of postrenal problems consists of treating the underlying cause of obstruction so that urine flow may be reestablished before permanent nephron damage occurs.

Acute renal parenchymal failure refers to intrinsic or primary damage to the nephrons, especially the tubular component. The most common cause of acute renal parenchymal failure is acute tubular necrosis (ATN), which results from an ischemic or toxic insult to the nephrons. Thus acute intrinsic renal failure and ATN have become almost synonymous terms. The most common cause of ischemic ATN is prolonged acute prerenal problems; the most common causes of toxic ATN are nephrotoxic drugs, toxic microbial products, and inflammatory mediators circulating in septicemia, septic shock, and MSOF, including endotoxin, tumor necrosis factor (TNF), interleukin-1 (IL-1), and prostaglandins.[3,5,7,10-12] Other causes of acute renal parenchymal failure include glomerulonephritis, pyelonephritis, interstitial nephritis, lupus nephritis, pregnancy-related conditions (septic abortion, eclampsia, postpartum hemorrhage, and abruptio placentae), cortical and papillary necrosis, intravascular hemolysis (transfusion reactions and disseminated intravascular hemolysis), nephrotic syndrome, and Goodpasture's syndrome.[3,5,7,10] Postischemic and toxic ATN that can occur as a result of MSOF is the specific focus of this chapter.

PATHOPHYSIOLOGY OF ACUTE TUBULAR NECROSIS

Fig. 12-2 is a schematic representation of the pathophysiology of ischemic and toxic conditions that can result in ATN. In MSOF, the ischemic event refers to prolonged hypoperfusion and ischemia of the kidneys as a result of prolonged low MAP (less than 50 to 70 mm Hg)[13] and/or maldistribution of circulating volume. The toxic event refers to toxic microbial products, endogenous mediators produced during septicemia and MSOF, and also to nephrotoxic drugs used to treat both syndromes (see box on p. 227).

Changes in renal hemodynamics, nephron alterations, and changes in cellular metabolism are related to the development of ATN.[14] Each of these changes is discussed in the following paragraphs.

Ischemic injury

Changes in renal hemodynamics. When the MAP falls below approximately 50 to 70 mm Hg, renal blood flow and perfusion pressure decrease. Renal autoregulatory ability is severely altered by intense sympathetic and renin-angiotensin activity. In response to sympathetic stimulation and angiotensin, the afferent arteriole constricts, glomerular blood flow decreases, glomerular hydrostatic pressure decreases, and, finally, the GFR decreases. Proximal tubular alterations result in decreased reabsorption of sodium in the proximal tubule and thus an increase in sodium in the distal tubule and the area of the macula densa. In response to the increased sodium in the distal tubule, tubuloglomerular feedback causes further afferent arteriole constriction that decreases glomerular blood flow and glomerular filtration pressure; this mechanism worsens tubular cell injury.[14] Adenosine, which is produced from ATP catabolism, may also act as a vasoconstrictor and potentiate the renal vascular constriction.[14] Prostaglandins have a controversial role in ATN. There may be either a decrease in prostacyclin synthesis[6] or an increase in thromboxane A synthesis by the injured renal cells. Prostacyclin acts as a vasodilator; thus its decrease would potentiate renal vasoconstriction. Thromboxane A acts as a vasoconstrictor; thus its increase in ATN would worsen renal vascular constriction.

Sympathetic stimulation and angiotensin production during ischemia also cause blood flow redistribution from the outer to the inner cortex.[4] Because the glomeruli and most of the tubular components are located in the cortex, the redistribution of blood further decreases blood flow through the glomerular capillary bed and worsens tubular ischemia.

The amount and degree of renal cell damage depend on the length of the ischemic episode. Research provides evidence that ischemia of 25 minutes or less causes reversible mild injury to renal

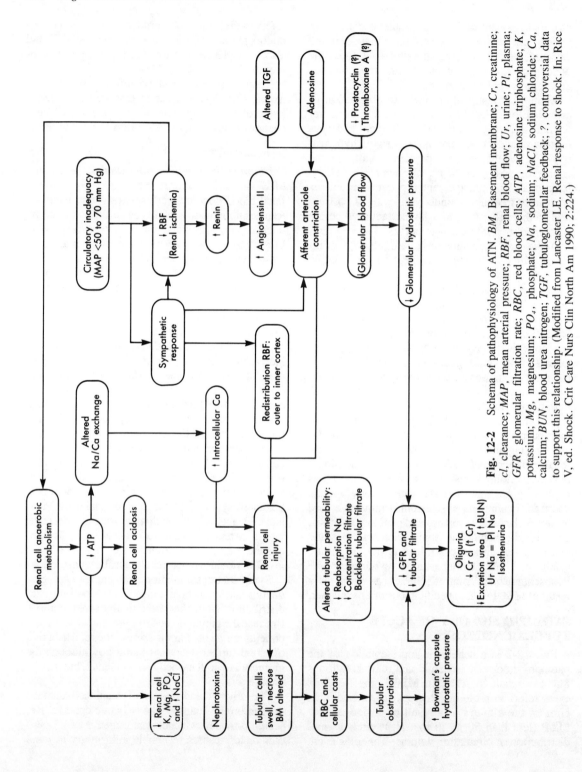

Fig. 12-2 Schema of pathophysiology of ATN. *BM*, Basement membrane; *Cr*, creatinine; *cl*, clearance; *MAP*, mean arterial pressure; *RBF*, renal blood flow; *Ur*, urine; *Pl*, plasma; *GFR*, glomerular filtration rate; *RBC*, red blood cells; *ATP*, adenosine triphosphate; *K*, potassium; *Mg*, magnesium; *PO₄*, phosphate; *Na*, sodium; *NaCl*, sodium chloride; *Ca*, calcium; *BUN*, blood urea nitrogen; *TGF*, tubuloglomerular feedback; *?*, controversial data to support this relationship. (Modified from Lancaster LE. Renal response to shock. In: Rice V, ed. Shock. Crit Care Nurs Clin North Am 1990; 2:224.)

NEPHROTOXIC DRUGS USED IN SEPTICEMIA AND MSOF

Amikacin	Kanamycin
Amphotericin B	Mefenamic acid
Cephaloridine	Neomycin
Cephalothin	Paromomycin
Cimetidine	Polymyxin B
Colistid	Salicylates
Colistimethate	Streptomycin
Contrast media	Sulfonamides
Corticosteroids	Tetracyclines
Edetate	Tobramycin
Ethacrynic acid	Vancomycin
Furosemide	Viomycin
Gentamicin	

From Lancaster LE. Renal response to shock. In: Rice V, ed. Shock. Crit Care Nurs Clin North Am 1990: 2, 225.

cells; ischemia of 40 to 60 minutes results in more severe damage, which may recover to some extent in 2 to 3 weeks; and ischemia lasting 60 to 90 minutes usually causes irreversible damage.[6]

In addition to the cellular damage related to the ischemia itself, cellular damage often continues during the period when the MAP and renal reperfusion are restored. Data show that "renal blood flow does not return to normal following resumption of circulation after a period of ischemia (the so-called 'no reflow' phenomenon)."[6] Studies show that renal blood flow remains reduced by as much as 50% following an ischemic event.[6] During reperfusion after a prolonged renal ischemic event, the formation of oxygen-derived free radicals further exacerbates cell damage.[4,6] See Chapters 3 and 5 for further information on reperfusion injury.

Changes in renal cell metabolism. As a result of decreased oxygenation of the renal cells, aerobic metabolism shifts to anaerobic metabolism, and the production of adenosine triphosphate (ATP) by the mitochondria decreases significantly, while the metabolic need for ATP continues.[4,6,13] Concomitant with the decrease in ATP, extracellular and intracellular acidosis develop, which further alters kidney function.[4,6,13] In addition, decreased ATP alters the Na/K pump and results in decreased renal cell potassium, magnesium, and inorganic phosphates and increased intracellular sodium and chloride.[4] Intracellular water increases along with

the increased sodium, which leads to cellular swelling and eventual cell death. Sodium/calcium exchange is abnormal because of low ATP, altered Ca-ATPase, and increased cell sodium. As a result, there is an increase in intracellular calcium, which seems to increase cell injury.[4]

Nephron alterations. As an outcome of prolonged tubular ischemia, tubular cells swell and become necrotic, altering the function of the tubular basement membrane. Tubular obstruction occurs from sloughed necrotic cells and cast formation. The tubular obstruction increases tubular hydrostatic pressure and Bowman's capsule hydrostatic pressure. Increased hydrostatic pressure in Bowman's capsule opposes the glomerular hydrostatic pressure, resulting in a decreased GFR. Injury to the basement membrane increases tubular permeability and allows tubular filtrate to leak back into the interstitium and peritubular capillaries. Back-leak of tubular filtrate further decreases the amount of tubular filtrate.*

Renal failure is the end result of the ischemic event. Postischemic ATN is usually associated with oliguria because of extensive nephron injury. In addition to oliguria, other clinical indications of ATN include decreased urea excretion (elevated blood urea nitrogen [BUN]); decreased creatinine clearance (elevated plasma creatinine); abnormal renal handling of sodium (usually decreased tubular sodium reabsorption with urinary sodium equal to plasma sodium); and inability to concentrate urine (urinary osmolality approximates plasma osmolality or 300 to 320 mOsm/kg H_2O, a condition called isosthenuria).†

Toxic injury

Whereas postischemic ATN begins with circulatory inadequacy that elicits the sympathetic response and stimulates renin-angiotensin production leading to tubular cell necrosis, toxins cause the initial injury to tubular cells seen in toxic ATN. In MSOF, toxic ATN occurs as a result of toxic microbial products of septicemia, endogenous inflammatory mediators, and nephrotoxic medications used to counteract the microorganisms responsible for the sepsis and the overall MSOF syndrome. Toxic mediators can also alter renal hemodynam-

---

*References 3, 5, 7, 8, and 10.
†References 3, 5, 7, 8, and 10.

ics, further exacerbating ischemic injury.

The pathophysiology following the toxic insult is similar to the pathophysiology of postischemic ATN; that is, there is tubular cell necrosis, cast formation, tubular obstruction, and altered GFR. The tubular basement membrane may not be injured in toxic ATN, or at least not as severely as in postischemic ATN; therefore the healing process with isolated toxic ATN is often more rapid than with postischemic ATN.[5,7] In addition, because of the lesser injury, nonoliguric renal failure is often associated with toxic ATN, although oliguria does occur in many instances. Unfortunately, both postischemic ATN and toxic ATN are present in MSOF. Many of the toxic mediators damaging the kidneys are also causing systemic abnormalities such as cardiovascular instability and maldistribution of volume that affect postischemic ATN.

In summary, renal responses to MSOF include:
1. Acute prerenal problems during the early stages of hypoperfusion
2. ATN related to profound ischemia during later stages of MSOF secondary to decreased cardiac output and decreased renal blood flow
3. ATN resulting from toxic microbial products of septicemia, endogenous inflammatory mediators, and the medications used to treat sepsis and the MSOF syndrome
4. ATN resulting from a combination of numbers 2 and 3

CLINICAL COURSE OF ACUTE TUBULAR NECROSIS

For the typical case of ATN, the clinical course follows four successive phases. Each phase is described in the following paragraphs. The assessment and management during each phase is described later in this chapter.

The *onset* or *initiating phase* is the time from the precipitating event until cell injury occurs.* This phase may correspond with acute prerenal failure, and it is a potentially reversible phase. The onset phase may last hours to days, depending on the causative factor, usually being shorter (hours) for postischemic ATN and longer (days) for toxic ATN.

If the onset phase is not reversed, the *oliguric-anuric* phase ensues and usually lasts about 1 to 2

weeks. Oliguria (output less than 400 mL/day) is more common in postischemic ATN, and nonoliguric renal failure (output over 400 mL/day, but not necessarily normal) is more common in toxic ATN.[5,7] Anuria (output less than 100 mL/day) is uncommon in ATN; it usually is related to bilateral acute postrenal obstruction.[5,7] During this phase, the GFR is significantly decreased, resulting in fluid overload, increased BUN and plasma creatinine, electrolyte abnormalities, metabolic acidosis, and alterations related to accumulation of uremic toxins. This constellation of alterations is called uremia or the uremic syndrome.

The *diuretic phase,* which lasts about 7 to 14 days, is associated with an increase in urine output and a gradual improvement in overall renal function. During the early diuretic phase, the urine output may double on successive days until the volume reaches 2000 to 3000 mL/day.[5,7] Initially the urine is comparable to the plasma filtrate, but then there are gradual increases in urea excretion and decreases in urinary sodium loss. The diuresis may be explained by the following factors:
1. Mobilization of urea causes an osmotic diuresis
2. The tubules can not reabsorb the glomerular filtrate and thus concentrate the urine
3. The edema fluid that collected during the oliguric-anuric phase is mobilized and adds to the glomerular filtrate
4. Excess intravenous fluid administration to replace the urine output also enhances diuresis[5]

During the late diuretic phase the BUN begins to fall and eventually stabilizes in a normal or near-normal range. Diuresis may continue during the late phase, electrolyte imbalances and acidosis begin to improve, and the GFR also begins to return to normal.

During the *recovery* or *convalescent* phase, recovery of renal function slowly occurs. GFR returns to 70% to 80% of normal within 1 to 2 years. In some cases, a mild to moderate residual renal damage may remain.[5,7]

ASSESSMENT AND THERAPEUTIC MANAGEMENT

Assessment and management of the patient with MSOF complicated by ATN requires assessment and treatment of MSOF and its underlying causes as well as assessment and treatment of the specific problems caused by ARF. Early intervention is

---

*References 5, 7, 8, 10, and 12.

Table 12-1 Typical Findings in Prerenal Problems and Intrinsic Acute Tubular Necrosis

Urine Parameter	Prerenal	ATN
Volume	Oliguria	Oliguria or nonoliguria
Urinary sediment	Normal (hyaline and granular casts)	RBC casts
		Cellular debris
Specific gravity	High	Low
Osmolality (mOsm/kg H_2O)	High	Low (isosthenuria)
Ratio osm urine to osm plasma	>1.5	<1.2
Urine Na (mEq/L)	Low (<20)	High (>20)
Urine urea (g/24 hr)	Low (15)	Low (5)
Urine creatinine (g/24 hr)	Normal (>1.0)	Low (<1.0)
Ratio urine creatinine to plasma creatinine	>15:1	<10:1

From Lancaster LE. Renal response to shock. In: Rice V, ed. Shock. Crit Care Nurs Clin North Am 1990:2, 227.

aimed at reversing prerenal failure and preventing ATN. If ATN develops, then the uremic syndrome and its complications must be assessed and treated. Although it is possible for a patient with ATN to develop any of the complications discussed, it is unlikely that any one patient will develop all the complications. Also, the specific clinical problems for an individual patient are the net sum of all pathophysiologic alterations and compensatory mechanisms for that particular patient. Because the patient with MSOF experiences multiple problems related to failure of various organs, each patient must be assessed and treated individually based on findings in his or her specific case.

Differential diagnosis of prerenal failure and acute tubular necrosis

Differentiating prerenal problems and actual ATN may present a challenge for the clinician. Because prerenal problems correspond with the onset phase of ATN, and because this is a reversible phase, it is essential for diagnosis and aggressive management to begin early in the course of prerenal problems.

Diagnosis requires an in-depth health history and physical examination, urinalysis, plasma analysis, and microscopic urine examination. The health history provides information about hypotensive episodes, nephrotoxic medications, and other disease processes that could precipitate prerenal or intrinsic renal failure. The physical examination discloses information about possible causes of the renal problem in addition to the systemic consequences of the renal failure.

Urinalysis and microscopic examination of the urine provide important data for differentiating prerenal failure from ATN. Table 12-1 summarizes typical urine and plasma findings in prerenal failure and ATN. The pathophysiologic basis of selected findings is discussed in subsequent paragraphs.

In prerenal problems, the urinary specific gravity and osmolality are high and the urinary sodium is low because of decreased renal blood flow and decreased GFR,* which the kidneys interpret as a state of dehydration. As a response, under the influence of aldosterone and ADH, maximal sodium and water are reabsorbed from the distal tubule and collecting duct into the peritubular capillary plasma. Thus a small amount (oliguria) of very concentrated urine with high specific gravity and high osmolality is excreted. Although maximal sodium is reabsorbed, the urine is concentrated because of urea or other solutes. In prerenal problems, urinary and plasma creatinine levels often show wide swings.[11]

In contrast to prerenal problems, ATN is characterized by altered renal ability to conserve sodium. Clinically, this is seen as a high urinary sodium (greater than 20 mEq/L).[5,7,10,15] The laboratory serum sodium varies, depending on the state of hydration. Oliguria is usually associated with postischemic ATN, whereas nephrotoxic ATN may or may not be associated with oliguria for reasons explained earlier in this chapter. The creatinine clearance is severely decreased, and the plasma creatinine rises at a rate of about 1 to 3 mg/dL/day.[11] The urine to plasma creatinine ratio is less than 10 to 1 in ATN.[5]

---

*References 3, 5, 7, 10, and 15.

Another distinguishing factor for prerenal problems and ATN is the response to therapy. In prerenal problems in which no actual nephron damage has occurred, the kidney's response to therapy aimed at correcting the underlying problem is often rapid with the return of normal urine output and normal blood chemistries.[5,7] For example, in shock, therapy consists of treating the basic cause of the shock state, which varies depending on whether the shock is related to volume depletion, altered myocardial contractility, or increased intravascular capacity. The use of diuretics (furosemide, ethacrynic acid, and mannitol) is controversial; however, they are often administered as adjuncts to other therapy.[16] Prophylactic diuretic therapy may be effective in patients with toxic ATN and, when used in the early stages of ischemic ATN, diuretics may reduce oliguria and increase solute excretion. Diuretics may also reduce the amount of dialytic therapy needed.[4,17] Many diuretics are nephrotoxic in high doses, especially in the context of decreased renal function; therefore they must be used cautiously. Calcium channel blockers may be used to prevent toxic intracellular calcium accumulation and lessen the degree of tubular necrosis.[4] Because some prostaglandins act as vasodilator agents and may partially counteract the vasoconstrictive effects of sympathetic stimulation and angiotensin, prostaglandin inhibitors (aspirin, ibuprofen, and indomethacin) may be contraindicated during the onset phase of ATN.[5,6]

In true ATN, which indicates actual nephron damage, response to therapy of the underlying problem is minimal, and the patient progresses to the oliguric-anuric phase. ATN requires additional therapy aimed at correcting alterations related to the inability of the kidneys to maintain their functions.

Oliguric phase

The oliguric phase of ATN represents severe nephron dysfunction and major alterations in the kidney's ability to maintain essential functions. Clinical manifestations during the oliguric phase are exhibited in almost every organ system and physiologic process. Table 12-2 summarizes the systemic alterations, including pathophysiologic basis of the signs and symptoms and management principles. These alterations related to uremia exacerbate the overall problems of MSOF.

Catabolism develops rapidly during shock states as well as during ATN. As catabolism increases so do BUN, acidosis, and hyperkalemia. Proper nutritional management is essential to correct catabolism and its complications. A diet high in calories but low in protein is recommended. The restricted protein intake must be of high biologic value (HBV) because in HBV-protein foods, all the essential amino acids are present in each food (meat, poultry, eggs, cheese, and milk), and less urea nitrogen is produced during metabolism than with low biologic value (LBV) proteins. In contrast, each LBV-protein food (bread, beans, and cereals) does not contain all the essential amino acids, and more urea nitrogen is liberated during metabolism than with HBV proteins. Typically, for the patient undergoing dialysis, the daily HBV protein intake is 1 g/kg of body weight, and for other patients with ATN the intake is limited to 40 g/day.[5,7,18]

If the patient cannot eat, total parenteral nutrition (TPN) is recommended. A TPN calorie-to-nitrogen ratio of greater than 450:1 is recommended to prevent body protein catabolism and BUN elevation. Insulin may be required to maintain normal blood glucose. During TPN therapy, potassium, phosphate, and magnesium must be monitored and alterations corrected.[5,7,18] Although phosphate and magnesium are usually elevated in renal failure, they may be low after the initiation of TPN.

About one third of all deaths in ATN occur as the result of infection, primarily of the lungs, urinary tract, and peritoneum.[5] It is imperative that an indwelling urinary catheter is NOT left in place because this is a major source of infection. An in-and-out catheterization may be done upon initial assessment to rule out bladder or urethral obstruction. Prophylactic antibiotic therapy is not recommended for infection control in ATN.[5] If an infection is suspected, culture and sensitivity to determine specific antibiotic therapy is required. All invasive procedures require strict sterile technique, and all invasive lines require impeccable care according to hospital protocol.

All drugs that are excreted by the kidneys require dosage adjustment based on the degree of renal function, and blood levels must be monitored closely to prevent toxic effects of the drugs. Data indicate that the half-life of a drug increases gradually as the creatinine clearance decreases until the creatinine clearance falls below about 30 mL/min.

Table 12-2 Systemic Manifestations of Acute Tubular Necrosis

Problem/manifestations	Pathophysiology	Management

Fluid overload as manifested by:
  Hypertension
  Pulmonary edema
  Congestive heart failure
  Pneumonia
  Peripheral edema
  Periorbital edema
  Sacral edema
  Ascites
  ↑ PCWP and ↑ CVP
	Decreased renal excretion of water, especially during oliguric phase of ATN	Decrease fluid intake
		Dialysis or CRRT

Hyperkalemia as manifested by EKG changes:
  Tall, tented T waves
  Depressed S-T segment
  Prolonged P-R interval
  Loss of P wave
  Wide QRS complex
  Cardiac arrest
	Decreased renal excretion of potassium ions
	Acidosis
	Catabolism
	Bleeding
	Blood transfusions
	Dietary intake
		Decrease intake
		Treat bleeding and catabolism
		Correct acidosis
		Use only fresh RBCs, and administer during dialysis
		Hypertonic glucose and insulin IV
		Calcium gluconate IV
		Cation-exchange resin (e.g., Kayexalate)
		Dialysis or CRRT

Metabolic acidosis manifested by:
  Kussmaul respirations
  Hyperkalemia
  Mental changes
	Decreased renal hydrogen ion excretion
	Decreased renal reabsorption of sodium ions
	Decreased bicarbonate regeneration
	Decreased ammonia synthesis and ammonium excretion
	Decreased excretion of titratable acids
	Catabolism
		Treat catabolism
		Alkaline medications
		Dialysis or CRRT

Pericarditis as manifested by:
Classic triad:
  Fever
  Chest pain
  Pericardial friction rub
EKG changes:
  S-T segment elevation with upward concavity
  Depressed P-R interval
  Low QRS voltage
	Pericardial membrane inflammation from uremic toxins	Dialysis or CRRT to decrease uremic toxins

Pericardial effusion and tamponade as manifested by:
  Paradoxical pulse > 10 mm Hg,
  ↑ JVP with pulsations
  ↓ systolic BP
  Narrow pulse pressure
  Muffled heart sounds
  Weak peripheral pulses
  ↓ LOC
	Bleeding and effusion of fluid into pericardial cavity due to pericarditis	Dialysis or CRRT
		Pericardiocentesis for rapidly developing effusion or tamponade

Hypertension (after shock syndrome is treated and ATN ensues)	Fluid overload and sodium retention Excess renin-angiotensin production	Dialysis or CRRT Restrict sodium and fluid intake Antihypertensives
Hypotension (during shock syndrome and onset of ATN)	Hypovolemia Septicemia Excess dialysis and fluid removal	Treat underlying shock syndrome Regulate fluid removal during dialysis or CRRT

From Lancaster LE. Renal response to shock. In: Rice V, ed. Shock. Crit Care Nurs Clin North Am 1990;2:228-229.

Continued.

Problem/manifestations	Pathophysiology	Management

Anemia as manifested by:
  ↓ Hct
  ↓ Hgb
  Shortness of breath
  Decreased activity tolerance
	Decreased renal erythropoietin production
	Shortened RBC life span due to uremic toxins
	Altered folic acid action
	GI bleeding
	Hemodialysis blood loss
		Iron and folic acid supplements
		Dialysis to remove uremic toxins
		Treat GI bleeding
		RBC transfusion when patient symptomatic with low Hct/Hgb

Potential for infection (NOTE: Urea is a hypothermic agent; therefore any temperature elevation in ATN is significant)	Decreased macrophage activity due to uremic toxins Invasive lines and procedures Nosocomial and iatrogenic causes	DO NOT use indwelling urinary bladder catheter Culture and sensitivity for specific microorganisms, and use specific antibiotics

Skin alterations as manifested by:
  Pale, yellow, dry, itching skin
  Purpura
  Uremic frost (only in terminal patients)
	Uremic anemia
	Deposition of pigments, uremic toxins, and calcium phosphate in skin and irritation of peripheral nerves
	Capillary fragility and platelet dysfunction
		Bath oils and lotions
		Dialysis or CRRT
		Correction of calcium phosphate imbalances

Glucose intolerance	Decreased peripheral sensitivity to insulin, but decreased half-life due to decreased renal excretion	Dialysis Monitor plasma glucose

Altered calcium and phosphate metabolism as manifested by:
  Hyperphosphatemia
  Hypocalcemia
  Metastatic calcifications
  Osteodystrophy (only if oliguric phase is very prolonged)
	Decreased renal excretion of phosphate
	Decreased renal synthesis of vitamin D
	Excess parathyroid hormone
	Deposition of calcium phosphate crystals in skin, soft tissues, and other structures
		Dialysis or CRRT
		Phosphate binding medications (e.g., Amphojel, Basaljel, Alucaps)
		Vitamin D supplements
		Calcium supplements

Altered gastrointestinal function as manifested by:
  Anorexia
  Nausea
  Vomiting
  Stomatitis
  Halitosis
  Gastritis with bleeding
  Diarrhea
  Constipation
	Mucous membrane inflammation due to uremic toxins
	Decomposition of urea in GI tract and ammonia release which irritates mucosa
	Capillary fragility and bleeding
	Electrolyte imbalances
		Dialysis or CRRT
		Mouth care
		Bulk laxatives prn

Altered neuromuscular-mental function as manifested by:
  Drowsiness
  Confusion
  Irritability
  Coma
  Tremors
  Twitching
  Convulsions
  Peripheral neuropathy (restless legs syndrome)
  Decreased concentration
  Altered perception
  Decreased mentation
	Uremic toxins' effect on nervous system
	Fluid and electrolyte imbalances
		Dialysis or CRRT

Beyond that point, the half-life of the drug increases rapidly with further decreases in creatinine clearance.[19] Thus the creatinine clearance and serum creatinine may be used as guides for altering drug doses in the patient with ATN.

Many drugs are removed from the plasma during hemodialysis and peritoneal dialysis. Such drugs require supplemental dosing after dialysis to maintain therapeutic plasma levels. Consultation with the dialysis team is important for determining which drugs as dialyzable and for deciding the appropriate supplementation dosage after dialysis.

Most patients with ATN will require dialytic therapy in addition to nutrition support, fluid management, and medications. Initiation of dialysis is indicated in the following situations:

1. Severe uremia as manifested by BUN greater than 100 mg/dL, serum creatinine greater than 10 mg/dL, and associated pericarditis, gastrointestinal bleeding, and mental changes
2. Hyperkalemia and severe catabolism that do not respond well to nutritional management and medications
3. Intravascular and extravascular fluid overload
4. Metabolic acidosis that cannot be controlled by medications[5]

Dialytic therapy may be provided as intermittent hemodialysis or peritoneal dialysis (PD) or as continuous renal replacement therapy (CRRT), such as continuous arteriovenous hemofiltration (CAVH) and slow continuous ultrafiltration (SCUF). Although hemodialysis is the most rapid, efficient form of therapy, it requires an access to the circulation and carries several complications, such as blood loss, hypotension, and disequilibrium from rapid osmolality changes.[20] Thus hemodynamically unstable patients are often unable to tolerate the procedure.[21]

PD requires an access to the peritoneal cavity for instillation of dialysate. Peritonitis is a frequent complication, and PD cannot be used for patients who have had recent abdominal surgery.[22,23]

CRRT therapy is suited for those patients who are hemodynamically unstable, especially those with myocardial failure, shock, or MSOF.[23-25] CRRT does, however, require a large indwelling vascular catheter, which can result in infection and emboli. CRRT allows for rapid removal of large volumes of fluid without rapid changes in vascular volume. CRRT also allows for TPN therapy without the complication of fluid overload.[23-25]

Diuretic phase

Although the diuretic phase heralds an improvement in renal function, the increased urine output does not indicate that the kidneys have regained the ability to control homeostasis. Dialytic therapy or CRRT may be necessary during this phase until the BUN and plasma potassium and sodium stabilize. Weight, blood pressure, pulse, and skin turgor are used as parameters for fluid replacement. A general rule for fluid replacement is to replace two thirds of the previous 12 hours of urine output during the subsequent 12 hours.[5] Drug doses and plasma drug levels must continue to be monitored during the diuretic phase.

Recovery phase

Regular assessment of renal function and supportive care are required during the recovery phase. Urinary tract infections and other insults to the already compromised kidneys must be prevented. Any condition that may precipitate prerenal failure and ATN must receive careful, early treatment.

Nursing diagnoses and collaborative problems

The nurse caring for the patient with ATN in the context of MSOF participates as a collaborative member of a multidisciplinary health care team. Care begins upon the patient's entry into the health care system and continues throughout the multidimensional spectrum of MSOF and the various phases of ATN. Nursing assessment, diagnoses, and interventions are an important part of this multidisciplinary, collaborative approach.

The box on p. 234 lists the most common nursing diagnoses and collaborative nursing problems that are encountered in the typical patient with ATN who may also be receiving dialytic therapy or CRRT. This list is not intended to be exhaustive or to describe the nursing care for any individual patient. Manifestations and treatment vary from patient to patient; thus individual patient assessment and care planning is imperative. Potential manifestations related to each diagnosis, assessment parameters, and interventions may be extrapolated from the information in this chapter.

CONCLUSION

When the MAP decreases below approximately 50 to 70 mm Hg, renal autoregulatory processes

---

NURSING DIAGNOSES RELATED TO ACUTE TUBULAR NECROSIS

Alterations in cardiac output (decreased) related to underlying shock syndrome, pericarditis, pericardial effusion and tamponade, electrolyte imbalances and dysrhythmias

Altered comfort: pain related to effects of uremic toxins on peripheral sensory nerves

Altered comfort: nausea and vomiting, related to gastritis secondary to uremic toxins

Altered comfort: pruritus, related to deposition of uremic toxins and calcium phosphate crystals in skin

Ineffective family coping related to a critically ill family member

Anxiety/fear related to uncertainty of prognosis

Fluid volume deficit related to fluid loss during diuretic phase of ATN

Fluid volume excess related to fluid retention during oliguric-anuric phase of ATN

High risk for infection related to altered immune processes in ATN, invasive lines and procedures, and nosocomial infections

Knowledge deficit about cause of illness, treatment regimen, and prognosis

Alterations in nutrition: less than body requirements, related to protein restriction during ATN and altered metabolism of nutrients

Impaired tissue integrity related to effects of uremic toxins on skin (dryness, altered circulation, pruritus, capillary fragility, and easy bruising)

Alterations in oral mucous membranes related to effects of uremic toxins on mucous membranes

---

From Lancaster LE. Renal response to shock. In: Rice V, ed. Shock. Crit Care Nurs Clin North Am 1990;2:231.

---

are no longer effective. Systemic maldistribution of volume and regional changes in renal blood flow secondary to circulating mediators also affect oxygen delivery to the kidneys. Decreased renal blood flow often leads to ATN and its related uremic syndrome. The patient with ATN typically experiences four successive phases as the ATN progresses and then eventually resolves; however, in the setting of MSOF, resolution is very infrequent. During the oliguric-anuric phase of ATN, multiple organ systems and physiologic processes are affected by the alterations occurring as the result of severely altered renal function. With appropriate treatment, such as fluid-electrolyte regulation, acid-base control, nutritional support, and renal replacement therapy, return to normal or near normal renal function is possible in some patients. Overall mortality is dependent on many underlying factors. The number of other organ systems involved, the presence of infection and other complications, and the severity of the underlying disease significantly affect the prognosis.

REFERENCES

1. Guyton AC. Textbook of medical physiology. 7th ed. Philadelphia: WB Saunders, 1986:395-400; 410-413.
2. Lancaster LE. Renal and endocrine regulation of water and electrolyte balance. In: Chambers J, ed. Common fluid and electrolyte disorders Nurs Clin North Am 1987;22:761-772.
3. Richard CJ. Comprehensive nephrology nursing. Boston: Little, Brown & Co, 1986:178-221.
4. Burke TJ et al. Renal response to shock. Ann Emerg Med 1986;15:1397-1400.
5. Eknoyan G. Therapy of the acute renal failure syndrome. In: Martinez-Maldonado M, ed. Handbook of renal therapeutics. New York: Plenum Medical Book Co, 1983:425-450.
6. Stahl W. Kidney in shock. In: Barrett J, Nyhus LM, eds. Treatment of shock: Principles and practice. 2nd ed. Philadelphia: Lea & Febiger, 1986:137-149.
7. Martin K. Pathophysiology of acute renal failure. In: Klahr S, ed. The kidney and body fluids in health and disease. New York: Plenum Medical Book Co, 1983:443-462.
8. Brezis M, Rosen S, Epstein FH. Acute renal failure. In: Brenner BM, Rector Jr FC. The kidney. 3rd ed. Philadelphia: WB Saunders, 1986.
9. Kellener SP, Berl T. Acute renal failure associated with hypovolemia. In: Brenner BM, Lazarus JM, eds. Acute renal failure. 2nd ed. New York: Churchill Livingstone, 1988: 233-250.
10. Solez K. Acute renal failure ("acute tubular necrosis," infarction, and cortical necrosis). In: Heptinstall RH, ed. Pathology of the kidney. 3rd ed. Boston: Little, Brown & Co, 1983:1069-1148.
11. Ayres SM, Schlichtig R, Sterling MJ. Care of the critically ill. 3rd ed. St Louis: Mosby–Year Book, 1988:276-283.
12. Lancaster LE, Baer C. Pathophysiology of acute renal dysfunction. In: Schoengrund L, Balzer P, eds. Renal problems in critical care. New York: John Wiley & Sons, 1985:21-46.
13. Haljamae H. Organ specific metabolic changes in shock. Prog Clin Biol Res 1988;264:17-26.
14. Gaudio K, Siegel NJ. Pathogenesis and treatment of acute renal failure. Pediatr Clin North Am 1987;34:771-787.
15. Rudnick MR et al. The differential diagnosis of acute renal failure. In: Brenner BM, Lazarus JM, eds. Acute renal failure. 2nd ed. New York: Churchill Livingstone, 1988:177-232.
16. Levinsky NG, Bernard DB. Mannitol and loop diuretics in acute renal failure. In: Brenner BM, Lazarus JM, eds. Acute renal failure. 2nd ed. New York: Churchill Livingstone, 1988:841-856.
17. Perry AG. Shock complications: Recognition and management. Crit Care Q 1988;11:1-8.

18. Mitch WE, Wilmore DW. Nutritional considerations in the treatment of acute renal failure. In: Brenner BM, Lazarus JM, eds. Acute renal failure. 2nd ed. New York: Churchill Livingstone, 1988:743-766.

19. Baer C. The pharmacologic aspects of renal failure. In: Lancaster LE, ed. Core curriculum for nephrology nursing. Pitman, NJ: American Nephrology Nurses' Assn, 1987: 157-184.

20. Lancaster LE. The patient with end stage renal disease. 2nd ed. New York: John Wiley & Sons, 1984.

21. Hakim RM, Lazarus JM. Hemodialysis in acute renal failure. In: Brenner BM, Lazarus JM, eds. Acute renal failure. 2nd ed. New York: Churchill Livingstone, 1988:767-808.

22. Nolph KD, Sorkin MI: Peritoneal dialysis in acute renal failure. In: Brenner BM, Lazarus JM, eds. Acute renal failure. 2nd ed. New York: Churchill Livingstone, 1988:809-838.

23. Price CA. Continuous renal replacement therapy: Conservative management of acute renal failure. Nephrol Nurs Update 1989;1:1-6.

24. Dirkes SM. Continuous arteriovenous hemofiltration (CAVH). Crit Care Nurs Currents 1989;7:1-4.

25. Paradiso C: Hemofiltration: An alternative to dialysis. Heart Lung 1989;282-290.

SUGGESTED READINGS

Anderson RJ, Schrier RW. Acute tubular necrosis. In: Schrier RJ, Gottschalk CW, eds. Diseases of the kidney. 4th ed. Boston: Little, Brown & Co, 1988:1413-1446.

Bonventure JV, Leaf A, Malis CD. Nature of the cellular insult in ischemic acute renal failure. In: Brenner BM, Lazarus JM, eds. Acute renal failure. 2nd ed. New York: Churchill Livingstone, 1988:3-44.

Finn W. Recovery from acute renal failure. In: Brenner BM, Lazarus JM, eds. Acute renal failure. 2nd ed. New York: Churchill Livingstone, 1988:875-917.

Kjellstrand CM, Berkseth RO, Klinkmann H. Treatment of acute renal failure. In: Schrier RW, Gottschalk CW, eds. Diseases of the kidney. 4th ed. Boston: Little, Brown & Co, 1988;1501-1540.

Madias ME, Donohoe JF, Harrington JT. Postischemic acute renal failure. In: Brenner BM, Lazarus JM, eds. Acute renal failure. 2nd ed. New York: Churchill Livingstone, 1988: 251-278.

Schrier RW et al. Pathophysiology of cell ischemia. In: Schrier RW, Gottschalk CW, eds. Diseases of the kidney. 4th ed. Boston: Little, Brown & Co, 1988:1379-1412.

Siegel NJ, Gaudio KM. Amino acids and adenine nucleotides in acute renal failure. In: Brenner BM, Lazarus JM, eds. Acute renal failure. 2nd ed. New York: Churchill Livingstone, 1988:857-874.

13 The Central Nervous System: Dysfunction and Exhaustion

Venita Dasch

Death from single organ failure is a rare occurrence in the critically ill patient because of advancement in resuscitative techniques and the interdependence of multiple organ systems. The exception to this phenomenon is seen in the mortality associated with head injury, which accounts for approximately half of all trauma-related deaths. The presence of a head injury increases patient mortality threefold.[1] Therefore it can be argued that virtually all patients who die in intensive care units, unless they experience sudden cardiac death or brain-stem herniation, die with some degree of multisystem organ failure (MSOF).

The syndrome of MSOF, however, is not simply the failure of two or more organ systems but a systemic deterioration sustained by the inflammatory response. Patient decline is progressive and often predictable, experienced initially as impaired function of the lungs followed by liver and kidney involvement. Continuing deterioration involves the gut, heart, and brain.[2]

Historically, patients who succumbed to this chain of events had the diagnosis of shock recorded as the mode of death. With the initiation of aggressive critical care intervention, many patients now survive the hypotensive episode associated with shock only to develop MSOF later in their course. Although hypotension may be the precipitating event, sepsis, cardiac arrest, trauma, and major surgery are other factors associated with the development of this catastrophic patient complication.

PATHOPHYSIOLOGY

The MSOF process and its precipitating factors negatively affect the central nervous system (CNS). Although the exact mechanism of damage

---

PATHOPHYSIOLOGIC DAMAGE TO THE CENTRAL NERVOUS SYSTEM

Associated with Sepsis
  Brain microabscesses
  Disordered amino acid transport and metabolism
  Altered neurotransmitter concentrations
  Reduced cerebral blood flow
Associated with Ischemia
  Glucose metabolic abnormalities
  Cellular acidosis
  ATP depletion
  Membrane damage
  Calcium shifts
  Excitatory amino acid neurotransmitter activity
Associated with Cerebral Reperfusion Injury
  Oxygen-derived free radical (ODFR) production
  Arachidonic acid metabolism
  No-reflow phenomenon

---

is poorly understood, sepsis, circulatory and microcirculatory perfusion deficits, and cerebral reperfusion injury are thought to be significant factors in this process (see box above).

Sepsis

The central nervous system is one of the first systems affected by sepsis. However, the exact mechanism of injury remains unclear. Current research directed at the etiology of CNS damage focuses on the development of brain microabscesses, disordered amino acid transport and metabolism, alterations in brain neurotransmitter concentration, and ischemia resulting from global or regional reduction in cerebral blood flow.

Brain microabscesses. Brain abscesses seeded by blood-borne contaminants most often originate at the junction of the white and gray matter. This rather poorly vascularized area is rich in end-arterioles, which are easily occluded by septic emboli, resulting in ischemia. Microabscesses can also threaten the integrity of the CNS by initiating hyperemia, edema, and petechial hemorrhages.[3]

The presence of brain microabscesses may occasionally be responsible for the septic encephalopathy noted in the patient with MSOF. Jackson et al[4] reviewed the neuropathologic records of 2172 patients. From this review, 12 patients were identified as having encephalopathies unexplained by metabolic, drug, or structural abnormalities. Of these 12 patients, eight were noted to have brain microabscesses during postmortem examinations.

In a similar review of 1728 consecutive autopsies, Pendlebury et al[5] found 24 cases of brain microabscesses. The primary site of infection was most commonly the lung. Although the overall incidence of brain microabscesses is relatively low in these studies, the actual frequency of occurrence and mortality associated with this lesion are unknown.

Disordered amino acid transport and metabolism. Disordered amino acid transport and metabolism are detected as increased plasma levels of aromatic and sulfur-containing amino acids in the patient with sepsis. Increased plasma levels of phenylalanine, tyrosine, glutamine, and the false neurotransmitter octopamine elevate shortly before death, indicating the liver's inability to metabolize these aromatic amino acids.[6] Specifically, increased phenylalanine and glutamine levels have been noted in the brain and cerebrospinal fluid (CSF) of the patient with sepsis. This alteration in brain amino acid content is thought to be independent of altered plasma levels and to actually reflect transport of neutral amino acids across the blood-brain barrier.[7] Accumulation of aromatic amino acids could play a role in the vasodilatation and altered cerebral function associated with sepsis.

Altered neurotransmitter concentration. Increased levels of serotonin and 5-hydroxyindoleacetic acid (5-HIAA) have been reported in rats with sepsis. The serotonin pathways generally result in inhibited behavioral and motor activity consistent with the encephalopathic changes associated with MSOF.[7]

Reduced cerebral blood flow. The effect of sepsis-induced alterations in cerebral blood flow was studied by Bowton et al[8] using the Xenon (Xe) washout technique in nine infected patients manifesting acute encephalopathies. This technique estimates cerebral blood flow (CBF) based on Xe clearance primarily by the superficial cortex. All patients had respiratory failure and one or more of the following: acute renal failure, acute hepatic dysfunction, and positive blood cultures.

Bowton et al found that all nine patients with sepsis had reduced CBF that was *not* related to changes in mean arterial pressure (MAP) or cerebral perfusion pressure (CPP). Furthermore the cerebral metabolic rate of oxygen measured after obtaining jugular bulb blood samples was significantly depressed at 1.1 mL/100 g/min. Augmentation or reduction in CBF did not alter the cerebral metabolic rate of oxygen. CO_2 reactivity remained intact.[8] Whether sepsis-induced encephalopathy is the result of hypoperfusion to the brain or the result of metabolic changes within the brain that reduce the cerebral metabolic rate of oxygen remains unclear.[8]

Perfusion deficits: cerebral ischemia

Perfusion deficits in the brain result when the metabolic demands of the cerebral cell exceed the available energy resources. When CNS damage is associated with hypotensive shock or cardiac arrest, its cause is well described. However, alterations in the microcirculation may actually be a more significant factor in the overall process of cerebral ischemia. The cause of microcirculatory disturbances remains under investigation.

Cerebral metabolic demands. Energy is required by the cerebral cell for maintaining synaptic transmission and cellular integrity. Synaptic transmission refers to the electrical activity of the neuron and has been termed *activation metabolism*.[9] Activation metabolism demands approximately 55% of the neuron's total energy requirements.[10] When cerebral perfusion falls below the threshold of activation metabolism, electrical silencing occurs. Maintenance of cellular integrity is termed *residual metabolism* and comprises 40% to 45% of the neuron's energy requirements. Violation of the lower ischemic threshold of residual metabolism results in irreversible cell damage.[9]

Ischemia results when residual metabolism is compromised by the perfusion or extraction deficits associated with sepsis and MSOF. This uncoupling of metabolic need to available energy resources forces adenosine triphosphate (ATP) production through anaerobic pathways. The result in the cerebral environment is lactic acid accumulation with concomitant intracellular acidosis. The exact mechanism by which acidosis produces cellular compromise is unknown. However, when intracellular pH falls below 5.5 or ATP is exhausted, irreversible cell damage occurs.[10] Cellular integrity is also affected by glucose metabolism, the maintenance of cellular membranes and ion gradients, the synthesis of neurotransmitters, and the presence of prostaglandins and oxygen-derived free radicals (ODFRs).[10]

Glucose metabolism. Glucose provides the energy for the synthesis of ATP from ADP and inorganic phosphates. In the initial step of glycolysis, glucose is converted to pyruvate, producing a net yield of 2 moles of ATP per mole of glucose.[11] In the presence of oxygen, pyruvate moves into the mitochondria and enters the tricarboxylic acid cycle (Krebs' cycle), producing 36 moles of ATP per initial mole of glucose.[12]

Without adequate blood flow, the supply of glucose is exhausted, rapidly depleting the ATP stores. Periods of incomplete ischemia resulting from decreased cerebral blood flow can actually be more damaging to the cerebral cell than the complete ischemia of circulatory arrest. When ischemia is incomplete, oxygen levels are inadequate to support aerobic metabolism. However, glucose delivery continues to the ischemic area. This continuing supply of glucose, anaerobically metabolized to lactate, produces large quantities of lactic acid, resulting in cellular acidosis.[10]

Cellular acidosis. Cellular acidosis decreases the uptake of calcium ions (Ca^{2+}) by the mitochondria; thus cytosolic Ca^{2+} levels increase. Increased Ca^{2+} activates enzymes such as phospholipases and proteases, which are capable of destroying cell membranes and intracellular organelles.[10] A pH of 6.0 to 6.4 also inhibits stage-3 mitochondrial respiration, which further blocks the synthesis of ATP from ADP and inorganic phosphate.[10]

ATP depletion. ATP is essential for all functions of the cerebral cell that require energy. During periods of complete ischemia, ATP is exhausted in 5 to 7 minutes. The depletion of ATP leads to calcium shifts, the synthesis of prostaglandins and ODFRs, and membrane damage.[13]

Membrane damage. The maintenance of ionic gradients in the cerebral cell is dependent on the Na^+/K^+ ATPase pump, which requires ATP as a source of energy. Depletion of ATP results in pump failure, followed by a massive influx of Na^+ and water, efflux of K^+, and membrane depolarization. Increased intracellular Na^+ concentrations result in cytotoxic edema and cell death. Increased extracellular K^+ concentrations alter the plasma membrane potential, resulting in intracellular Ca^+ shifts.[10]

Calcium shifts. Calcium enters the cerebral cell through voltage-dependent and NMDA receptor-controlled channels during periods of ischemia. Large calcium influx results in cytotoxic edema and cell death. Ca^{2+} has also been implicated in damage of the mitochondrial membranes by two processes. First, massive Ca^{2+} influx can activate enzymes, including phospholipases and proteases, capable of destroying cell membranes. Phospholipase A_2 hydrolyzes phospholipids within the cell and mitochondrial membranes, releasing free fatty acids (particularly arachidonic acid) and their metabolites. Second, calcium inhibits adenine nucleotide translocase, thus preventing mitochondrial oxidative phosphorylation and ATP production.[10]

Excitatory amino acid neurotransmitters. The excitatory neurotransmitters, glutamate and aspartate, may have a role in the ischemic process. The evidence to support their role is based on the concept of *selective vulnerability,* which refers to a heightened susceptibility to ischemia experienced by specific brain regions.[10]

Glutamine occurs in increased concentrations in areas of ischemia. Also, postsynaptic receptors for the excitatory neurotransmitters glutamate and aspartate occur primarily in those areas of the brain that are known to be particularly vulnerable. One of these receptors, the NMDA receptor, is coupled to an ion chain. Repeated stimulation of the NMDA receptor opens the ion chain, allowing an accumulation of Na^+ and Ca^{2+}, which produces osmotic swelling, membrane damage, and cell death.[10]

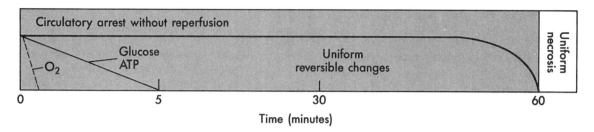

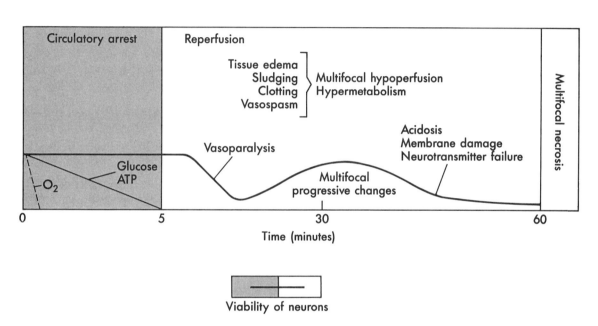

Viability of neurons

Fig. 13-1 Diagram of hypothetical events in the brain following total circulatory arrest (no blood flow). *Vertical axes:* Viability of brain tissue, from preischemic normal *(left)* to postischemic brain death *(right)*. *Top:* Without reperfusion, brain damage becomes clearly irreversible (necrosis) after only 30 to 60 minutes of no flow (complete ischemia). *Bottom:* With reperfusion after no flow for at least 5 minutes, secondary changes are provoked, which adds to the initial insult, resulting in multifocal necroses. (From Safar P. Hosp Pract 1981;16:67.)

Cerebral reperfusion injury

Cerebral reperfusion injury refers to ischemic damage occurring after circulation has been restored to the brain compromised by complete or incomplete perfusion deficits (Fig. 13-1). Damage during cerebral reperfusion results from the accumulation of free fatty acids, prostaglandins, and ODFRs.

Free fatty acids. Free fatty acids normally enter the tricarboxylic acid cycle for the synthesis of ATP. Their conversion to ATP, however, is ATP dependent. During periods of ischemia, sepsis, trauma, or any process that results in Ca^{2+} influx into the cell, phospholipase A_2 is activated and hydrolyzes phospholipids in the cell membrane. Large accumulations of free fatty acids result, which can alter oxidative phosphorylation, encourage flux of K^+ and Ca^{2+} into the cytosol, produce cerebral edema, and increase arachidonic acid metabolism.[10]

Arachidonic acid metabolism. During ischemia, sepsis, or trauma, arachidonic acid accumulates. The three major arachidonic acid metabolites are leukotrienes (LT), thromboxane (TX), and prostaglandins (PG). In the vasculature, a balance most likely exists between PGI_2 (a potent vasodilator) and TxA_2, a potent vasoconstrictor and platelet aggregator. Formation of leukotrienes within the CNS occurs with both ischemia and cerebral reperfusion injury. The leukotrienes have been shown to cause vasoconstriction of the cerebral circulation.[14]

During ischemia of the cerebral vessel wall, there is an inactivation of PGI_2 synthetase (enzyme necessary to form PGI_2), resulting in diminished synthesis of PGI_2. TxA_2 synthetase necessary for TxA_2 formation is affected less severely because only a small proportion of systemic platelet content is in the brain during periods of ischemia (platelets are a major source of TxA_2). The ensuing imbalance shifts the metabolism of arachidonic acid toward an increased synthesis of TxA_2, resulting in vasoconstriction and platelet aggregation.[10]

Oxygen-derived free radicals. Free radicals are highly reactive, unstable molecules generated during normal oxidative phosphorylation and ATP production. Free radicals are normally tightly bound within the mitochondrial membrane, posing no threat to cellular integrity. Their exact impact on neuronal cell death is currently under investigation.[10]

During periods of ischemia, the tissue enzyme xanthine dehydrogenase is converted to xanthine oxidase. The oxidase enzyme, along with other products produced in the ischemic tissue, combines with oxygen to form oxygen-derived free radicals (ODFRs), such as the superoxide radical, hydrogen peroxide, and the hydroxyl radical. Because oxygen must be present for ODFR generation, free radicals are found in higher concentrations after periods of incomplete ischemia or during reperfusion after ischemia, when more oxygen is present. Accumulation of the superoxide radical has been shown to change phospholipid and protein structure.[10] See Chapters 3 and 5 for figures and an in-depth explanation of reperfusion injury.

Furthermore, during ischemia the increase in free-iron concentration encourages the conversion of the superoxide radical to the more unstable and toxic hydroxyl radical. Hydroxyl radicals can damage protein, cause breakdown of DNA strands, and initiate lipid peroxidation of polyunsaturated fatty acids in the cell membrane. The by-products of lipid peroxidation, aldehydes and hydrocarbon gases, damage membranes and disrupt ionic gradients. The result is vasogenic and cytotoxic edema, disruption of the blood-brain barrier, and inflammation. These by-products can also alter phospholipase activity, increasing the release of arachidonic acid and the subsequent formation of prostaglandins.[10]

When reperfusion occurs subsequent to circulatory arrest, cerebral reperfusion injury has been identified by two processes: postischemic hypoperfusion and the no-reflow phenomenon. Morphologic support for the occurrence of injury during the reperfusion period notes a watershed pattern of cerebral damage consistent with incomplete ischemia instead of the expected diffuse patterns of global ischemia.[10]

Postischemic hypoperfusion. Postischemic hypoperfusion occurs after periods of complete global ischemia and is noted clinically as a 15- to 20-minute period of hyperemia followed by the initiation of vasospasm-induced hypoperfusion. Hyperemia results from the loss of autoregulation during the ischemic process and from the difference in blood viscosity of the stagnant blood versus the blood in the microcirculation. Vasospasm, lasting 6 to 24 hours, is thought to be a response to calcium activation and increased production of TxA_2.[10]

No-reflow phenomenon. The no-reflow phenomenon, lasting 1 to 3 days, is seen more rarely than postischemic hypoperfusion and refers to the continued decrease in cerebral blood flow despite normal MAP and CPP. Damaging processes identified in this phenomenon are edema, vasospasm, increased blood viscosity with red-cell sludging, hypermetabolism, membrane damage, intracellular or mitochondrial calcium shifts, and the release of ODFRs.[13]

CLINICAL PRESENTATION AND ASSESSMENT

The CNS is one of the first systems affected by the MSOF syndrome, and its clinical decline is the least understood. Complicating the picture are EEG changes consistent with metabolic or anoxic encephalopathy, such as slowing and triphasic waves. However, a period of clinical hypoxia is frequently not present, and researchers have been unsuccessful in isolating a metabolic reason for these findings. Furthermore, some patients with profound EEG abnormalities, such as burst suppression, recover normal neurologic function.[15] An even more puzzling phenomenon is the inconsistent morphologic findings during postmortem examination that do not always reflect the profound neurologic deterioration experienced by the patient.[2]

CNS failure

CNS failure in the MSOF process is defined as a decreased level of consciousness ranging from confusion to coma that cannot be explained by structural, drug, or metabolic abnormalities. Typically, the patient loses interest in his surroundings and becomes restless and easily distracted. Muscle stiffness and meningism occur, but CAT scan is normal, and there are no localizing signs.[2] If deterioration continues, drowsiness, confusion, and coma follow (see box below).

These early neurologic changes noted in the patient with MSOF are consistent with the neuroendocrine activities associated with stress or trauma. Immediately following the onset of injury, the patient is quiet, lethargic, and disinterested in his surroundings. This primal response of withdrawal attempts to maximize the beneficial effects of the

---

CLINICAL CONDITIONS AND ASSESSMENT PARAMETERS

Emotional Response to Sympathetic Stimulation
  Increased wariness
  Poor eye contact
  Increased concentration
  Restlessness
  Resistance to fatigue
  Insomnia
  Perceptual inaccuracies
Clinical Evidence of CNS Dysfunction
  Altered concentration
  Confusion
  Coma
  Rigidity and postural action tremors
  EEG abnormalities
  Increased CSF protein
Indicators of Neuroendocrine Exhaustion or
  Failure
  Glucose intolerance
  Failure to mount a febrile response
  Neurogenic pulmonary edema
  Low T_3 syndrome

---

neuroendocrine response to injury and increase the possibility of survival without treatment. The initiator is most likely the production of beta-endorphins, enkephalin, and interleukin-1 (IL-1).[16]

Neuroendocrine response

Following the initial response, the neuroanatomic pathways are activated by two processes. First, sensory impulses are relayed directly to the cerebral cortex and are processed to memory. If the event is perceived as stressful, signals are sent to the limbic system, where unpleasant emotions are generated, and to the ascending reticular activating system, which increases the level of arousal. Second, signals are sent to the hypothalamus by way of the cerebral cortex or the direct thalamic pathways. Stimulation of the thalamus without cortex involvement explains why some patients demonstrate physical responses to stress but deny feelings of fear or anxiety.[17]

Thalamic stimulation from cortical or direct thalamic routes activates the neural and hormonal responses originating in the hypothalamus. This results in increased muscle tone through activation of the gamma motor neurons, stimulation of the sympathetic nervous system, and the release of hormones from the anterior and posterior pituitary gland (Fig. 13-2). This prepares the patient for the "fight or flight" response to stress.[17]

Sympathetic stimulation results in increased wariness, poor eye contact, increased concentration, restlessness, and resistance to fatigue. Insomnia occurs, inducing perceptual inaccuracies, changes in time sense, memory alterations, and communication difficulties that further compound perceptual disturbances.[17]

Current research

In a study of encephalopathy associated with septic illness, Young et al[15] noted similar neurologic alterations. Over a 31-month period, they observed all patients at their institution who had positive microbial cultures from either blood or a deep surgical site and a rectal or oral temperature greater than 38.5° C when the culture was taken. From this population, 69 patients were admitted to the study and classified as severely encephalopathic (SE), mildly encephalopathic (ME), or nonencephalopathic (NE).

Young et al[15] described the neurologic changes in these patients as diffuse, ranging from altered

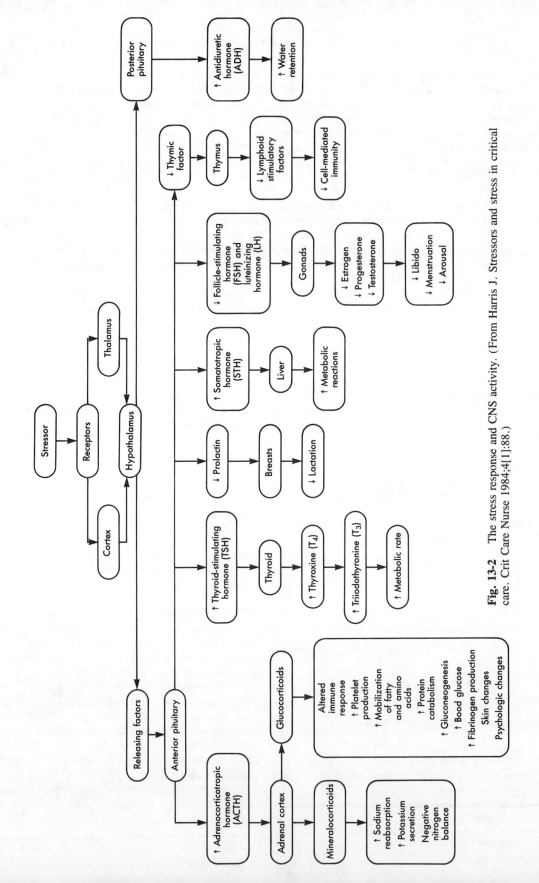

Fig. 13-2 The stress response and CNS activity. (From Harris J. Stressors and stress in critical care. Crit Care Nurse 1984;4[1]:88.)

concentration and intermittent confusion to coma in the patient with a severe encephalopathy. Rigidity and postural-action tremor were present in some of the patients in each category. EEG findings were likewise variable, with the degree of EEG abnormality correlating to the degree of encephalopathy and reflecting changes consistent with metabolic derangement. However, the researchers were unable to identify a metabolic abnormality capable of causing the degree of encephalopathy.

The patients who were classified as SE in the study experienced delirium, stupor, or coma. Cerebrospinal fluid results on the SE patients only showed an increase in protein concentration. Glucose and cell counts were normal. The increase in protein concentration could reflect increased permeability of the blood-brain barrier induced by cytokines and other vasoactive mediators released from activated macrophages and neutrophils in sepsis. Gram-negative bacterial endotoxin may directly damage the endothelium or trigger the release of other damaging mediators, such as tumor necrosis factor (TNF) and IL-1 from activated macrophages. These mediators alter the microcirculation, including capillary permeability, in extracerebral organs and probably in the brain as well. The resultant increase in interstitial fluid impairs diffusion between cells and capillaries.[15]

In summary, much of the early clinical evidence of failure can be explained by neuroendocrine responses to stress and trauma. However, the exact cause of the profound changes of stupor and coma remain unclear. Current research is directed to a myriad of microcirculatory and chemical alterations that affect the viability and functional ability of the cerebral cell.

IMPACT ON THE MSOF PROCESS

Nervous system dysfunction is a frequent occurrence in the patient with sepsis and MSOF and is predictive of a poor prognosis. The impact of CNS failure on the MSOF process is observed not only in increased patient mortality but also in increased length of stay and recovery time in the ICU. Pine et al[18] used the inability to follow commands as an indicator of CNS dysfunction in 106 patients with sepsis. They noted a mortality rate of 100% when CNS failure accompanied sepsis, compared to a 10% mortality when sepsis accompanied damage to any other single organ.

Mortality in MSOF increases with the length of

hospital stay. Young et al[15] compared recovery time in patients with mild or severe encephalopathies. Mild encephalopathy usually cleared in 6 weeks, while a severe encephalopathy took 6 weeks to 3 months to clear.

In association with its impact on hospital stay and mortality, CNS dysfunction affects the MSOF process in three areas: septic encephalopathy, critical illness polyneuropathy, and neuroendocrine exhaustion or failure.

Septic encephalopathy

Many studies have been reported comparing mortality in patients with sepsis who exhibit either nonencephalopathic or encephalopathic symptoms. Sprung et al[19] studied 1333 patients with sepsis using an altered sensorium as the indicator of neurologic dysfunction. They stated that the overall incidence of altered mental status was 23%. Mortality ranged from 49% for the encephalopathic group to 26% for patients with normal mental status. In the previously mentioned study by Young et al,[15] mortality occurred at a rate of 0% for the patients without encephalopathies, 35% for patients with mild encephalopathies, and 56% for patients with severe enccphalopathies.

It is obvious from these data that encephalopathy is associated with increased mortality. However, what is not obvious is the cause-and-effect relationship between these two variables (encephalopathy and mortality). Such alterations as failure to mount a febrile response within the first 24 hours, hypotension, and thrombocytopenia occur in direct relationship to severity of encephalopathy and mortality.[19] However, these alterations are also reflective of patients with severe and progressive MSOF. These patients are simply more severely ill, and the presence of a specific neurologic precursor to the MSOF process has not been identified.[19,20]

More likely, the increased mortality in MSOF associated with septic encephalopathy is due to the overall effects of critical illness, such as immobility, increased ICU stay, respiratory failure, mechanical ventilation, and loss of power and purpose.[1]

Critical illness polyneuropathy

Profound weakness and muscle wasting have long been identified as components of sepsis and MSOF. The resultant increased recovery time and difficulty weaning from the ventilator common to patients with sepsis and MSOF were thought to be exclusively related to catabolic myopathy. However, research and results from postmortem examinations have shown axonal degeneration of the phrenic nerve and denervation atrophy of the diaphragm and intercostal muscles in the patient with MSOF.[21] Therefore current thinking includes denervation atrophy as a second cause of weakness and muscle wasting in the patient with MSOF. The exact cause has not been identified, but a basic defect generated by the inflammatory response is one theory.

This syndrome has been termed critical illness polyneuropathy and includes primary axonal degeneration of motor and sensory fibers and denervation atrophy of limb and skeletal muscles. Witt et al[21] performed electrophysiologic studies on 43 patients who were diagnosed with sepsis and MSOF. Of the 43 patients, 30 (70%) had an abnormal nerve function index. Of these 30 patients, 15 (50%) had clinical signs of polyneuropathy such as difficulty weaning from the ventilator, distal weakness of limb muscles, and reduced deep-tendon reflexes. Electrophysiologic studies showed alterations consistent with a primary axonal degeneration of both sensory and motor fibers.

Witt et al[21] found no relationship between the development of polyneuropathy and the number of failed organs, total number of antibiotics, aminoglycoside antibiotic blood levels, nutritional factors, water or electrolyte disturbances, indices of kidney or liver failure, or elevation of muscle enzymes. They did, however, find a positive relationship between lowered serum albumin and the development of polyneuropathy. In combination, the presence of lowered serum albumin, days in ICU, and elevated serum glucose accounted for 47% of all potential variables affecting the altered nerve function index.

Three theories have been postulated to explain the impact of these variables on the development of critical illness polyneuropathy.[21] First, hyperglycemia common in sepsis increases microvascular resistance, which reduces the nerve microcirculation. The resultant hypoxia could compromise mitochondrial function and impair axonal transport of structural proteins, thereby inducing the axonal degeneration typical of polyneuropathy. Second, low serum albumin is associated with in-

creased microvascular permeability. A shift of albumin out of the intravascular compartment into the peripheral blood-nerve barrier could increase edema and, hence, hypoxia. The third theory focuses on alterations of circulation. Maldistribution of circulating volume is common in sepsis and MSOF because blood is shunted from peripheral tissues to more central areas, such as the heart, brain, liver, and kidneys. Since blood vessels supplying the peripheral nerves lack autoregulation, they would be particularly susceptible to perfusion deficits during this process.

Critical illness polyneuropathy affects the MSOF process by increasing patient mortality and doubling or tripling recovery time.[15] Witt et al[21] noted the effect of polyneuropathy on mortality in their study of 43 patients with sepsis and MSOF. All three patients classified with severe polyneuropathy (an absence of voluntary or reflex-induced movement in all four limbs) died (100% mortality) compared to a 53% overall mortality in this study.

Neuroendocrine exhaustion or failure

The neuroendocrine system plays an important role in the hormonal response to injury and stress. However, the concept of neuroendocrine exhaustion as an affecting factor on the MSOF process is an area of extensive research. Normally in response to stress, the hypothalamus activates a multitude of processes by way of the sympathetic nervous system and direct stimulation of the anterior and posterior pituitary (Fig. 13-2). The sympathetic nervous system triggers the adrenal medulla to secrete epinephrine and norepinephrine. Epinephrine causes vasoconstriction, hypertension, slight tachycardia, and enhancement of the clotting mechanism in preparation for impending blood loss. In preparation for impending volume loss, norepinephrine causes sodium retention and potassium excretion. The posterior pituitary gland secretes antidiuretic hormone (ADH), further improving vascular volume.[17]

The release of ACTH stimulates the adrenal cortex to increase glucocorticoid release, which increases platelet and fibrinogen production, protein catabolism, gluconeogenesis, blood glucose, and free fatty acid generation necessary to supply the increased energy needs of the stressed individual. Temperature increases in response to the increased metabolic rate and the activity of endogenous pyrogens (TNF and IL-1)[22] and exogenous pyrogens (viruses, bacteria, and endotoxin).[17]

During critical illness, numerous complications continually stimulate or damage the neuroendocrine system. Exhaustion or failure is the ultimate result. Neuroendocrine exhaustion or failure is highly suspected with the occurrence of four processes: glucose intolerance, failure to mount a febrile response, neurogenic pulmonary edema, and low T_3 syndrome (see box on p. 241).

Glucose intolerance. Both insulin and growth hormone induce anabolic activity. Insulin plays an important role in controlling glycogenolysis, gluconeogenesis, and lipolysis. Growth hormone stimulates amino acid transport and protein synthesis. During sepsis, this balance is disrupted by factors such as increased gluconeogenesis and catecholamine-driven glycogenolysis, resulting in hyperglycemia.[23] Increased blood glucose is associated with increased intracellular lactate levels, lowered pH, and decreased cerebral blood flow during postischemic reperfusion.

Failure to mount a febrile response. Increased temperature normally accompanies an infectious process because pyrogenic substances circulate to the hypothalamus and stimulate the thermosensitive neurons to produce fever. The new temperature is then recognized as the "normal" temperature, and it is maintained by shivering and peripheral vasoconstriction.[17]

The failure to mount a febrile response within the first 24 hours of an infectious process heralds a poor prognosis and has been associated with increased mortality in the patient with sepsis.[19] The mechanism of failure is unclear, but microscopic lesions of the hypothalamus secondary to ischemic damage or other sources has been suggested. Duff and Durum[24] noted that the T-cell proliferation responses to IL-1 and IL-2 are much greater at 39° C than at 37° C. Therefore fever may play an important role in the host response in sepsis.

Neurogenic pulmonary edema. Neurogenic pulmonary edema results in hypoxemia and could be a factor in the initial respiratory dysfunction associated with trauma, sepsis, and MSOF. Although the overall occurrence is relatively low, it is a well-established complication in processes associated with severe head injury accompanied by increased intracranial pressure.

The causative factors are massive catecholamine release and specific lesions of the hypothalamus and medulla; however, the exact mechanism of injury remains unclear. Massive catecholamine release triggered by medullary ischemia results in peripheral vasoconstriction, which may redistribute blood from systemic to pulmonary vessels. Direct endothelial damage and increased pulmonary microvascular permeability may result. Specific lesions of the hypothalamus can also produce neurogenic pulmonary edema, and transection of sympathetic efferents in the hypothalamus can halt this process.[25]

Low T_3 syndrome. Triiodothyronine (T_3) and thyroxine (T_4) are biologically active thyroid hormones that increase metabolic activity and stimulate the metabolism of carbohydrate, fat, and protein. Approximately 90% of the thyroid hormone produced by the thyroid gland is T_4. The remaining 10% is produced in the form of T_3, although much of the T_4 is converted to T_3 in the blood and peripheral tissue.[26]

Low T_3 syndrome has been identified in many chronic and acute illness states. In sepsis, low T_3 levels occur concurrently with high catecholamine levels and a decrease in the norepinephrine/epinephrine ratio. This clinical picture is associated with increased mortality. As thyroid hormone levels return to normal, catecholamine levels also normalize.

The occurrence of this hormonal imbalance is thought to be an indicator of hypothalamic and pituitary dysfunction or suppression and alteration of peripheral metabolism and release of T_4.[27] It has not been elucidated whether low T_3 levels stimulate catecholamine production to fuel the metabolic processes normally dependent on T_3 or whether massive catecholamine discharge associated with sepsis triggers the conversion of T_3 to the inactive T_3.

THERAPEUTIC MANAGEMENT

There are no proven organ-specific treatments at this time for the CNS failure that accompanies sepsis and MSOF. Many isolated interventions have been and continue to be reviewed. However, it is unlikely that any one treatment will make an impact on so complex a process as MSOF. Much remains to be discovered concerning the effect of cerebral resuscitation on the *incomplete* ischemia associated with sepsis and MSOF.

Isolated treatments

Intracranial pressure (ICP) monitoring and hyperventilation. The CNS dysfunction associated with MSOF is caused by a multitude of cellular phenomena, and increased intracranial pressure is rarely seen in this patient population. Therefore ICP monitoring and hyperventilation are not effective treatment methods unless increased intracranial pressure exists.

Sedation. The hypermetabolic effects of MSOF are compounded in the patient who is also agitated from septic encephalopathy. Agitated patients often have the greatest oxygen consumption (Vo_2), increasing up to 200% in some cases. Sedation, with or without chemically induced muscle paralysis, can significantly reduce both Vo_2 and carbon dioxide production (Vco_2) in the restless and agitated patient. The value of sedation and paralysis to decrease metabolic demands must be weighed against the increased muscle wasting and negative nitrogen balance associated with inactivity.[25]

Beta-blockade. Beta-blockade is experimental and focuses on decreasing the profound catecholamine discharge common to sepsis and MSOF. Adrenergic blockade with propranolol has been shown to decrease Vo_2 by approximately 25% and decrease catecholamine levels.[25]

Control of hyperglycemia. Hyperglycemia has been shown to correlate with poor patient outcome following cardiac arrest. In a retrospective study of patients surviving cardiac arrest, patients who awakened had significantly lower blood glucose levels than patients who remained comatose. Furthermore, in the patients who awakened, those without neurologic deficit had significantly lower blood glucose levels than those with lingering neurologic deficit.[10] Whether strict control of serum glucose levels by insulin administration can improve neurologic outcome in focal ischemia is currently under investigation.

Hormone replacement. Hormone replacement to restore thyroid levels has been studied in patients suffering from burns and sepsis. Becker et al[28] noted a reduced thyroid level in this population, and Vaughan et al[29] showed decreased hormone levels correlated with decreased mental function and increased mortality in burn patients. However, T_3 replacement has not been shown to alter the metabolic or mortality rate of these patients.[27]

Conversely, Hesch et al[30] reported improvement in dopamine-dependent patients with septic shock after T_3 replacement. Furthermore, the thyroid-releasing hormone protirelin has been associated with improvement after experimental endotoxemia, hemorrhagic shock, and spinal trauma,[31] although its mechanism of action has not been defined.

In summary, the most effective management strategy for CNS dysfunction in MSOF focuses on prevention of the MSOF syndrome, which carries a mortality of 40% to 90%. Baue[32] lists five factors crucial to achieving this goal: (1) control of the injury, (2) excision of necrotic tissue, (3) improvement of blood flow and oxygen consumption, (4) support of metabolism, and (5) early and thorough prevention or treatment of infection.

Cerebral resuscitation

Cerebral resuscitation refers to brain-oriented resuscitative therapy that extends the traditional methods of cardiopulmonary resuscitation to include treatment methods that optimize the neuronal recovery of the brain during and after cardiac arrest (see box below). It focuses not only on the initial cessation of cerebral blood flow, but also on the secondary events such as cerebral edema, hypoperfusion, hypermetabolism, and membrane damage.[13] The application of cerebral resuscitation research to the incomplete ischemic processes associated with MSOF is not as defined as its application to the global ischemia occurring in cardiac arrest. The following discussion presents the brain-oriented resuscitative therapies currently being examined as discussed in the comprehensive text on the subject by Safar and Bircher.[13]

TREATMENT METHODS IN CEREBRAL RESUSCITATION[13]

Hypoperfusion
   Hypertensive therapy
   Hemodilution
   Intracarotid hemodilution
   Calcium channel blockade
Hypermetabolism
   Hypothermia
   Barbiturates
Membrane Damage
   Barbiturates
   Free radical scavengers
   Steroids
   Calcium channel blockade

Brain-oriented resuscitative therapies

Brain-oriented resuscitative therapy begins immediately after the restoration of circulation. In the first step, the critical care team attempts to determine and treat the specific cause of the arrest. This step has been termed "gauging" and encompasses the actions of assessment and critical care triage.

In the second step, termed "human mentation," the patient is evaluated for salvageability. An attempt is made to determine the patient's outcome in terms of survival and overall performance capability. Although there is a lack of reliable prognostic indicators of long-term recovery after severe brain insult, the team critically evaluates the severity and duration of the insult, the speed and quality of emergency resuscitation, and the early initiation and quality of brain-oriented resuscitative therapy. There is a tremendous need for clinical research to determine reliable measures that would predict long-term patient outcome as well as to determine legal and ethical ways to terminate resuscitation efforts in cases of brain death.

The final step of brain-oriented resuscitative therapy is intensive care and multiple organ support. The goal is to initiate effective multisystem methods of care that particularly benefit the recovery of the cerebral neuron. It is important to note that brain-oriented resuscitative therapy addresses the neuronal compromise occurring after circulatory arrest and should not be confused with literature on cerebral insult resulting from infarction or trauma. There are important distinctions between the focal ischemia of cerebral infarction or embolism and the global ischemia common in shock states or cardiac arrest. There are also significant differences between the incomplete ischemia of shock and the total cessation of blood flow common in cardiac arrest. Furthermore, in considering therapeutic measures there is a distinction between protective measures instituted before and during the arrest, and resuscitative measures initiated after the arrest.

Because of the current nature of research into brain-oriented resuscitative therapy, many of the methods of care are still experimental or under investigation (Table 13-1). Results from animal experiments and clinical studies on brain resuscitative measures indicate that a combination of therapies

Table 13-1   Potential Brain Resuscitation Therapies

Treatment	Ready for clinical trials after cardiac arrest	Cardiac arrest		Brain infarct		Cerebral trauma Acute ICP rise Cerebral edema	
		Animal	Man	Animal	Man	Animal	Man
Moderate, brief, induced hypertension	Yes	+		(+)	(+)		
Hemodilution (IV)	Yes	(+)		+	(+)	(+)	
Intracarotid hypertensive hemodilution ("flush")		+					
Heparinization	?	0		—	—	—	—
Cardiopulmonary bypass	Yes	+		—	—	—	—
Barbiturate high dose	*	(+)	0*	+		(+)	(+)
Barbiturate anesthetic dose		(+)		+		+	+
Phenytoin (Dilantin)	Yes	(+)					
Immobilization and IPPV during coma		(+)	(+)	(+)		+	+
Osmotherapy	Yes			(+)		+	+
Hypothermia			(+)	+		(+)	(+)
Calcium entry blocker	Ongoing*	+	*	(+)			(+)
Free radical scavenger		(+)					

From Safar P, Bircher NG. Cardiopulmonary cerebral resuscitation. Philadelphia: WB Saunders, 1988:259.
*International collaborative randomized clinical study (Resuscitation Research Center, University of Pittsburgh) 1979–1989.
Key: +, Reduces brain damage; (+), possibly reduces brain damage; —, may be harmful; 0, studies showed no effect; *(blank)*, not studied for effect on outcome.

rather than a single agent will be necessary to ameliorate the brain damage of total circulatory arrest. The following review outlines the present clinical and experimental therapies specific to the major pathologic events of hypoperfusion, hypermetabolism, and membrane damage that occur during the postresuscitation syndrome (see box on p. 246).[13]

Hypoperfusion. Hypoperfusion, seen as focal areas of no-reflow, constitutes the first phase of reperfusion failure after circulatory arrest (Fig. 13-1). This state can be partially counteracted by induced transient hypertension and normovolemic hemodilution.

Hypertensive therapy. Hypertensive therapy involves raising the mean arterial blood pressure to between 130 and 140 mm Hg for 5 to 15 minutes after normal heart rhythm is established, or, in the absence of normal heart rhythm, placing the subject on cardiopulmonary bypass. It is achieved by intravenous fluids and/or vasopressors. Transient, moderate hypertension may help overcome the initial sludging and stasis in the cerebral microcirculation seen in the no-reflow phenomenon. Prolonged hypertension is not recommended, since it increases the risk of brain damage from vasogenic changes.

Hemodilution. Hemodilution is a therapeutic measure to decrease blood viscosity, which increases as volume shifts from the vascular compartment to the interstitium during a period of cerebral ischemia. This increase in viscosity is thought to play a role in no-reflow states. Combinations of crystalloid and colloid solutions have been used. Normovolemic hemodilution to a hematocrit of 25% to 30% looks promising in cerebral infarction and experimental contusion and has been shown to possibly reduce brain damage after circulatory arrest.

Intracarotid hemodilution flush. An intracarotid hemodilution flush with dextran 40 has also been used in combination with transient hypertension and heparinization with good results in animal studies. In intracarotid hemodilution, drugs and fluids are infused directly into the carotid artery instead of intravenously. The following substances have been recommended for further study for possible addition to the initial flush reperfusion fluid: heparin, streptokinase, calcium channel blockers, and free radical scavengers.

Intravenous heparin has not been shown effective in animal studies. However, if prolonged stasis during circulatory arrest promotes clotting, heparin or streptokinase should be evaluated as part of the initial flush perfusion fluid.

Calcium channel blockers and a combination of free radical scavengers may help protect neurons against biochemical cascades (calcium influx and ODFR production) that produce membrane damage and cell necrosis during reperfusion. Calcium channel blockers decrease cerebral vasospasm and are believed to improve cerebral blood flow and diminish blood cell sludging during the postreperfusion period. This effect is gained by reducing the intraneuronal liberation of the free calcium that seems to accumulate during ischemia and reperfusion. Most calcium channel blockers do not cross the blood-brain barrier, but they may be effective in the postreperfusion period when the blood-brain barrier is already disrupted.

The use of osmotherapy is well documented for the cerebral edema that develops after neurosurgery and head injury. The value of this treatment for promoting reperfusion is unclear and warrants more investigation.

Hypermetabolism. Hypermetabolism is believed to result from a chaotic and disorganized renewal of the brain's metabolic processes during the reperfusion stage. Catecholamine synthesis, especially norepinephrine and dopamine, is increased. This hypermetabolic state results in neuronal destruction when cerebral perfusion cannot meet the metabolic needs of the brain.

Hypothermia. Hypothermia reduces metabolism and cerebral blood flow and is the most potent, protective pretreatment measure for cerebral ischemia. Although drugs can lower metabolic needs, only hypothermia can stop all metabolic activity. Hypothermia (core temperature below 35° C) decreases the metabolic rate of oxygen by 50% to 75%, also reducing cerebral edema and intracranial pressure. Studies have shown that temperatures of 30° C during 30 minutes of circulatory arrest and 20° C during 60 minutes of circulatory arrest protect against postischemic brain damage.

Animal studies of hypothermia induced after cardiac arrest have not been accepted because of the difficulty in controlling the complications of increased incidence of dysrhythmias, shock, increased blood viscosity with reduced blood flow, and increased susceptibility to infection and stress ulcers. Protective external head and brain cooling during prolonged CPR is feasible, but its effect has not been demonstrated. Hypothermia is achieved by surface cooling and control of shivering with various drugs, such as phenobarbital or chlorpromazine. The recommended duration of this treatment is 3 to 12 hours, but may be extended to 72 hours. One technique is to lower the core temperature to between 30° C and 32° C for 3 to 6 hours and then gradually rewarm. The danger to the patient significantly increases if the temperature is below 28° C. However, in persons with healthy cardiovascular systems, such as children after near-drowning, short-term moderate hypothermia is justified. This cooling and rewarming must be accompanied by the use of therapies that block the body's natural defenses to cooling. These therapies include neuromuscular-blocking agents, controlled ventilation, drugs to prevent dysrhythmias (such as lidocaine), and drugs to prevent hypothermia-induced shivering and to aid in vasodilatation (such as chlorpromazine, thiopental, or pentobarbital). These drugs must be titrated as necessary to control shivering while avoiding hypotension.

Barbiturates. Barbiturates are known to reduce the cerebral metabolic rate of oxygen up to 50% of normal by reducing neuronal activity. When thiopental or pentobarbital plasma levels reach 3 to 5 mg/dL, the EEG activity is silenced, and the brain is considered to be at rest. Barbiturates also suppress seizure activity and narrow the differential between perfusion and metabolic need. The multifocal ischemia of the cerebral postresuscitation syndrome might benefit from the activity and metabolic depressant effects of barbiturates. However, clinical studies have been inconclusive, and at this time barbiturates are not recommended for routine use in a patient after cardiac arrest. They can be selectively used in anesthetic doses for seizure prophylaxis, seizure control, sedation, and intracranial pressure control. Barbiturates decrease formation of free fatty acids and scavenge free radicals, which are known to play a part in membrane damage.

Miscellaneous agents. Miscellaneous drugs can be substituted for barbiturates. Phenytoin effectively controls seizure activity and also reduces the energy requirements of the neuron by stabilizing the flux of ions across the membrane. Halothane reduces cerebral metabolism but increases cerebral blood flow and intracranial pressure, worsening focal ischemia. Isoflurane shows potential for cerebral protection.

Membrane damage. Stabilization of the cell membrane is important in protecting the blood-brain barrier and the prevention of cytotoxic (intracellular) and vasogenic (extracellular) edema. Barbiturates, free radical scavengers, steroids, and calcium channel blockers have all been investigated for their membrane-stabilizing effects. The use of steroids is controversial and not recommended, since documentation of their brain-saving effect is limited, and their use in sepsis and MSOF is contraindicated.

CONCLUSION

Failure of the central nervous system is a significant component in the very complex MSOF process. Clinical evidence of failure ranges from confusion to coma and from generalized weakness to profound respiratory failure. The mechanisms of failure are complex; therefore much of the research is preliminary and experimental. Great caution must be used in applying results of individual studies to all types of CNS ischemic events and dysfunction. Research studies on complete, incomplete, global, and focal ischemia differ in their findings on pathophysiologic mechanisms and extent of damage. Furthermore, significant differences exist between treatments focusing on cerebral protection in the preischemic period and treatments instituted for cerebral preservation after ischemia has already developed.

Within the framework of recent developments, however, there is one common theme. CNS failure or exhaustion is directly related to increased mortality, recovery time, and expense for the patient with MSOF. More than any other single occurrence, CNS failure heralds a poor prognosis in the patient with MSOF.

REFERENCES

1. Baue AE. Central nervous system failure. In: Baue AE, ed. Multiple organ failure: Patient care and prevention. St Louis: Mosby–Year Book, 1990:405-410.
2. Duff JH. Multiorgan failure in critically ill or injured patients. In: Sibbald WJ, ed. Synopsis of critical care, 3rd ed. Baltimore: Williams & Wilkins, 1988:273-278.
3. Davis L, Reed W. Infections of the central nervous system. In: Rosenberg RN, ed. Comprehensive neurology. New York: Raven Press, 1991:215-288.
4. Jackson AC et al. The encephalopathy of sepsis. Can J Neurol Sci 1985;12:303-307.
5. Pendlebury WW et al. Disseminated microabscesses of the central nervous system [Abstract]. Neurology 1983;33(Suppl 2):223.

6. Baue AE. Metabolic failure. In: Baue AE, ed. Multiple organ failure: Patient care and prevention. St Louis: Mosby–Year Book, 1990:374-395.

7. Bowton DL. CNS effects of sepsis. Crit Care Clin 1989;5:785-792.

8. Bowton DL et al. Cerebral blood flow is reduced in patients with sepsis syndrome. Crit Care Med 1989;17:399-403.

9. Astrup J. Energy-requiring cell functions in the ischemic brain: Their critical supply and possible inhibition in protective therapy. J Neurosurg 1981;56:482-497.

10. Milde LN. Pathophysiology of ischemic brain injury. Crit Care Clin 1989;5:729-753.

11. Rehncrona S. Molecular mechanisms for ischemic brain damage and aspects of protection. Acta Neurochir 1986; 36(suppl):125-128.

12. Aitkenhead A. Cerebral protection. Br J Hosp Med 1986; 35:290-298.

13. Safar P, Bircher NG. Cardiopulmonary cerebral resuscitation, 3rd ed. London, WB Saunders, 1988:229-278.

14. Sprague RS et al. Proposed role for leukotrienes in the pathophysiology of multiple systems organ failure. Crit Care Clin 1989;5:315-329.

15. Young GB et al. The encephalopathy associated with septic illness. Clin Invest Med 1990;13:297-304.

16. Baue AE. Surgical homeostasis: Metabolic and neuroendocrine responses to injury. In: Baue AE, ed. Multiple organ failure: Patient care and prevention. St Louis: Mosby–Year Book, 1990:3-29.

17. Shekleton ME, Litwack K. Critical care nursing of the surgical patient. Philadelphia: WB Saunders, 1991:69-73.

18. Pine RW et al. Determinants of organ malfunction or death in patients with intra-abdominal sepsis: A discriminant analysis. Arch Surg 1983;118:242-249.

19. Sprung CL et al. Impact of encephalopathy on mortality in the sepsis syndrome. Crit Care Med 1990;18:801-805.

20. Bolton CF, Young GB. Sepsis and septic shock: Central and peripheral nervous systems. In: Sibbald WJ, Sprung CL, eds. New horizons: Perspectives on sepsis and septic shock. Fullerton: Society of Critical Care Medicine, 1986:157-171.

21. Witt NJ et al. Peripheral nerve function in sepsis and multiple organ failure. Chest 1991;99:178-184.

22. Pinsky MR, Matuschak GM. Multiple systems organ failure: Failure of host defense homeostasis. Crit Care Clin 1989;5:199-220.

23. Vary TC, Linberg SE. Pathophysiology of traumatic shock. In: Cardona VD, Hurn PD, Mason PJB, Scanlon-Schilpp AM, Veise-Berry SW, eds. Trauma nursing: From resuscitation through rehabilitation. Philadelphia: WB Saunders, 1988:127-159.

24. Duff GW, Durum SK. Fever and immunoregulation: Hyperthermia, interleukin I and II and T cell proliferation. Yale J Biol Med 1987;55:437-442.

25. Demling R, Riessen R. Pulmonary dysfunction after cerebral injury. Crit Care Med 1990;18:768-774.

26. Alspach JG, ed. Core curriculum for critical care nursing, 4th ed. Philadelphia: WB Saunders, 1991:616-617.

27. Baue AE. Neuroendocrine system failure. In: Baue AE, ed. Multiple organ failure: Patient care and prevention. St Louis: Mosby–Year Book, 1990:396-404.

28. Becker RA et al. Free T_4, free T_3, and reverse T_3 in critically ill, thermally injured patients. J Trauma 1980;20:713-721.

29. Vaughan GM et al. Alterations of mental status and thyroid hormones after thermal injury. J Clin Endocrinol Metab 1985;60:1221-1225.

30. Hesch RD et al. Treatment of dopamine-dependent shock with triiodothyronine. Endocr Res Commun 1981;8:229-237.

31. Faden AI, Jacobs TP, Holaday JW. Thyrotropin-releasing hormone improves neurologic recovery after spinal trauma in cats. N Engl J Med 1980;1063-1067.

32. Baue AE. Prevention of multiple organ failure. In: Baue AE, ed. Multiple organ failure: Patient care and prevention. St Louis: Mosby–Year Book, 1990:487-500.

14 Pancreatitis

Janice McMillan

Acute pancreatitis is an inflammatory response resulting from premature activation of pancreatic enzymes. The pathologic changes range from mild edema to extensive hemorrhage, necrosis, and abscess formation. The process is usually self-limiting; however, severe pancreatitis occurs in 25% of all cases and can affect virtually every organ system in the body.[1] Pancreatitis has an overall mortality rate of 10%.[2]

The pancreas plays a more causal role in MSOF than do many of the other individual organs. Severe pancreatitis often leads to the development of regional and systemic inflammation, a common setting for the development of MSOF. Intense activation of inflammatory mediators with concomitant changes in distribution of circulating volume, oxygen supply and demand, and metabolic alterations leads to systemic abnormalities and damage to organs distant from the site of inflammation.

ANATOMY AND PHYSIOLOGY

The pancreas is an elongated gland about 12 to 15 cm long that has both endocrine and exocrine functions.[3,4] The pancreas lies anterior to the first and second lumbar vertebrae and posterior to the stomach. It consists of three sections: the head, body, and tail (Fig. 14-1). The head, or right end of the pancreas, lies within the curvature of the duodenum. The left portion is the tail, which extends to the spleen. The intervening portion is the body that lies horizontally across the abdomen. Adjacent organs are easily involved in the course of acute pancreatitis because of the retroperitoneal location of the pancreas. The absence of a well-developed pancreatic capsule allows the inflammatory process to spread freely and affect such organs as the duodenum; terminal common bile duct; splenic artery and vein; spleen; mesocolon; greater omentum; small-bowel mesentery, celiac, and superior mesentery ganglia; lesser omental sac; posterior mediastinum; pararenal spaces; and the diaphragm.[5]

Endocrine function

The pancreas is composed of two types of tissues: the acinar cells and the islets of Langerhans. The acinar cells secrete digestive juices into the pancreatic duct, which drains into the duodenum. The islets of Langerhans, also called pancreatic islets, secrete insulin and glucagon directly into the blood. One million to two million islets populate the pancreas, and they are centered around small capillaries into which cells secrete their hormones.[6] The pancreatic islets contain three distinct cells: alpha, beta, and delta cells. Alpha cells, which constitute about 25% of the total islet cells, secrete glucagon. Glucagon has several functions, but the major effect is increasing blood glucose concentration. The beta cells comprise 60% of all islet cells and secrete insulin. The delta cells, which comprise 10% of the total islet cells, secrete somatostatin. Somatostatin depresses insulin and glucagon secretion and decreases gastrointestinal motility. This extends the time food stores are assimilated into the blood and prevents rapid exhaustion of food supplies. Somatostatin is the same chemical substance as growth hormone release inhibiting hormone. There is at least one other type of cell, the PP cell, which secretes a hormone of uncertain function called pancreatic polypeptide.[6]

Exocrine function

The endocrine role of the pancreas focuses mainly on glucagon and insulin secretion, while the exocrine role focuses on normal digestive and absorptive processes. Acinar cells are arranged in groups called acini. Acinar cells produce 1500 to 3000 mL of pancreatic juice daily.[7] This juice con-

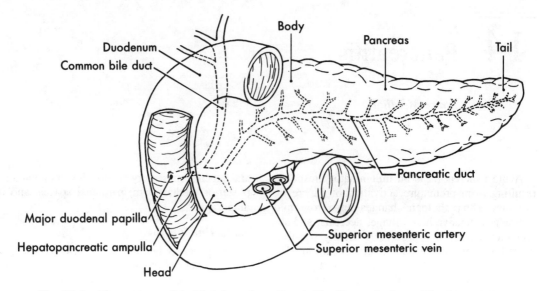

Fig. 14-1   The pancreas. (Modified from Swan R, ed. The Human Body on File. New York: Facts on File, Inc., 1983;8.03.)

Table 14-1   Pancreatic Secretions

Secretion	Function
Endocrine	
Insulin	Decreases blood glucose
Glucagon	Increases blood glucose
Somatostatin	Depresses insulin/glucagon secretion; decreases gastrointestinal motility
Exocrine	
Trypsin	Protein digestion
Chymotrypsin	Protein digestion
Elastase	Protein digestion
Nuclease	Protein digestion
Amylase	Carbohydrate digestion
Lipase	Fat digestion
Bicarbonate ions	Neutralization of acid chyme

tains enzymes for digesting proteins, carbohydrates, and fats. It also contains water and large quantities of bicarbonate ions that neutralize the acid chyme emptied by the stomach into the duodenum. The enzymes in pancreatic juice include proteolytic enzymes, which include trypsin, chymotrypsin, elastases, and nucleases and serve to break down proteins; pancreatic amylase, which hydrolyzes carbohydrates; and pancreatic lipase, which degrades fat (Table 14-1).

ETIOLOGY

Acute pancreatitis has a number of causes, but the most common are biliary tract disease in women and alcohol abuse in men.

Biliary tract disease

Gallstones are present in two thirds of reported cases of pancreatitis; however, only about 5% of patients with gallstones develop pancreatitis.[8] It is unclear how gallstones lead to pancreatitis, but it may be that stones impacted in the ampulla of Vater cause bile reflux, which leads to pancreatitis. Gallstone pancreatitis occurs two times more often in women than in men.[5]

Alcohol abuse

Alcohol abuse is the leading cause of pancreatitis in men. These patients usually develop chronic pancreatitis from the damage sustained to the pancreas. The pathogenesis of alcohol pancreatitis remains unclear. One hypothesis is that protein plugs form in the pancreatic ducts and cause partial outflow obstruction.[8] A second mechanism by which alcohol may cause pancreatic damage is increased gastric acid secretion from alcohol ingestion. This leads to increased pancreatic secretion. Increased secretion leads to atony and edema of Oddi's sphincter, which results in reflux of duodenal contents into the pancreas.[4,7,8]

Lipid abnormalities

Lipid abnormalities, specifically hypertriglyceridemia, can cause pancreatitis. These patients usually have familial hyperlipoproteinemia of Frederickson types I, IV, or V.[8,9] Women taking oral contraceptives can develop type IV or V hyperlipemia and pancreatitis.[9] The mechanism by which elevated triglycerides lead to pancreatitis is unclear; however, local lipolysis results in an excess of fatty acids that causes inflammation and damage to capillary membranes and can result in pancreatitis. Patients with lipemia-associated pancreatitis usually do not have elevated serum amylase values. Recurrences can usually be prevented by maintenance of a low-fat diet, weight reduction, and treatment with triglyceride-lowering agents.

Idiopathic and drug-related causes

Approximately 8% to 25% of patients with acute pancreatitis will have pancreatitis from no ascertainable cause. Some cases of idiopathic pancreatitis may actually be related to pancreas divisum, a hereditary pancreatic duct abnormality, which has recently been identified.[9]

It is difficult to pinpoint whether a true connection exists between drug administration and pancreatitis or if it is an idiosyncratic reaction. Glucocorticosteroids, thiazide diuretics, furosemide, tetracycline, estrogens, methyldopa, and immunosuppressive drugs are a few of the drugs that have been associated with the development of pancreatitis.[8,9] Other causes of acute pancreatitis are listed in the box at right.

PATHOPHYSIOLOGY HYPOTHESES
Autodigestion

Many immunologic and etiologic factors have been implicated in the pathogenesis of acute pancreatitis, but confusion remains over the mechanism by which these factors initiate pancreatitis. The most popular hypothesis for the development of acute pancreatitis is autodigestion. The pancreas protects itself from autodigestion by synthesizing proteolytic enzymes and phospholipase A as inactive zymogens (proenzymes) that are activated through enzymatic splitting of a peptide chain only after reaching the intestine. The other digestive

---

CAUSES OF ACUTE PANCREATITIS

Biliary tract disease (gallstones)
Alcohol
Gastric disease (duodenal ulcer)
Metabolic disorders
    Hyperlipidemia
    Hyperparathyroidism
    Renal failure
    Hypercalcemia
Drugs (thiazide diuretics, furosemide, estrogens, tetracycline, valproic acid, salicylates, corticosteroids, immunosuppressive agents, and methyldopa)
Infections (mumps, viral hepatitis, mycoplasma, coxsackie virus)
Trauma
Tumors
Pregnancy (third trimester)
Surgery
Hereditary pancreatitis
Scorpion venom

---

enzymes (amylase, lipase, and nuclease) are synthesized in active form. The enzymes stored in zymogen granules are isolated by a phospholipid membrane in the acinar cell. Trypsinogen is activated to trypsin by enterokinase, which is secreted by the intestinal mucosa when chyme comes into contact with the mucosa. For unclear reasons, in acute pancreatitis, trypsinogen is activated to trypsin within the pancreas. Trypsin activates all known pancreatic zymogens that are involved in autodigestion. These activated enzymes cause proteolysis, edema, hemorrhage, coagulation necrosis, fat necrosis, parenchymal cell necrosis, and vascular damage. Thus, to prevent autodigestion of the pancreas, it is important that the proteolytic enzymes remain as inactive zymogens until they have been secreted into the intestine.

A second safeguard against autodigestion is trypsin inhibitor. Trypsin inhibitor is a substance that is secreted by the same cells that secrete proteolytic enzymes into the acini of the pancreas. Since trypsin activates the other pancreatic proteolytic enzymes, trypsin inhibitor also prevents the subsequent activation of other enzymes. If the pancreas becomes damaged or a pancreatic duct becomes blocked, secretions can back up and may pool. This increased concentration of pancreatic secretions may overpower the effect of trypsin inhibitor. The proteolytic enzymes are activated, since trypsin inhibitor is ineffective. Acute pancreatitis develops as a result of the autodigestion of the pancreas.

The events that trigger the sequence of enzymatic reactions that initiate acute pancreatitis are unknown. It is probable that more than one etiologic mechanism is responsible. As previously stated, the most popular hypothesis is autodigestion. However, obstruction, reflux of duodenal contents, and bile reflux have also been considered as mechanisms for initiating pancreatitis.

Obstruction

Some investigators hypothesize that acute pancreatitis results from obstruction to the outflow of pancreatic juice. Permanent decompression of a choledochocele has prevented recurrent pancreatitis attacks in several patients, presumably by removing intermittent pancreatic outflow obstruction.[10] Evidence against obstruction as the major cause of acute pancreatitis exists, since ligation of the pancreatic duct or its occlusion by tumor generally does not result in acute pancreatitis. In addition, sphincterotomy and sphincteroplasty have been performed in patients with recurring episodes of acute pancreatitis with disappointing results.[5]

Duodenal reflux

Another theory is that reflux of duodenal contents leads to pancreatitis, since acute pancreatitis developed in animals after the creation of a closed duodenal loop. Normally defense mechanisms prevent duodenal reflux, such as Oddi's sphincter, the mucosal fold at the transmural portion of the duct, and a normal pressure gradient between the pancreatic duct lumen and the duodenum. Arguments against reflux of duodenal contents causing acute pancreatitis include the finding of a normal Oddi's sphincter and pancreatic duct resting pressure in the majority of patients with acute pancreatitis; the absence of ill effects after sphincteroplasty, which allows intermittent reflux; and the research findings showing that similar animals with ligated pancreatic ducts did not develop duodenal reflux and pancreatitis. Thus duodenal regurgitation may be a contributing factor toward development of pancreatitis in some patients, but there is not enough evidence to support this as applicable to the ma-

jority of patients with pancreatitis.

Bile reflux

One of the older hypotheses is the bile reflux, or common channel, hypothesis, which applies to pancreatitis associated with cholelithiasis. It was initially hypothesized that the presence of an impacted gallstone in the ampulla of Vater allowed bile to reflux into the pancreatic duct through a common channel.[5,7] However, bile reflux has not been found to cause pancreatitis in animals, and a common channel allowing bile to reflux is present in only 18% of the population.[11]

Summary

Many investigators hypothesize that obstruction or ligation of the pancreatic duct with associated reflux leads to pancreatic edema but not pancreatitis. Autodigestion remains the most common hypothesis explaining the development of acute pancreatitis. Although a variety of factors, such as endotoxins, exotoxins, viral infections, ischemia, anoxia, and direct trauma to the pancreas, have been considered, the exact mechanism by which autodigestion is initiated remains unclear. Fig. 14-2 depicts a schematic diagram of the development of acute pancreatitis.

CLINICAL PRESENTATION AND ASSESSMENT

No single diagnostic sign or symptom of acute pancreatitis exists. Diagnosis is based upon typical clinical features and laboratory findings and remains a clinical interpretation. The clinical presentation of acute pancreatitis changes as the disease progresses. In the initial 2 to 3 hours after onset, symptoms are suggestive of acute cholecystitis; after 6 to 8 hours, the symptoms are suggestive of a perforated ulcer; and after 2 to 3 days, the abdominal distention and ileus that develop are suggestive of intestinal obstruction. In addition, elevation of serum amylase occurs in all of these conditions.

Physical assessment

Abdominal pain is the most common symptom of acute pancreatitis. The pain may vary from mild, dull discomfort to severe, constant pain. The pain is located across the midepigastrium and periumbilical region and may radiate into the back or

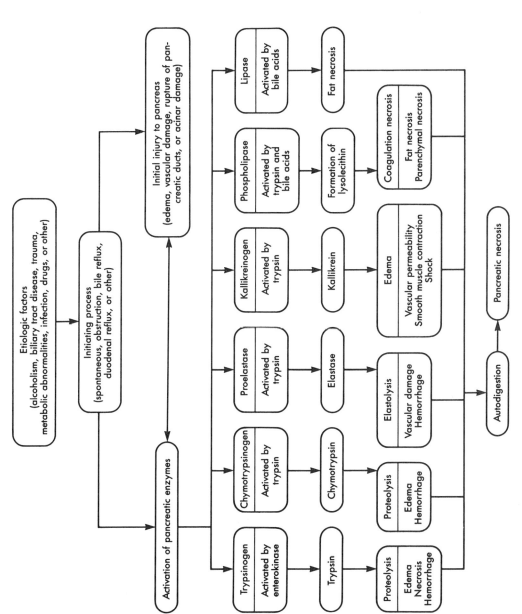

Fig. 14-2 Schematic diagram depicting the development of acute pancreatitis. (Modified from Cruetzfeldt W, Schmidt H. Scand J Gastroenterol 1970;5[suppl 6]: 47-62.)

flanks because of the retroperitoneal location of the pancreas. The pain is worse in the supine position and is relieved by sitting with the thighs and spine flexed. Factors that cause the pain of acute pancreatitis include chemical peritonitis; extravasation of blood, inflammatory exudate, and pancreatic enzymes into the retroperitoneal space; obstruction and distention of the pancreatic ducts; edema and stretching of the pancreatic capsule; obstruction of the duodenum from edema of the head of the pancreas; and obstruction of the extrahepatic biliary tract.[7]

On physical examination, the abdomen is initially soft, with tenderness developing in the upper abdomen. Bowel sounds are diminished but present. During the first 2 days, abdominal distention develops because of the combined effects of the paralytic ileus and accumulation of intraperitoneal fluid. Nausea and vomiting are common and occur because of gastric and intestinal hypomotility, the ileus, and chemical peritonitis. The patient's temperature is usually between 37.7° and 38.3° C (100° and 101° F) as a result of injured tissue products and inflammatory mediators entering the circulation.

Hypotension occurs in approximately 30% to 50% of pancreatitis patients.[5,7] Shock results from a combination of factors, including the following: hypovolemia secondary to plasma exudation in the retroperitoneal space, leading to a retroperitoneal burn, fluid accumulation in an atonic intestine, vomiting, and hemorrhage; increased formation and release of kinin peptides that cause stimulation of smooth muscle, vasodilatation, increased vascular permeability, and enhanced leukocyte migration; systemic effects of proteolytic and lipolytic enzymes released into the circulation; and impaired myocardial contractility from release of kinin peptides.[5,7] The systemic effects in pancreatitis result from absorption of activated pancreatic enzymes and the products of pancreatic digestion into the blood.

Blue-brown discoloration of the flanks (Grey Turner's sign) or in the periumbilical area (Cullen's sign) may occur as a late sign of severe pancreatitis. These signs indicate the presence of hemorrhagic pancreatitis and retroperitoneal dissection of blood into these areas. The blue-brown discoloration may not appear until a week or two of progressive pancreatic destruction has occurred.

Laboratory findings

Diagnosis of acute pancreatitis is usually based on the clinical presentation, a history of the precipitating cause, and an elevated serum amylase concentration. Serum amylase is the single most important test for the diagnosis of acute pancreatitis. Serum amylase levels are usually greater than twice the upper limit of normal (normal is 80 to 150 Somogyi units). Serum amylase levels do not always reflect the severity of the pancreatitis.

Relying on serum amylase values to diagnose pancreatitis has drawbacks. Amylase levels rise within a few hours of developing pancreatitis; however, amylase is rapidly metabolized and cleared by the kidneys. Serum amylase levels return to normal within 24 to 48 hours; thus, if the patient is examined several days after the onset of symptoms, the serum amylase will be normal. Serum amylase may be falsely low in patients with hypertriglyceridemia and may be elevated in patients with renal insufficiency, cerebral trauma, intraabdominal disease, burns, and ketoacidosis. Serum amylase is more specific if isoenzymes are determined because serum amylase is composed of pancreatic and salivary isoamylase. An elevated serum amylase along with an elevated pancreatic isoamylase makes the diagnosis of pancreatitis likely; however, numerous intestinal disorders can cause elevated pancreatic isoamylase levels.

Urine amylase levels are increased in patients with pancreatitis. Urine amylase clearance may remain elevated for 9 to 15 days after an episode of acute pancreatitis.[7] A reversible renal tubular defect is believed to be the mechanism for decreased amylase reabsorption and increased renal clearance of amylase. However, many of the conditions that can elevate serum amylase levels can also affect urine amylase levels; thus elevated urine amylase is not specific to pancreatitis.

Other laboratory tests that may be helpful in diagnosing pancreatitis are serum lipase levels, serum immunoreactive trypsin levels, serum glucose, serum calcium, and a white blood cell count. Serum lipase levels remain elevated much longer than amylase levels, but lipase levels can be elevated in a variety of conditions and are not specific for acute pancreatitis. Trypsin is not specific for any one type of pancreatic disease. It can be elevated with acute pancreatitis as well as with pancreatic carcinoma.

Transient hyperglycemia is often present in the early stages of acute pancreatitis because of altered pancreatic islet cell function. There is decreased release of insulin from the beta cells, increased release of glucagon from alpha cells, and increased output of glucocorticoids and catecholamines. A sustained fasting hyperglycemia of greater than 200 mg/dL is a poor prognostic sign because it reflects pancreatic necrosis.[5] Hypocalcemia may occur 2 to 3 days after the onset of pancreatitis and can be due to an altered response to parathyroid hormone, hypoalbuminemia, and calcium deposition in fatty necrotic areas in the abdominal cavity. Leukocytosis of 10,000 to 25,000 cells/mm^3 is often present secondary to the inflammatory process.[5]

The presence of methemalbumin may be an indicator of severe pancreatitis. Pancreatic enzymes break down retroperitoneal hemoglobin into heme, which oxidizes to hematin and then combines with serum albumin to form methemalbumin.[12] However, the presence of methemalbumin is not specific to pancreatitis because it may be present with upper abdominal trauma, bleeding gastric ulcer, bone fractures, and retroperitoneal hematoma.[7]

Radiologic studies

Radiologic studies are helpful in confirming the presence of pancreatic disease, detecting complications, and establishing the presence of alternative conditions. Plain films of the abdomen may show a sentinel loop (a distended small intestinal loop near the pancreas), a paralytic ileus, the colon cutoff sign, or evidence of other causes for the patient's abdominal pain such as free intraperitoneal air indicating mesenteric infarction. A chest x-ray may show a pleural effusion or interstitial fluffy infiltrates similar to those seen with pulmonary edema but without associated cardiomegaly. These infiltrates are indicative of respiratory failure associated with severe pancreatitis.

The most useful radiologic studies are an abdominal ultrasound and an abdominal CT scan. An ultrasound can show gallstones, enlargement or abnormal texture of the pancreas, enlargement or distention of the common bile duct, a pancreatic mass, or an accumulation of free fluid in the abdomen. The disadvantage with ultrasound is its inability to penetrate bowel gas, which means a normal scan does not rule out acute pancreatitis. CT scanning with contrast provides better imaging of the pancreas and is indicated if complications are suspected. CT scanning is contraindicated if the patient is allergic to contrast medium or has compromised renal function. Neither ultrasound nor CT scan can determine if pseudocysts (if present) are infected, nor can they detect common bile duct stones impacted in the ampulla of Vater.

Dynamic pancreatography is a relatively new technique that is being used to determine the severity of acute pancreatitis. Pancreatography is performed by rapidly injecting large volumes of contrast material (100 to 200 mL) IV and then rapidly performing CT scanning of the pancreas to determine the rate and pattern of pancreatic perfusion.[12] Some studies have shown a positive correlation between lack of perfusion on dynamic scanning and the presence of pancreatic necrosis at the time of surgery.[12,13] Unfortunately, pancreatography is not helpful in detecting pancreatic abscess formation, since these patients have normal to slightly decreased perfusion. Thus the specificity of pancreatography is unclear.

Diagnosis

The diagnosis of acute pancreatitis can usually be made when the physical examination of a patient yields abnormal findings (severe, constant abdominal pain; fever; and nausea and vomiting), abnormal laboratory values (elevated serum amylase, elevated serum lipase, and increased amylase clearance) and abnormal radiologic studies. Pancreatitis severity can be predicted by using Ranson's criteria. Ranson[14] identified 11 risk factors that aid in identifying patients who are at risk for major complications or death. Five of the factors are identifiable at the time of admission. These include the patient's age, WBC, glucose, LDH, and SGOT. The other six factors look at changes that occur during the first 48 hours after admission. These include changes in hematocrit, BUN, calcium, PaO$_2$, base deficit, and the amount of fluid sequestered. The major difficulty in using Ranson's criteria is that it takes 48 hours to determine whether a patient has severe pancreatitis. Ranson's risk factors and the impact of their presence on mortality are shown in the box on p. 258.

Progression

The initial stages of acute pancreatitis are characterized by interstitial edema. The disease can

Risk Factors for Quantifying the Severity of Acute Pancreatitis and the Impact of Their Presence on Mortality[14-16]

Risk Factors		Mortality	
At admission	*During initial 48 hours*	*Number of factors*	*Mortality*
Age > 55 years	Hct decreases > 10 percentage	<3	< 1
WBC > 16,000/mm³	points	3 to 4	15
Serum LDH > 350 u/L	BUN rises > 5 mg/dL	5 to 6	40
SGOT > 250	Arterial Po₂ <60 mm Hg	7 +	100
Sigma Frankel u/dL	Base deficit >4 mEq/L		
	Estimated fluid sequestration >6 L		

Modified from Ranson JHC. Risk factors in acute pancreatitis. Hosp Pract 1985;20(4):69-73.

progress from acute edematous pancreatitis to necrotizing pancreatitis, which is characterized by coagulation necrosis of glandular elements and their surrounding fatty tissue. The factors determining the progression are unknown, but pancreatic elastase may mediate the thrombotic occlusion of blood vessels. Hemorrhagic pancreatitis occurs when blood collects within the pancreas or the surrounding retroperitoneal spaces from ruptured blood vessels.

Acute pancreatitis very rarely progresses to chronic pancreatitis. Chronic pancreatitis is characterized by continuing inflammation that leads to irreversible structural changes and by permanent impairment of exocrine and endocrine pancreatic function. The clinical distinction between acute and chronic pancreatitis can be difficult to make, especially in the early stages of exacerbation of chronic alcoholic pancreatitis; thus the patient should be treated for acute pancreatitis.

COMPLICATIONS

Pancreatic phlegmon, pancreatic abscess, pseudocysts, or obstructive jaundice may occur. A pancreatic phlegmon is a mass of inflamed pancreas that often contains patchy areas of necrosis. Abscesses can occur with more severe cases of pancreatitis and are usually associated with infection within the peripancreatic collection of fluid. Gram-negative intestinal flora are the most common infecting microorganisms.[17] Patients with abscesses have abdominal pain, high fever, leukocytosis, and vomiting. Abscesses can be detected on abdominal CT scan, abdominal ultrasound, or a plain film of the abdomen that shows extraluminal gas collection. Prompt recognition and surgical intervention to drain the abscess are needed because there is a high mortality associated with undrained abscesses.

Pseudocysts are pockets of pancreatic enzymes that develop within the retroperitoneal space. These pseudocysts are frequently palpable as an upper abdominal mass and can be documented on ultrasound, abdominal CT scan, or barium study of the upper gastrointestinal tract. Obstructive jaundice is usually secondary to edema of the head of the pancreas, causing obstruction of the extrahepatic biliary tree. In the absence of choledocholithiasis, jaundice is transient, with serum bilirubin levels returning to normal in 7 to 10 days.

MULTISYSTEM INVOLVEMENT

Patients with acute hemorrhagic or acute edematous pancreatitis develop multiple organ problems. These multisystem problems begin with the lungs and circulation and progress to other organs.

Pulmonary damage

Pleural effusions, atelectasis, pneumonia, and mediastinal abscess may develop. ARDS develops in approximately 20% of patients with acute pancreatitis.[7] Injury to the lungs occurs from pancreatic enzymes reaching the pleural fluid from passage through pores in the diaphragm and exudation from thoracic lymphatic channels. Alveolocapillary membrane integrity is lost, and pulmonary edema occurs. Pulmonary surfactant may be damaged by circulating free fatty acids, phospholipase A, or other vasoactive substances.[5,18] The pulmonary edema results from a reversible disruption of the alveolocapillary membrane with loss of the normal size selectivity for diffusion of plasma proteins. Therefore both proteins and fluid move into the interstitium and alveoli.

Other factors associated with pancreatitis contribute to the development of pulmonary complications. Abdominal pain alters the breathing pattern, resulting in a decreased tidal volume and increased rate of breathing. Abdominal distention and inflammation under the diaphragm elevate the diaphragm and decrease expansion. Cardiovascular demands increase ventilation needs. All of these factors contribute to respiratory failure.

Circulatory abnormalities

Patients with severe pancreatitis develop a hyperdynamic circulatory state, which is characterized by decreased peripheral vascular resistance and an increase in the shunt fraction of the pulmonary circulation. This results in an elevated cardiac index and a decrease in the arteriovenous oxygen gradient.[19] A retroperitoneal burn occurs from exudation of blood and plasma protein into the retroperitoneal space and causes hypovolemia. The retroperitoneal inflammatory process demands a hyperdynamic circulation and vigorous fluid restoration. Trypsin activates the kallikrein-kinin system. The kinin peptides cause vasodilation, increased vascular permeability, and leukocyte migration. Shock develops from the combination of hypovolemia, the effects of the kinin peptides, and the systemic effects of proteolytic and lipolytic enzymes.

In addition, impaired myocardial contractility can contribute to the shock state. Controversy remains concerning the presence of myocardial depression in pancreatitis. A myocardial depressant factor, which is believed to be a small peptide produced by the action of trypsin, phospholipase A, and lysosomes on compartmentalized protein, has been implicated in some of the hemodynamic alterations occurring in patients with pancreatitis.[18] It is thought that myocardial depressant factor enhances splanchnic vasoconstriction and depresses myocardial contractility. It also affects the role of calcium in myocardial contractility and electrical excitation. Although some studies have found ev-

idence of myocardial depression, others have not.[20-23]

DIC

Disseminated intravascular coagulation can occur from the release of pancreatic proteolytic enzymes into the blood. Elastase dissolves elastic fibers, which increases vascular permeability. Activation of kinin peptides also causes vasodilatation and increased vascular permeability. Hypovolemia contributes to cell aggregation and the development of microthrombi. Fibrin-related antigen levels rise with an increase in the platelet count and fibrinogen levels. Impaired clot lysis and consumption of clotting factors occur, which result in DIC.

Altered renal function

Altered renal function can develop and range from mild impairment to anuria. Acute renal failure results from renal tubular necrosis secondary to hypovolemia and shock. Renal artery thrombosis and renal vein thrombosis also contribute to the renal failure.

Metabolic complications

Metabolic complications include hyperglycemia, hypocalcemia, and hyperlipidemia. Hyperglycemia is usually transient and occurs because of excess glucagon release from alpha cells and damage to insulin-secreting beta cells. Since the hyperglycemia is transient, diabetes mellitus usually does not develop, but it may if the pancreatitis becomes chronic. The cause for hypocalcemia is uncertain. Calcium deposition in areas of fat necrosis, release of glucagon, hypomagnesemia, and inadequate parathyroid function may contribute to hypocalcemia. Serum calcium levels usually remain low for 7 to 10 days. Tetany rarely occurs. Hyperlipidemia occurs in about 12% to 25% of all patients with pancreatitis.[7] The mechanism for hyperlipidemia in pancreatitis remains unclear. Lipemia usually precedes pancreatitis rather than lipemia being a manifestation of pancreatic inflammation. Local lipolysis with liberation of cytotoxic free fatty acids may be the factor that triggers pancreatitis.

THERAPEUTIC MANAGEMENT

Treatment of acute pancreatitis focuses on halting the progression of damage to the pancreas, preventing or treating local complications, and treating systemic complications. Treatment remains symptomatic and supportive because there is no specific therapy that halts the process of autodigestion.

Suppression of pancreatic activity

In order to halt the process of pancreatic injury, attempts are made to correct the initiating factor if possible, decrease the activity of the pancreas, and inhibit the activity of damaging pancreatic enzymes. Pancreatic enzyme synthesis and pancreatic secretions are suppressed by keeping the patient NPO and utilizing nasogastric suctioning. Various pharmacologic agents such as anticholinergics, antacids, cimetidine, glucagon, calcitonin, somatostatin, prostaglandin synthetase inhibitors, inhibitors of trypsin and phospholipase A_2, and infusions of fresh frozen plasma have been used in attempts to reduce pancreatic enzyme synthesis and secretion.[3,5,9,15] None of the pharmacologic agents has proven valuable in suppressing pancreatic secretions in clinical trials. There has also been no evidence that prophylactic treatment with antibiotics prevents infectious complications except in cases of gallstone pancreatitis.[24]

Supportive care

Supportive care of acute pancreatitis consists of administering analgesics, restoring and maintaining intravascular volume and electrolyte balance, and constantly assessing physical findings and vital signs for indications of complications. Meperidine hydrochloride (Demerol) is the analgesic of choice because it causes less spasm of Oddi's sphincter than does morphine. Albumin, plasma, dextran, or whole blood may be required to restore intravascular volume. Total parenteral nutrition is indicated if the patient remains NPO for several days. Additional supportive measures include administering IV calcium to combat severe hypocalcemia, correcting magnesium deficits, and administering low doses of regular insulin if hyperglycemia exists.

Surgical intervention

Surgical intervention is indicated when the diagnosis of pancreatitis is uncertain, the patient's condition worsens despite medical therapy, acute cholecystitis is present, or an abscess is suspected.[25] Peritoneal lavage and peritoneal dialysis have been performed to try to remove necrotic debris and activating enzymes from the peritoneal cavity in patients with severe pancreatitis. Neither of these two treatments has been found to decrease mortality rates.[26-27]

CONCLUSION

Approximately 25% of all patients with pancreatitis will develop life-threatening, multisystem complications.[1] Whether pancreatitis causes MSOF or is a result of the changes and damage occurring in an existing state of MSOF, the intense inflammation stimulated by the pancreatitis process and enzyme damage greatly increases the morbidity and mortality associated with critical illness. Since no specific therapy for acute pancreatitis is available, the major objective of therapeutic management is to support the patient until the acute phase of the disease subsides.

REFERENCES

1. Fan ST et al. Prediction of severity of acute pancreatitis: An alternative approach. Gut 1989;30:1591-1595.
2. Williamson RCN. Early assessment of severity in acute pancreatitis. Gut 1984;25:1331-1337.
3. Ermak TH, Grendell JH. Anatomy, histology, embryology, and developmental anomalies. In: Sleisenger MH, Fordtran JS, eds. Gastrointestinal disease: Pathophysiology, diagnosis, management. 4th ed, vol 2. Philadelphia: WB Saunders, 1989:1765-1777.
4. Fain JA, Amato-Vealey E. Acute pancreatitis: A gastrointestinal emergency. Crit Care Nurse 1988;8(5):47-61.
5. Seorgel KH. Acute pancreatitis. In: Sleisenger MH, Fordtran JS, eds. Gastrointestinal disease: Pathophysiology, diagnosis, management. 4th ed, vol 2. Philadelphia: WB Saunders, 1989:1814-1841.
6. Guyton AC. Textbook of medical physiology. 8th ed. Philadelphia: WB Saunders, 1991:718,855.
7. Greenberger NJ. Gastrointestinal disorders: A pathophysiologic approach. 4th ed. St Louis: Mosby–Year Book, 1989;253-300.
8. Creutzfeldt W, Lankisch PG. Acute pancreatitis: Etiology and pathogenesis. In: Berk JE, ed. Bockus gastroenterology. 4th ed. Philadelphia: WB Saunders, 1985:3971-3992.
9. Sabesin S. Countering the dangers of acute pancreatitis. Emerg Med 1987;19(17):70-96.
10. Venu RP et al. Role of endoscopic retrograde cholangio-pancreatography in the diagnosis and treatment of choledochocele. Gastroenterology 1984;87:1144-1149.
11. DiMagno EP, Shorter RG, Taylor WF. Relationships between pancreaticobiliary ductal anatomy and pancreatic ductal and parenchymal histology. Cancer 1982;49:361-368.
12. Steinberg WM. Predictors of severity of acute pancreatitis. Gastroenterol Clin North Am 1990;19:849-860.
13. Bradley EL, Murphy F, Ferguson C. Prediction of pancreatic necrosis by dynamic pancreatography. Ann Surg 1989;210:495-504.
14. Ranson JHC. Risk factors in acute pancreatitis. Hosp Pract 1985;20(4):69-73.

15. Moody FG. Pancreatitis as a medical emergency. Gastroenterol Clin North Am 1988;17:433-443.

16. Switz DM. Pancreatitis. In: Shoemaker WC, Ayres S, Grenvik A, Holbrook PR, Thompson WL, eds. Textbook of critical care. 2nd ed. Philadelphia: WB Saunders, 1989:732-736.

17. Collins AS. Gastrointestinal complications in shock. Crit Care Nurs Clin North Am 1990;2:269-277.

18. Baue AE. Multiple organ failure: Patient care and prevention. St Louis: Mosby–Year Book, 1990:415-417.

19. Beger HG et al. Hemodynamic data pattern in patients with acute pancreatitis. Gastroenterology 1986,90:74-79.

20. Ito K et al. Myocardial function in acute pancreatitis. Ann Surg 1981;194(1):85-88.

21. Goldfarb RD et al. Canine left ventricular function during experimental pancreatitis. J Surg Res 1985;38:125-133.

22. Altimari AF et al. Myocardial depression during acute pancreatitis: Fact or fiction? Surgery 1986;100:724-731.

23. Cobo JC et al: Sequential hemodynamic and oxygen transport abnormalities in patients with acute pancreatitis. Surgery 1984;95:324-330.

24. Byrne JJ, Treadwell TL. Treatment of pancreatitis: When do antibiotics have a role? Postgrad Med 1989;85:333-339.

25. Poston GJ, Williamson RCN. Surgical management of acute pancreatitis. Br J Surg 1990;77:5-12.

26. Mayer AD et al. Controlled clinical trial of peritoneal lavage for the treatment of severe acute pancreatitis. N Engl J Med 1985;312:399-404.

27. Stone HH, Fabian TC. Peritoneal dialysis in the treatment of acute alcoholic pancreatitis. Surg Gynecol Obstet 1980;150:878-882.

Special Considerations and Management

Pediatric patients require special consideration because of their limited reserves and anatomic and developmental differences. Previous management in both the adult and pediatric patient has focused on supporting individual organs. More recent interventions aggressively target the initial resuscitation and pathophysiologic changes. Newer investigational therapies must move farther up the cascade to control primary events such as overwhelming activation of the inflammatory/immune response, sympathetic activation, and extensive endothelial damage. There lies the greatest chance of reversing the vicious cycle *before* organ damage occurs.

SECTION FOUR

Special Considerations and Management

15 The Pediatric Patient

Patricia A. Moloney-Harmon and Sandra J. Czerwinski

Multisystem organ failure (MSOF) has been studied and well defined in adult populations. To date, the only available data concerning pediatric patients with MSOF were published by Wilkinson et al in 1986 and 1987.[1,2] Because of the limited information available about infants and children with MSOF, it is difficult to describe and define this syndrome for these patients and to make accurate comparisons between child and adult populations. Table 15-1 provides the specific criteria that Wilkinson et al[1] established to define MSOF in children, but diagnostic criteria will vary from study to study. Certain conditions that are frequently associated with the development of MSOF in adult patients are also seen in children (see box below), but no studies have been published to validate the relationship between these conditions and the development of MSOF in pediatric patients. In adults and children, however, MSOF is an acute and potentially reversible process that occurs in a significant number of patients admitted to the intensive care unit (ICU).

Mortality rates for children with MSOF are considerably higher than those reported for critically ill children without MSOF. The studies by Wilkinson et al[1,2] documented mortality rates of 54%, which are similar to mortality rates reported by Faist et al[3] for young, healthy, adult patients with multiple injuries. As with adult populations, the mortality rate in pediatric patients increases as the number of organs involved increases. These system failures can occur progressively, in sequence, or at the same time. However, pediatric patients with simultaneous organ failures have a higher mortality rate than those with progressive or sequential failures (when the same number of organ systems is involved). Wilkinson et al[1] reported a 75% mortality rate for both medical and surgical pediatric patients when four or more organ systems are involved. This would indicate that the maximum number of organ system failures is a simple reliable indicator of severity of illness and mortality in children.[4]

Respiratory failure is the most frequent organ failure seen in infants and children, followed by cardiovascular, neurologic, hematologic, and renal

---

EVENTS REPORTED TO TRIGGER MSOF

Advanced age	Intraabdominal infection	Poor nutrition
Alcoholism	Liver cirrhosis	Sepsis
Atherosclerotic cardiovascular disease	Malignancy	Shock
Burns	Multiple transfusions	Splenectomy
Chronic renal failure	Neurologic trauma	Steroids
Emergency surgery (specifically abdominal)	Pancreatitis	Vascular procedure
GI bleeding	Polytrauma	Others

From Toro-Figuera L. Multiple organ system failure. In: Levin DL, Morriss FC, eds. Essentials of pediatric intensive care. St Louis: Quality Medical Publishing, Inc., 1990:186.

Table 15-1 Criteria for Failure of Specific Organ Systems

Organ system	Criteria	Organ system	Criteria
Cardiovascular	MAP < 40 mm Hg (infants < 12 months) MAP < 50 mm Hg (children ≥ 12 months) HR < 50 beats/min (infants < 12 months) HR < 40 beats/min (children ≥ 12 months) Cardiac arrest Continuous vasoactive drug infusion for hemodynamic support	Neurologic	Glasgow coma scale < 5 Fixed, dilated pupils Persistent (> 20 min) intracranial pressure (> 20 mm Hg or requiring therapeutic intervention)
Respiratory	RR > 90/min (infants < 12 months) RR > 70/min (children ≥ 12 months) Pao_2 < 40 mm Hg (in absence of cyanotic heart disease) $Paco_2$ > 65 mm Hg Pao_2/Fio_2 < 250 mm Hg Mechanical ventilation (> 24 hr if postoperative) Tracheal intubation for airway obstruction or acute respiratory failure	Hematologic	Hemoglobin < 5 g/dL WBC < 3000 cell/mm^3 Platelets < 20,000/mm^3 Disseminated intravascular coagulopathy (PT > 20 sec or aPTT > 60 sec in presence of positive FSP assay)
		Renal	BUN > 100 mg/dL Serum creatinine > 2 mg/dL Dialysis
		Gastrointestinal	Blood transfusions > 20 mL/kg in 24 hr because of GI hemorrhage (endoscopic confirmation optional)
		Hepatic	Total bilirubin > 5 mg/dL and SGOT or LDH more than twice normal value (without evidence of hemolysis) Hepatic encephalopathy ≥ grade II

From Wilkinson JD et al. Mortality associated with multiple organ system failure and sepsis in pediatric intensive care. J Pediatr 1987; 111:325.
Abbreviations: *FSP*, fibrin split products; *HR*, heart rate; *LDH*, lactic dehydrogenase; *MAP*, mean arterial pressure; *PT*, prothrombin time; *aPTT*, activated partial thromboplastin time; *RR*, respiratory rate.

system involvement. No data are available on the incidence of hepatic or gastrointestinal failure, but these systems can be involved. A specific sequence of organ system failure has not been identified for children, and no specific combination of organ system failures has been found to raise mortality. Additionally, sepsis was not as strongly associated with MSOF in children as in adult populations. Wilkinson et al[2] reported that more than 50% of pediatric critical care patients developed MSOF in the absence of documented sepsis.

This chapter will focus on the assessment and collaborative management of pediatric patients with MSOF. Medical and nursing interventions are directed toward supporting individual organ systems before failure occurs. Nurses play a key role in assessing these system failures, identifying abnormalities early, and minimizing complications.

It is essential that nurses understand the differences in anatomy, physiology, and response to illness between children and adults as well as the systemic consequences of nursing interventions.

PATHOPHYSIOLOGY

The pathophysiology of MSOF in children is a complex process. When conditions such as sepsis or trauma disrupt the normal physiologic equilibrium, compensatory mechanisms work to regain homeostasis. However, when these mechanisms fail or become exhausted, a variety of physiologic, hemodynamic, metabolic, and inflammatory/immune dysfunctions occur.

Maldistribution of circulating blood volume is a common cause for the hemodynamic changes seen in the child with MSOF and results in an oxygen supply deficit. Compensatory mechanisms respond that attempt to restore normal circulation and use fuel stores to meet cellular oxygen demands. When the normal circulatory pattern cannot be restored quickly, the compensatory mechanisms and fuel stores are quickly exhausted. Cellular oxygen needs then go unmet.

The cellular hypoxia that results from decreased oxygen supplies damages the cell structure, which interferes with the cells' ability to extract and use oxygen. At the same time that oxygen supply is low or underused, the initial event that triggered the MSOF has greatly increased the body's need for oxygen. The greater demand goes unmet, and further cellular hypoxia results.

As the cells receive an inadequate oxygen supply, their metabolic activity becomes dysfunctional. The process that supplies energy to the cells requires oxygen. When oxygen is not present, the energy transfer is less efficient, and lactic acid is released. The buildup of lactic acid and inefficient metabolism cause generalized cell damage, unmet cellular energy needs, and cell death. Children normally have higher metabolic rates, and conditions such as sepsis or trauma increase them even more. The hypermetabolic state quickly depletes the child's limited energy reserves, and the anaerobic metabolic process cannot meet the increased energy demand. Liver failure occurs, and the hypermetabolism cannot be maintained. Cellular energy production becomes even further decreased, oxygen supply is further compromised, and cellular damage continues.

The normal inflammatory/immune response (IIR) is a multifaceted series of events that results in phagocytic activity and the release of mediators that are directed toward destroying the invading pathogen.[3] When the IIR is altered, the balance between mediators is lost, and the child's optimal protection is disrupted. Uncontrolled phagocytosis and mediator activity serve to intensify the IIR. The generalized systemic consequences that result are capillary vasodilatation, increased capillary permeability, smooth muscle contraction, heightened coagulation and fibrinolytic activity, enhanced macrophage and lymphocyte function, myocardial depression, and many others[4] (see Chapter 3).

The child's inability to meet cellular and metabolic needs leads to organ dysfunction, systemic disruption, and death. The generalized systemic effects elicit different reactions from individual organ systems. The remainder of this chapter focuses on the effect of systemic disruptions on the individual organ systems and the specialized nursing care to support the child with MSOF.

IMPAIRED GAS EXCHANGE

Respiratory failure is generally one of the first system failures seen in children.[1,5] It is classified according to both anatomic and physiologic parameters; however, the anatomic classification system is particularly useful in directing early ICU interventions (see box on p. 268). Regardless of the cause of respiratory failure, the end result is that the metabolic oxygen needs of the tissues will not be met, and carbon dioxide excretion will be inadequate.

Anatomic and physiologic differences

Children have little respiratory reserve because of a number of anatomic and physiologic factors that are peculiar to the pediatric respiratory system.[6] Narrow airways result in high airflow resistance, and decreased cartilaginous support of the airways causes early airway closure during forced expiration. The soft compliant chest walls, more horizontal positioning of the ribs, decreased curvature of the diaphragm, and the large abdomen that pushes up on the diaphragm and restricts lung expansion will not allow generation of high intrathoracic pressures.

In addition, infants are at risk for respiratory muscle fatigue because of the immaturity and structure of respiratory skeletal muscles. These factors all predispose infants and children to respiratory dysfunction and failure regardless of the underlying condition.

Pathophysiology

Respiratory dysfunction in MSOF is frequently manifested as adult respiratory distress syndrome (ARDS). As in adults, this syndrome results from injury to the child's alveolocapillary membrane and pulmonary endothelial damage that leads to increased pulmonary capillary permeability and leakage of fluid into the interstitium and alveoli. The lung damage may result from direct injury such as that sustained from aspiration, inhalation of toxic gases, or pulmonary infections; or it may also be the result of indirect injury from shock, sepsis, or

---

CAUSES OF RESPIRATORY FAILURE: ANATOMIC CLASSIFICATION

Central nervous system

Sedative overdose
Head trauma
Intracranial bleeding
Apnea of prematurity

Peripheral nervous system

Spinal cord injury
Guillain-Barré syndrome
Myasthenia gravis
Phrenic nerve paralysis

Respiratory muscles

Muscular dystrophies
Muscle wasting of cachexia
Respiratory muscle fatigue because of increased
   work of breathing

Chest wall and pleurae

Flail chest
Kyphoscoliosis
Pneumothorax
Hemothorax
Empyema
Chylothorax

Airways

Upper airways
   Epiglottitis
   Croup
Lower airways
   Foreign body aspiration
   Asthma
   Bronchiolitis

Parenchyma

Pneumonia
Pulmonary edema
Adult respiratory distress syndrome

Pulmonary blood flow

Pulmonary emboli
Persistent fetal circulation

From Witte M. Acute respiratory failure. In: Blumer J, ed. A practical guide to pediatric intensive care. 3rd ed. St Louis: Mosby–Year Book; 1990:98.

trauma.[7] The common denominators generally are hypotension, inflammation, and extensive tissue damage. Clinically, the child with ARDS exhibits hypoxemia that does not respond to increasing amounts of inspired oxygen, decreased pulmonary compliance, respiratory alkalosis, dyspnea, tachypnea, and the appearance of diffuse, fluffy infiltrates on chest x-ray films without evidence of cardiogenic causes.

Therapeutic management

Successful therapeutic management of the child with ARDS depends on recognizing its basic cause and implementing effective supportive therapy. The goal of therapy is to deliver adequate oxygen to meet the metabolic needs of tissues. Close observation of the child's general appearance is critical when assessing respiratory status. Nurses must be alert for signs of fatigue, diaphoresis, restlessness, and poor perfusion, which may indicate impending respiratory failure. Frequent nursing assessments of respiratory rate and effort, adequacy of breath sounds, and effectiveness of chest wall movements are important if the child is breathing spontaneously. Increased dyspnea, decreased respiratory rate, diminished breath sounds, altered level of consciousness, or paradoxical respirations may indicate increasing respiratory dysfunction and the need for more ventilatory support. Rapid intervention for deteriorating respiratory status is essential to correct hypoxemia and decrease the work of breathing.

Endotracheal intubation, mechanical ventilation, and the use of positive end-expiratory pressure (PEEP) will often be required to support the child's failing respiratory system. A variety of mechanical ventilation modes can be used successfully with children. Infants are frequently ventilated using time-cycled or pressure-cycled modes that limit inspiration and cause cycling from inspiration to expiration based on a preset time or pressure. Both of these modes provide a continuous flow of gas that reduces the infant's work of breathing and energy expenditure. These modes of ventilation are not as useful in older children, since they may not provide adequate flows for children weighing more than 15 kg.

Volume-cycled ventilation is used in many critically ill children. A preset tidal volume is delivered without regard for changes that occur in the child's lung compliance or airway resistance. High inflating pressures will be required to deliver the prescribed tidal volume in children with decreased compliance or increased airway resistance, which may lead to barotrauma.[8] Volume-cycled ventilation can be pressure limited to prevent the use of excessive inflating pressures that may be necessary to deliver the preset volume. This safety feature minimizes the risk of creating excessively high airway pressures and makes this mode of ventilation a good option even for small children.

Most volume ventilators that are currently used with children are equipped with options such as assist control, intermittent mandatory ventilation (IMV), synchronized IMV (SIMV), and pressure support, all of which allow the child to breathe independently between ventilator breaths. If these independent breaths are synchronized with positive pressure ventilations, the child will not have to work as hard to open the demand valve, and the risk of hypoventilation will be reduced. The combination of SIMV and pressure support will meet this requirement.

Pressure controlled ventilation is being used more frequently in the management of pediatric patients. This mode of ventilation allows the preset inspiratory pressure to be reached early in inspiration and maintained throughout the inspiratory effort. The advantage of this mode is that the sustained inspiratory pressure will keep the partially collapsed alveoli open.

All patients with acute respiratory failure require supplemental oxygen; however, the dose and duration must be carefully monitored since prolonged exposure to high levels of inspired oxygen can be toxic to lung tissue. Positive end-expiratory pressure (PEEP) is used routinely in ventilatory management of children and can effectively reduce the

---

GUIDELINES FOR INITIATING POSITIVE-PRESSURE SUPPORT

Provision of adequate alveolar ventilation
  Select rate—physiologic norm for age
  Select tidal volume—12 to 15 mL/kg
  Select PIP—15 to 20 cm H_2O, increase as needed
  Select inspiratory time (I:E ratio)—age-specific norm generally resulting in I:E ratio = 1:2
  Obstructive diseases—prolong E time, avoid prolonged I time
  Immediately assess for signs of adequate ventilation (chest excursion and breath sounds)
  Measure $Paco_2$; adjust IMV rate and/or tidal volume as needed to maintain between 35 and 45 mm Hg
  Decrease IMV rate to level tolerated as determined by $Paco_2$
Maintenance of adequate oxygenation
  Fio_2—1.0
  PEEP 3 cm H_2O, or higher level if needed, anticipating hemodynamic effects
  Immediately assess for signs of adequate oxygenation (color) and circulatory depression (hypotension and diminished peripheral pulses)
Measure Pao_2
  Decrease Fio_2, maintaining Pao_2 > 70 mm Hg
  Restrictive disease (low FRC, low compliance)—increase PEEP as needed to achieve Pao_2 > 70 mm Hg at Fio_2 = 0.4 to 0.5
  Consider direct monitoring of cardiac output if PEEP > 15 cm H_2O
  Decrease PEEP while maintaining Pao_2 > 70 mm Hg

From Boegner E. Modes of ventilatory support and weaning parameters in children. Clin Issues Crit Care Nurs 1990; 1:382. Abbreviations: *PIP*, peak inspiratory pressure; *I*, inspiratory; *E*, expiratory; *IMV*, intermittent mandatory ventilation; *PEEP*, positive end-expiratory pressure; *FRC*, functional residual capacity.

need for increasing concentrations of inspired oxygen (see box above). PEEP can be particularly useful with children who have ARDS since they frequently require high concentrations of oxygen to meet their cellular needs.

Management of children with respiratory failure

includes continuous electrocardiogram recordings; an arterial line for continuous measurement of blood pressure; and a pulmonary artery catheter to help evaluate fluid status, measure cardiac output, and monitor pulmonary capillary wedge pressures. Judicious fluid management, careful measurement of intake and output, and daily weighing will also be necessary. Serial chest x-ray examinations will document the progress of the disease. There is no specific drug therapy for ARDS, but generally antibiotics (based on Gram's stain and culture reports) and bronchodilators are included. Paralytic agents may be used with ventilated patients and should be given in conjunction with sedation. Evaluation of the effectiveness of sedation is more difficult in the unconscious child, but vital sign parameters are valid indicators and should be closely monitored during neuromuscular blockade.

Continuous nursing assessments of the ventilated child are critical and must include observations for signs of pneumothorax or pneumomediastinum resulting from barotrauma associated with high PEEP. Monitoring vital signs, color, level of consciousness, breath sounds, chest wall movements, ventilator settings, arterial blood gases, oxygen saturation, and end-tidal carbon dioxide levels should be done at least every 1 to 2 hours. Careful attention to peak inspiratory pressures can alert the nurse to the child's decreasing lung compliance and narrowing airways. Meticulous pulmonary hygiene is critical, and frequent suctioning is necessary to maintain patency of the narrow endotracheal tubes required to intubate children. Hyperoxygenation is required before suctioning, and the procedure must be accomplished using strict aseptic technique and caution, since the child is often immunologically and hemodynamically unstable. Elevating the head of the bed 15 to 30 degrees, frequent position changes, and chest physiotherapy are all important to ensure good pulmonary care.

Nurses must provide adequate rest periods and accomplish numerous interventions at the same time when possible. Limb restraints are required to prevent the child from accidentally removing essential equipment, and parents must understand the rationale for the restraints. Attention to light and noise levels is an important nursing function, and their adverse effects must be minimized without risking patient safety.

ALTERATION IN CARDIAC OUTPUT: DECREASED

The limited pediatric data available indicate that cardiovascular failure is seen clearly and relatively frequently in children with MSOF.[1] It is unclear, however, if the cardiovascular changes lead to generalized organ disruption or if the cardiovascular system is compensating for organ damage that has already occurred. As in adults, the child's myocardium can be damaged by ischemia, inflammatory mediators, and acidosis.

Cardiac output in children

Hemodynamic function is determined by cardiac output (CO) and vascular resistance. If the hemodynamic conditions change, alteration in CO and/or vascular resistance should occur. CO is the product of heart rate and stroke volume, and pediatric CO is greatly affected by the child's heart rate and body surface area. Heart rates in children tend to vary over a wide range and decrease with age as shown in Table 15-2. Conversely, stroke volume is relatively fixed in infants and young children and increases with age; therefore children respond to stress and increased metabolic needs by increasing their heart rates rather than by augmenting their stroke volume.[9]

To effectively maintain optimal CO and achieve maximal cardiac index in critically ill children, the heart rate should be maintained within the high

Table 15-2 Heart Rate Limits

Age	Low (beats/min)	High (beats/min)
0 to 24 hours	100	180
1 to 7 days	100	180
8 to 30 days	100	200
1 to 3 months	100	200
3 to 6 months	100	200
6 to 12 months	100	200
1 to 3 years	80	160
3 to 5 years	80	150
5 to 8 years	70	120
8 to 12 years	60	120
12 to 16 years	50	120

From Allen E. Basic minimal intensive care monitoring. In: Blumer J, ed. A practical guide to pediatric intensive care. 3rd ed. St Louis: Mosby Year Book, 1990:14.

normal range for age. Although this sustained high rate places the child at an increased risk for myocardial ischemia, it is much less of a concern than for adult patients. Children are better able to compensate for the increased myocardial oxygen consumption (MVo_2) that results from the increased heart rate by increasing oxygen delivery to the myocardium (MDo_2). Although it is not a common event, myocardial ischemia can occur in children of all ages during rapid heart rates. Other conditions frequently associated with myocardial ischemia include shock, thoracic trauma, head injury, asthma, and tachydysrhythmias (see box below).

When CO is inadequate, cellular hypoxia, altered cellular metabolism, and decreased energy production result.[10] This state of circulatory dysfunction is clinically described as shock. It is generally caused by a reduced CO, maldistribution of circulating volume, or both and if allowed to proceed uninterrupted, it will result in death.

Shock

The causes of shock in children are the same as in adults; however, the frequency with which they occur is different. Generally, the classifications of shock are hypovolemic (lack of vascular volume), distributive (altered vascular tone), and cardiogenic (pump failure).[10]

Shock occurs in a wide variety of clinical settings, often without any associated illness or obvious predisposing factors. The outcome is often better for children than for adults, because the child is generally healthy before the onset. Although shock occurs in children of all ages, some populations are more vulnerable to specific types. Neonates, children with congenital heart disease, and oncologic and urologic patients are at greater risk to develop septic shock. Organisms responsible for septic shock vary with the age of the patient. β-Hemolytic streptococci and *Haemophilus influenzae*, which are generally not associated with septic shock in adults, are seen frequently in infants and young children. Also, children with congenital heart disease are more likely to develop cardiogenic shock.

Hypovolemic shock. Hypovolemic shock is the most common cause of shock in children.[10] It results from decreased intravascular volume generally related to water and electrolyte losses, hemorrhage, third space losses, or pathologic renal losses.[11] These losses result from a variety of insults including trauma, gastrointestinal hemorrhage, renal disease, and burns. The decreased circulating volume results in reduced venous return and preload and therefore decreased stroke volume and CO. Although a child's circulating blood volume is larger relative to weight than an adult's circulating blood volume (80 mL/kg), a child can become hypovolemic with a minimal amount of fluid loss because his or her total circulating volume is small. The hypovolemia often results from vomiting and diarrhea because much of the child's total fluid volume is extracellular. Early symptoms usually include cool extremities, decreased peripheral perfusion, tachycardia, and decreased urine output.

CAUSES OF MYOCARDIAL ISCHEMIA IN CHILDHOOD

Neonatal ischemic heart disease
    Asphyxia neonatorum
    Increased demand
        Persistent transitional circulation
        Pulmonary hypertension (respiratory distress syndrome and meconium aspiration)
Congenital heart disease
    Cyanotic heart disease
        Total anomalous pulmonary veins
        Transposition of great vessels
    Obstructive disease
        Aortic or pulmonary stenosis
    Anomalous coronary arteries
Increased demand
    Catecholamine-induced ischemia (isoproterenol treatment of asthma)
    Head injury
Vascular disease
    Kawasaki disease
    Infantile periarteritis nodosa
    Embolism
    Atheroma (rare)
    Trauma
Trauma and head injury

From Rogers MC, Wetzel RC, Deshpande JK. Unusual causes of pulmonary edema, myocardial ischemia, and cyanosis. In: Rogers MC, ed. Textbook of pediatric intensive care. Baltimore: Williams & Wilkins, 1987:378.

Cardiac output is decreased, but blood pressure is usually normal because of the child's efficient vasoconstrictive mechanisms. If volume loss is not corrected, the symptoms worsen; the child becomes hypotensive, anuric, and mentally confused, and cardiac failure results.[9]

Distributive shock. Distributive shock, the second most common type of shock to occur in children, is associated with an abnormal distribution of circulating volume.[12] As a result, tissues are inadequately perfused even with normal or high CO. This shock occurs during anaphylaxis, drug toxicity, neurologic injury, and sepsis. These children may show signs and symptoms of virtually every other type of shock.

Septic shock may result from decreased intravascular volume, maldistribution of intravascular volume, and impaired myocardial function, all of which occur at different times during its course. Critically ill children with severe burns or multiple trauma frequently develop septic shock. Surgery, invasive devices, antibiotics, immunosuppression, hypothermia, and critical illness are all risk factors in septic shock.[13] Although the cause is usually bacterial, viral pathogens and their toxins can also cause septic shock. As in the adult, the child's clinical course can move from the high cardiac output, hyperdynamic stage when the child looks well perfused (although tissue hypoxia may be present in some organ beds) to the uncompensated stage when the child is cold, cyanotic, listless, anuric, and manifesting the signs and symptoms of cardiogenic shock. Adequate fluid resuscitation is vital to prevent decompensation and low CO.

Cardiogenic shock. Cardiogenic shock does not occur frequently in children; however, it can result from congenital heart disease, trauma, ischemia, sepsis, hypothermia, and drug toxicity. In neonates, the usual cause of cardiogenic shock is a congenital heart defect that is characterized by outflow obstruction or systemic pulmonary shunts.[12] It may also result from cardiac dysrhythmias such as paroxysmal atrial tachycardia or atrioventricular block, cardiomyopathies, or metabolic imbalances.[11]

Therapeutic management

The successful management of cardiovascular dysfunction is aimed at perfusing vital organs and preventing or correcting metabolic abnormalities resulting from cellular hypoperfusion. The goals of therapy are to establish and maintain the appropriate oxygen and substrate delivery to meet metabolic needs of the child without increasing MVO_2 and to support the child until homeostasis is restored and healing begins.

Assessment

Nursing assessments must focus on the child's volume status. Heart rate, blood pressure, temperature, systemic perfusion, color, level of consciousness, quality of pulses, and core temperature should be monitored continuously. An important consideration for children in shock is that blood pressure is often the last parameter to change; therefore careful consideration must be given to early changes in the systemic perfusion. Prompt identification of arrhythmias is necessary, and interventions should include correction of hypoxia, acidosis, hypocalcemia, hypokalemia, or hyperkalemia, and the use of cardioactive drugs such as atropine, isoproterenol, digoxin, verapamil, and lidocaine.[9] The use of pacemakers and cardioversion may also be necessary to increase the heart rate and maximize CO. Blood pressure monitoring should be accomplished using an intraarterial line if possible. This continuous display with beat-to-beat analysis of waveform and continuous display of pulse pressure is critical. This device also is valuable in the ongoing analysis of arterial blood gases. If a manual cuff is used, particular attention must be given to cuff size. The cuff should be two thirds to three fourths of the upper-arm size and should completely encircle the child's arm only once. Monitoring peripheral and core temperature is helpful in assessing peripheral perfusion, and differences in these parameters could indicate a compromised CO. Evaluation of serial arterial blood gases, electrolytes, electrocardiogram, isoenzymes, and body weight is also essential to the assessment.

Decreased cardiac output often can be improved by increasing preload. Children have a larger daily fluid requirement than adults, but their total fluid requirement is smaller as illustrated in Tables 15-3 and 15-4.

Volume replacement

Volume replacement of 10 to 20 mL/kg over 10 to 15 minutes is a priority for the child in shock.

Table 15-3 Pediatric Maintenance Fluid Requirements

Body weight (kg)	Water maintenance (mL/24 hr)	Electrolyte maintenance
< 10	100 mL/kg	
10 to 20	1000 mL + 50 mL for each kg above 10 kg	
> 20	1500 mL + 20 mL for each kg above 20 kg	3 mEq of sodium + 2 mEq of potassium for each 100 mL of fluid

Recommended maintenance fluid is D5 + ¼ NS with 20 mEq of KCl/L. Do not routinely use D5W in children.

From Blumer J. Pediatric emergency guidelines. In: Blumer J, ed. A practical guide to pediatric intensive care. 3rd ed. St Louis: Mosby–Year Book, 1990:cover.

Table 15-4 Fluid Resuscitation Requirements in Neonates and Children in Shock*

IV fluid	Amount	Rate
First D5NS	10 to 20 mL/kg	Over 5 to 10 min
Then NS or R/L	10 to 20 mL/kg†	Over 5 to 20 min
5% albumin or hetastarch	10 mL/kg for every 40 mL of crystalloid given	Over 5 to 20 min

From Blumer J. Pediatric emergency guidelines. In: Blumer J, ed. A practical guide to pediatric intensive care. 3rd ed. St Louis: Mosby–Year Book, 1990:cover.
*Physical examination: lethargic, cool extremities, mottled skin, slow capillary refill, tachycardic, and hypotensive.
†Give repeated IV boluses until vital signs improve and peripheral perfusion improves.

Additional replacement must be based on an ongoing assessment of the child's vital signs, level of consciousness, systemic perfusion, urine output, and hemodynamic parameters. Urine output should be measured at least hourly and should exceed 0.5 to 1.0 mL/kg/hr if renal function is normal. Urine output of less than 0.5 mL/kg/hr suggests decreased renal perfusion.[14] Accurate intake/output,

Table 15-5 Normal Pressure Values for Children

Pressure	Value (mm Hg)
Central venous pressure	4 to 12
Systolic pulmonary artery pressure	20 to 30
Diastolic pulmonary artery pressure	< 10
Mean pulmonary artery pressure	< 20
Pulmonary capillary wedge pressure	4 to 12

Modified from Smith J, Giblin M, Koehler J. The cardiovascular system. In: Smith J, ed. Pediatric critical care. New York: J Wiley & Sons, 1983:100.

including blood loss from laboratory work, must be recorded.

Pulmonary artery catheters are often used and allow the nurse to monitor filling pressures and calculate hemodynamic indices (Table 15-5). These data provide valuable information about the child's volume status, myocardial function, and ventricular afterload.

Pharmacologic support

Pharmacologic support with inotropic and/or vasopressor agents such as dopamine, dobutamine, and isoproterenol may be necessary to increase cardiac output. Children receiving these agents should always be managed using invasive hemodynamic monitoring techniques. Combining inotropic drugs with vasodilators such as sodium nitroprusside will decrease afterload and increase cardiac output without the adverse peripheral vasoconstrictor effects. Table 15-6 lists the various vasoactive agents with the appropriate range of doses used in children. Aggressive intervention must take place to restore adequate cardiovascular function. If restoration of function is delayed or does not occur, additional organ dysfunction will occur, resulting in MSOF.

ALTERATION IN TISSUE PERFUSION: CEREBRAL
Primary vs. secondary injury

Cerebral injuries are often classified as primary and secondary. The primary injury occurs during the initial event and results in neuronal death at the time of injury. Secondary injury occurs after the primary injury and is caused by the inability of the

Table 15-6   Vasoactive Agents Used in Children

Agent	Site of action	Dose (μg/kg/min)	Effect
Dopamine	β	1 to 3	Renal vasodilator Inotrope
	α > β	5 to 20	Peripheral vasoconstriction Increased PVR Dysrhythmias
Dobutamine	β₁	1 to 20	Inotrope Vasodilatation Lowered PVR Weak alpha activity Tachycardic and extrasystolic
Isoproterenol	β₁ and β₂	0.05 to 2.0	Inotrope Vasodilatation Lowered PVR Increased MVo_2 Dysrhythmias
Epinephrine	β > α	0.05 to 1.0	Dysrhythmias Tachycardia Decreased renal flow Increased MVo_2 Dysrhythmias
Norepinephrine	α > β	0.05 to 1.0	Profound constrictor Inotrope Increased MVo_2, SVR
Sodium nitroprusside	Vasodilator—arterial greater than venous	0.5 to 10	Rapid onset, short duration Increased ICP V/Q mismatch Cyanide toxicity
Nitroglycerin	Vasodilator—venous greater than arterial	1 to 20	Decreased PVR Increased ICP

From Wetzel RC. Shock. In: Rogers MC, ed. Textbook of pediatric intensive care. Baltimore: Williams & Wilkins, 1987:514.

cerebral vasculature to deliver adequate oxygen and glucose to the neurons; ischemia, hypoxia, anoxia, or metabolic derangements result.[15] Interventions must be directed at limiting secondary injury since very little can be done about the primary injury. The resulting cerebral ischemia and secondary injury cause swelling of the cerebral tissue and increased intracranial pressure (ICP). An infant's skull does have open sutures that do allow for some compensation as cerebral edema occurs. Eventually, however, if edema continues, ICP will rise.

Assessment

Nursing management must focus on preventing secondary injury. Assessment must begin with an evaluation of airway, breathing, and circulation.[16]

Adequate ventilation must be ensured in order to restore perfusion and oxygen delivery. Inadequate ventilation leads to increased $Paco_2$, which elevates the ICP. The respiratory assessment should focus on rate and rhythm and abnormal breathing patterns that might indicate changes in sensorium and ICP. The abnormal patterns may negatively affect the child's oxygenation and alter cerebral blood flow and ICP. Breath sounds must be evaluated frequently in order to detect signs of neurogenic pulmonary edema, which is often associated with intracranial hypertension. Careful observation of the color and temperature of extremities, capillary refill, color of nailbeds and mucous membranes, pulses, blood pressure, and heart rate is valuable in assessing the child's perfusion. Changes in these

---

MODIFIED GLASGOW COMA SCALE FOR INFANTS

Eye opening

No response	1
Response to pain	2
Response to voice	3
Spontaneously	4

Verbal response

No response	1
Moans to pain	2
Cries to pain	3
Irritable cries	4
Coos and babbles	5

Motor response

No response	1
Abnormal extension	2
Abnormal flexion	3
Withdraws to pain	4
Withdraws to touch	5
Normal spontaneous movements	6
Maximum score	**15**

From Davis RJ et al. In: Rogers MC, ed. Textbook of pediatric intensive care. Baltimore: Williams & Wilkins, 1987:658.

---

parameters could indicate shock or increasing ICP.

The classic Cushing's triad, which consists of bradycardia, increasing systolic blood pressure, and widening pulse pressure, frequently indicates increasing ICP and impending herniation. This phenomenon is not often seen in infants and does not provide a reliable assessment of ICP in this group of patients.

After the ABCs are evaluated, a thorough ongoing neurologic assessment is necessary using the Glasgow coma scale. This tool is used to pinpoint the patient's level of consciousness and identify high-risk patients. The scale provided in the accompanying box has been modified for use with children. Scores of less than 9 suggest very severe injury and are associated with high mortality. These patients will need airway support and are potential candidates for ICP monitoring and other invasive hemodynamic monitoring.[17]

Pupil size and reactivity, cranial oculovestibular reflexes, and oculocephalic reflexes should be evaluated frequently. Cortical function may be assessed by giving the child simple directions and assessing his ability to follow them. Look for changes in muscle tone and posture. Decorticate postures are associated with cortical or hemispheric dysfunction, and decerebrate postures correlate with high pontine and midbrain lesions. Flaccidity indicates severe low brainstem dysfunction and may signal imminent death.

Seizures are often associated with severe head injuries, diffuse cerebral edema, and acute subdural hematoma and should be treated aggressively.[18,19] Seizure activity leads to increased cerebral blood flow and ICP. Immediate control can be established using diazepam (0.1 to 0.3 mg/kg) or phenobarbital (20 to 30 mg/kg). Phenytoin (5 mg/kg/day) can be given for long-term control, since posttraumatic seizures may occur for 1 to 2 years after injury.[20]

Normal ICP limits for children are 10 to 15 mm Hg and less than 10 mm Hg for infants.[21] Cerebral perfusion pressure must be greater than 50 mm Hg. ICP can be assessed in infants by palpating the anterior fontanel. A bulging fontanel is often associated with increased ICP; however, this is a very subjective measurement. Invasive ICP monitoring techniques provide a much more objective measurement.

Current techniques for monitoring ICP include intraventricular devices, subarachnoid monitors, epidural monitors, and intraparenchymal devices. Intraventricular catheters provide a very reliable measurement of ICP and allow for removal of small amounts of cerebrospinal fluid (CSF) to treat rising ICP. These devices, however, are associated with greater morbidity because of their position in the ventricle. Subarachnoid devices are simple to use and relatively noninvasive, but they often significantly underestimate ICP and do not allow the removal of large amounts of CSF to lower ICP.[20] Epidural catheters are used minimally with children, and the new intraparenchymal devices are used least.

Control of ICP

Many methods may be used to control ICP, and expert nursing care is critical to successful management. Temperature control is very important, and antipyretics and cooling blankets are frequently required to treat hyperthermia. If a blanket is used, continuous temperature monitoring and interventions to reduce shivering will be necessary. The head of the bed should be elevated to 30 degrees and the patient's head kept midline to facilitate venous drainage. Isometric muscle contractions increase intrathoracic and intraabdominal pressures, thus decreasing cerebral venous drainage and increasing cerebral blood volume and ICP.[22] These contractions can be caused by hip and knee flexion, abnormal posturing, shivering, and pushing on the footboard. Nursing care must be directed at preventing isometric contraction by log rolling the child when turning, avoiding footboards and using high-top tennis shoes, controlling posturing with pancuronium or vecuronium, and reducing shivering with chlorpromazine (Thorazine). Rest periods should be provided between activities, and procedures should be accomplished as quickly as possible. Certain activities such as suctioning, using the bedpan, coughing, chewing, and conversations that center around the child but do not include the child have been shown to increase ICP.[23] Noxious stimuli, including loud noises, painful procedures, and nontherapeutic touch, are also associated with elevating ICP, especially during rapid eye movement (REM) sleep.[24] Purposeful touch, on the other hand, decreases ICP,[25] and families should be encouraged to talk with and touch the child as much as possible. Since suctioning causes increased ICP, it should be preceded by adequate oxygenation and limited to 10 seconds. Drugs such as lidocaine and thiopental given before suctioning may prevent an acute rise in ICP during the procedure.

In general, children with a cerebral injury should be fluid restricted. Two thirds of normal maintenance is adequate for minor cerebral injuries, and one half to one third of normal maintenance is adequate for more severe injuries. This restriction should be implemented upon a hemodynamically stable patient, with an adequate blood pressure, urine output, and peripheral perfusion.[17] Hypotonic fluids should be avoided, with lactated Ringer's solution or half-normal saline being appropriate fluids to use.

Diuretics are useful in reducing ICP and are usually given in conjunction with fluid restrictions. Osmotic diuretics such as mannitol are commonly used in children to treat ICP and reduce brain bulk. Unfortunately, mannitol can draw fluid from uninjured tissue as well as damaged cells, causing fluid and electrolyte imbalances. Mannitol is given in a wide dose range from 0.25 to 2.0 g/kg. Side effects of high-dose therapy are significant and include hyperosmolality, hemolysis, renal failure, and rebound intracranial hypertension. Lower doses of 0.25 g/kg are recommended and associated with fewer problems. Serum osmolality should be evaluated at least every 6 hours and should not exceed 320 mOsm/L. If the child does become hyperosmolar, administration of hypotonic solutions to reduce the osmolality can exacerbate the cerebral edema.

Loop diuretics such as furosemide and ethacrynic acid are also used in the management of ICP, but their role is less defined. These drugs reduce swelling by limiting the amount of sodium available for reabsorption into the cerebrospinal fluid. They are often administered with other agents in order to increase the effectiveness of therapy. The recommended dose of furosemide is 0.5 to 1.0 mg/kg every 4 to 6 hours. Serum sodium and potassium levels must be closely monitored in any patient receiving loop diuretics. Daily weights are also necessary.

Steroids are often used in the management of ICP, but the benefit is unclear. There is no clear evidence of their value in improving outcome, and considerable risks are associated with their use. If used, the patient must be monitored for gastrointestinal bleeding, immunosuppression, and glucose intolerance.[17]

Another controversial therapy involves barbiturates such as pentobarbital. The purpose of this treatment, which is generally used as a last resort, is to decrease cerebral metabolic rate and demand for oxygen. In addition to decreasing ICP, barbiturate coma also suppresses cardiovascular, respiratory, immunologic, and liver function. A loading dose of 2.0 to 5.0 mg/kg is given with a continuous infusion of 1.0 to 3.0 mg/kg/hr to maintain a serum level of 20 to 40 µg/mL.[2] The use of barbiturate coma eliminates the clinician's ability to evaluate the child's neurologic status by physical examination, and as a result the EEG will be invalid.

One of the most effective means of controlling ICP is by manipulating the arterial carbon dioxide ($Paco_2$) level. It is important that $Paco_2$ be maintained between 25 and 35 mm Hg so that excessive cerebral blood flow will be prevented. Lowering

$Paco_2$ below 25 mm Hg can cause additional cerebral ischemia, and the resulting respiratory alkalosis can interfere with tissue oxygenation. CO_2 levels should be continuously monitored with end-tidal CO_2 monitors and frequent arterial blood gases.

ALTERATION IN FLUID VOLUME: DEFICIT

Although hematologic failure occurs less frequently in children than in adults,[1] it is a common problem in critically ill children. Normal coagulation in children and adults is the result of an organized series of events that involves the blood vessels, platelets, plasma proteins, and fibrinolytic system. Each component plays a vital role in the coagulation process, and a deficiency of, or damage to, any of these coagulation components can result in uncontrolled and abnormal hemostasis, blood loss, and fluid volume deficit.

Thrombocytopenia

The normal platelet count for children and adults is 150,000 to 400,000/mm^3 and thrombocytopenia is defined as a count less than 150,000/mm^3. In neonates, the normal platelet count is lower, and thrombocytopenia is defined as less than 100,000/mm^3.[26] Inadequate quantities or defective platelets will alter hemostasis and result in bleeding. Certain drugs that are frequently used to treat children, such as antibiotics, antihistamines, nonsteroidal antiinflammatory agents, phenothiazines, and vinca alkaloids, have been known to cause platelet dysfunction. Even so, the most common cause of bleeding in critically ill children is not defective platelet function but inadequate quantities of platelets.

Children experience a variety of bleeding disorders. Some are congenital coagulation disorders, such as hemophilia or Christmas disease, in which essential plasma proteins are deficient. More commonly, children develop acute acquired bleeding disorders generally associated with platelet defects or plasma protein dysfunction or deficiencies. Idiopathic thrombocytopenic purpura (ITP), thrombocytopenia resulting from certain diseases, autoimmune disorders, and bone marrow failure syndromes are disorders caused by platelet defects (see box above). Disseminated intravascular coagulation (DIC), liver failure, and vitamin K deficiency

---

ETIOLOGY OF THROMBOCYTOPENIA

Decreased production
  Bone marrow suppression (chemotherapy)
  Aplastic anemia
  Malignancy
  Congenital amegakaryocytosis
Accelerated destruction or loss (nonimmune)
  Congenital
    TORCH infections
    Giant hemangioma
  Acquired
    HUS, thrombotic thrombocytopenic purpura
    Infection
    DIC
    Necrotizing enterocolitis
    Massive transfusion
    Hypersplenism
Accelerated destruction or loss (immune)
  Infection
  Idiopathic thrombocytopenic purpura
  Neonatal passive immunization
  Autoimmune disorders
  Drug-induced

From Gordon JB et al. Hematologic disorders in the pediatric intensive care unit. In: Rogers MC, ed. Textbook of pediatric intensive care. Baltimore: Williams & Wilkins, 1987:1199. Abbreviations: *TORCH*, toxoplasmosis, rubella, cytomegalovirus, herpes; *HUS*, hemolytic-uremic syndrome; *DIC*, disseminated intravascular coagulation.

---

are examples of disorders caused by plasma protein dysfunction or deficiencies.

ITP usually occurs in a healthy child after a viral infection. The child's physical appearance is generally normal except for petechiae, ecchymosis, and hemorrhage from the nose or mouth. Occasionally acute intracerebral bleeding occurs, but generally the child is not acutely ill and recovers spontaneously within several weeks. Hemolytic-uremic syndrome is a serious disorder that causes decreased platelets. It is usually characterized by acute renal failure and hemolytic anemia. Children with this syndrome are hypertensive, volume overloaded, and anemic.

Bacterial and viral infections, especially in neonates, also result in low platelet counts. These children do not hemorrhage, although they have significant thrombocytopenia. Children with bone marrow failure also have platelet production problems and usually bleed more profusely than other children with equivalent platelet counts. Whatever the cause, treatment is aimed at correcting the underlying process and restoring normal platelet counts and functions.

DIC

Plasma proteins and the fibrinolytic system have similar functions in adults and children. The end-product of coagulation is fibrin clot formation, and the function of the fibrinolytic system is to dissolve the clot and restore blood flow. Normally, these activities occur with exact precision; however, diffuse endothelial or organ destruction can lead to severe disruption of the process. DIC is characterized by uncoordinated coagulation and fibrinolysis.[27] The pathophysiology for children and adults is the same (see Chapter 4). Excessive amounts of thrombin are produced; the coagulation factors, fibrinogen, and platelets are consumed; and the fibrinolytic system is continuously activated. The result is a clinical picture of hemorrhage and microthrombosis that can lead to organ ischemia and high mortality.

DIC is not a primary disease, but results from an underlying illness or injury (see box below). DIC is present in nearly all critically ill patients. It is often low grade and causes little clinical change because the spleen, liver, and bone marrow can compensate by increasing production of platelets and clotting factors and normalizing hemostasis.

DISORDERS ASSOCIATED WITH DISSEMINATED INTRAVASCULAR COAGULATION

Sepsis
Shock
Severe (penetrating) head injury
Thermal injuries
Snake bite
Fresh-water drowning
Acute promyelocytic leukemia
Necrotizing pneumonitis
Transfusion reactions

From Kedar A, Gross S. Disseminated intravascular coagulation. In: Blumer J, ed. A practical guide to pediatric intensive care. 3rd ed. St Louis: Mosby–Year Book, 1990:518.

In MSOF, however, these hematologic organs often suffer damage themselves, and they cannot adequately compensate for the disrupted coagulation. Birth depression (Apgar score < 3 at 1 minute and < 7 at 5 minutes) and sepsis are the most common causes of DIC in the newborn.[26] Necrotizing enterocolitis (NEC) and respiratory distress syndrome also may be associated with DIC in the neonate.

The treatment of DIC centers on identifying and treating the underlying disease process. Correction of the associated shock, acidosis, and electrolyte imbalances is critical. Laboratory findings in children are similar to adults. Blood component replacement therapy is controversial, but packed red blood cells, platelets, fresh frozen plasma, coagulation factors, and cryoprecipitate transfusions are often essential to treat hypovolemia and replace clotting components. Exchange transfusions have been used in infants with limited success. Heparin and antithrombin III infusions have been used with adults and children in an attempt to inhibit thrombin activity. These treatments are often unsuccessful and, in fact, may cause more bleeding. Other options are becoming available but are still considered investigational with children.

Liver disease

Liver disease and vitamin K deficiency should also be considered when managing coagulopathies in children. Bleeding may be the first sign of liver disease, which is often accompanied by hepatomegaly, jaundice, and other obvious signs of liver failure. Treatment is often not necessary, but serious bleeding may occur. Vitamin K deficiency may result because of inadequate nutritional status, and the onset may be rapid. Children who have illnesses that inhibit fat absorption, such as biliary atresia and cystic fibrosis, are at risk for vitamin K deficiency. Children who ingest rat poison or take certain drugs such as phenytoin, vitamin E, or aspirin are also at risk for vitamin K deficiency. Replacement therapy to restore vitamin K levels can be given orally, intramuscularly, or intravenously.

Assessment

Nursing assessments are essential for early detection of hematologic dysfunction. Prolonged bleeding from venipuncture sites; oozing from wounds and catheter insertion sites; bleeding from gums and teeth; blood in gastric contents, urine, and stools; and petechiae and ecchymosis are critical nursing observations. Careful monitoring of laboratory values such as white blood count, hematocrit, platelet count, prothrombin time, and fibrin split products provides valuable information. Since thrombocytopenia is frequently present in acute DIC, the nurse must be alert for signs of bleeding and must avoid damage to the skin and mucous membranes. Meticulous skin and mouth care are essential. Accurate intake and output records are necessary, as is continuous monitoring of vital signs. Good pulmonary hygiene is mandatory; however, caution must be used to prevent bleeding. An accurate assessment of the child's response to blood product transfusion is necessary. Documentation of the need for blood products can help assess the progression of the hematologic failure. Nursing and medical interventions are generally aimed at supporting the child until the underlying illness is reversed.

ALTERATION IN FLUID VOLUME: EXCESS

Renal failure occurs in more than 40% of adult patients with MSOF.[28-31] The study by Wilkinson et al documents renal failure in only 8% of the children with MSOF.[1] Even so, renal dysfunction and failure are problems often seen in critically ill children that complicate their management and increase their mortality. The mortality of children for all renal failure is much less than that of adults. Most acute renal failures in children are potentially reversible with optimal management.[32] In spite of this, the impact of renal failure in critically ill children is still great. It occurs suddenly, and normal compensatory mechanisms are often unable to respond quickly enough to prevent life-threatening complications.[33] Critical illness itself adds stress to the kidneys because they work to maintain homeostasis and rid the body of by-products of tissue breakdown. Interventions for critical illness such as volume replacement, transfusions, and drug therapies place added burden on the kidneys and often have toxic side effects.[32]

Acute renal failure

When acute renal failure (ARF) does occur in children, oliguric failure, which is defined as a urine output less than 0.5 mL/kg/hr, is most com-

monly seen. ARF can be caused by many things, including hypovolemia, peripheral vasodilatation and hypotension, renal vasoconstriction, nephrotoxins, or primary parenchymal renal disease (see box on p. 280).

Causes are usually categorized as prerenal, intrarenal, and postrenal. Prerenal and postrenal failures are reversible with rapid correction of the precipitating event. These conditions can, however, progress to intrarenal failure if not corrected, and the damage may be irreversible.

Assessment and management

The clinical picture and management of ARF are similar regardless of the cause or age of the patient. Patients are at risk for volume overload, hypertension, peripheral edema, skin breakdown, and infection. Electrolytic disturbances such as hyperkalemia, hyponatremia, hypernatremia, hyperphosphatemia, hypocalcemia, and hypermagnesemia are frequently seen. A severe metabolic acidosis often develops because the kidneys are unable to excrete hydrogen ions, and azotemia develops slowly as evidenced by rising blood urea nitrogen and creatinine levels.

Hypertension is commonly associated with ARF. It may be due to volume overload, especially with parenchymal renal disease. Moderate hypertension can generally be controlled by careful fluid management and efforts to decrease fluid overload. If significant hypertension persists, parenteral medication should be considered. These medications should be administered in a controlled setting with the ability to accurately monitor mean blood pressure. A rapid intravenous push of 5 mg/kg of diazoxide has a direct arterial vasodilating effect, with a peak effect in 5 minutes after administration and a duration of 4 to 12 hours. Sodium nitroprusside administered at 0.5 to 8.0 µg/kg/min has an immediate onset and acts by reducing afterload and preload and dilating arteries. Hydralazine administered at 0.1 to 0.2 mg/kg may be used in moderately severe hypertension.

Low-dose dopamine at 1 to 5 µg/kg/min is used to increase renal flow and improve urine ouput in children with ARF. Renal vasodilatation may persist up to 15 µg/kg/min. Higher doses, however, are associated with renal vasoconstriction. Diuretics such as mannitol or furosemide may be used in an effort to avert ARF or improve urine output.

CAUSES OF ACUTE RENAL FAILURE

Prerenal disease
True volume depletion
Hemorrhage
Dehydration
Third-space sequestration

Vasodilatation
Sepsis
Antihypertensives

Edematous states
Heart failure
Hepatic disease (hepatorenal syndrome)
Hypoalbuminemia (nephrosis and protein-losing enteropathy)

Renal ischemia
High doses of vasopressor agents
Bilateral renal artery stenosis (exacerbated by ACE [angiotensin converting enzyme] inhibitors)
Nonsteroidal antiinflammatory drugs
Cyclosporin A
Renal artery thrombosis (in neonates related to umbilical artery catheter)

Intrarenal disease ("fixed" renal failure)
Postischemic: any prerenal insult, if prolonged, can result in "fixed" renal failure

Nephrotoxins
Aminoglycoside antibiotics and amphotericin B
Radiocontrast material
Chemotherapy (cisplatin and others)
Heme pigments (myoglobinuria and hemoglobinuria)

Primary renal disease
Hemolytic uremic syndrome
Glomerulonephritis (primary and secondary)
Interstitial nephritis (drug related and infectious)

Postrenal disease
Obstruction
Urethral or bladder neck
Ureterovesicle junction
Ureteropelvic junction
(Can be congenital or related to stones, blood clots, or extrinsic compression such as masses and retroperitoneal fibrosis)

From Stork J. Acute renal failure. In: Blumer J, ed. A practical guide to pediatric intensive care. 3rd ed. St Louis: Mosby–Year Book, 1990:430.

Hyperkalemia may require emergent interventions. As a rule, a potassium level of 6.0 mEq/L or above should be treated. Efforts to decrease potassium may include calcium chloride administered at 20 mg/kg IV as first-line therapy for patients with ECG changes. Another therapy to decrease potassium levels is to administer 1 to 2 mEq/kg IV of sodium bicarbonate or 1 to 2 g/kg IV of glucose with insulin at 0.2 unit/g of glucose. If the child continues to be hypercatabolic or has marked elevation of uremic toxins, dialysis may be indicated.

Anticipation is a critical component in the management of renal failure. Maintaining an adequate intravascular volume is vital. Ongoing nursing assessments must focus on the child's state of hydration to recognize dehydration or fluid overload. Dry mucous membranes, postural changes in heart rate and blood pressure, "tenting" of the skin, and a sunken fontanel may indicate dehydration. Peripheral edema, rales, liver enlargement, gallop,

or hypertension may be associated with volume overload. Careful fluid management is required and includes frequent assessment and accurate documentation of intake and output, since these children are often restricted or receiving fluid challenges or diuretics. Diapers must be weighed to measure urine output if a catheter is not in place. All output must be measured, including blood loss, gastrointestinal drainage, and stool. Daily weights should be recorded using the same scale each day for accuracy. The child's response to all interventions must be documented in order to assess their effectiveness. Frequent monitoring of blood pressure, pulmonary capillary wedge pressures, cardiac output, and urine specific gravity are important measures. A continuous electrocardiogram (ECG) should be displayed to watch for changes associated with hyperkalemia. Serial assessment of laboratory data such as serum and urine creatinine, blood urea nitrogen, and serum and urine electrolytes is a vital nursing function.

HIGH RISK FOR INJURY RELATED TO HEPATIC FAILURE
Pathophysiology

Hepatic failure in the child with MSOF is defined as a total bilirubin of greater than 5 mg/dL, SGOT or LDH more than twice normal value (without evidence of hemolysis), and hepatic encephalopathy of greater than or equal to grade II.[2] The mechanism of hepatic injury in the child with MSOF has been described as a primary mechanism that occurs even when the tissues are well perfused. This mechanism is felt to be mediated by the liver macrophage (Kupffer cell).[4] A stimulus such as endotoxin stimulates the Kupffer cell, which then releases mediators such as prostaglandins or IL-1. These mediators injure the surrounding hepatocytes and cause cell dysfunction or death. Ischemic damage may also play a role in cellular dysfunction.

Assessment and management

The overall goal of therapy for the child with hepatic failure is to support the child until hepatic regeneration can occur. Nursing and medical management of the child with hepatic dysfunction therefore revolves around preventing and treating complications such as hepatic encephalopathy, cerebral edema, gastrointestinal bleeding, infection, respiratory failure, and hepatorenal syndrome. Assessment includes monitoring for abnormal signs and symptoms associated with liver disease. Encephalopathy, jaundice, ascites, and bleeding disorders are commonly seen. Basic monitoring should include hourly observation of pulse, respirations, blood pressure, level of consciousness, urine output, and central venous pressure. Arterial blood gases should be routinely measured and a toxicology screen drawn to rule out other causes of coma.

Hepatic encephalopathy. Serial neurologic examinations are necessary to provide a clinical picture of the degree of encephalopathy, which reflects the severity of liver failure. Table 15-7 describes the stages in the development of hepatic coma. Other conditions that can worsen the encephalopathy include excessive protein load, respiratory alkalosis, hyponatremia, hypoglycemia, infection, upper intestinal bleeding, and administration of medications that alter the level of consciousness.[34]

Cerebral edema associated with hepatic encephalopathy is the cause of death in as many as 40% of the patients with hepatic failure.[34] The etiology is poorly understood, but both edema and encephalopathy appear to be related, since patients who develop deeper levels of encephalopathy proceed to cerebral edema if the process is not stopped. Cerebral edema associated with hepatic encephalopathy has the same clinical picture as cerebral edema associated with any condition and is treated the same way.

Ammonia intoxication has long been suspected as one of the major problems in hepatic encephalopathy. Serial measurement of serum ammonia levels provides a guide to the effectiveness of therapy for hyperammonemia. The degree of elevation of the ammonia level does not correlate well with the grade of encephalopathy, but changes in the ammonia level will reflect changes in the encephalopathic picture.[35]

The child with liver failure will require a decrease in dietary protein to 0.5 to 1.0 g/kg/day to attempt to keep ammonia levels within normal lim-

Table 15-7 Stages in Development of Hepatic Failure

Stage	Mental stage	Tremor	EEG findings
I (prodrome)	Euphoria, mild confusion, slurred speech, and disorder in sleep	Slight	Normal
II	Drowsiness	Present, easily elicited	Abnormal, generalized slowing
III	Asleep or stuporous most of the time; arousable confusion is pronounced	Usually present with cooperation	Slowing delta wave
IV	Not arousable, except sometimes in pain	Usually absent	Slowing delta wave

From Halpin TJ. Acute hepatic failure. In: Blumer JL, ed. A practical guide to pediatric intensive care. 3rd ed. St Louis: Mosby–Year Book, 1990:136.

its.[36] Another therapy is to decrease intestinal bacteria ammonia production and absorption. This is accomplished by administering 1 mL/kg/dose of lactulose 3 to 6 times/day to maintain one to two soft stools per day and administering 125 to 500 mg of neomycin 4 times/day through a nasogastric tube. Gastrointestinal bleeding should be treated immediately, since blood in the gastrointestinal tract will cause an increased serum ammonia.

Liver function studies. Serum transaminase levels (ALT and AST) will increase with liver dysfunction 10 to 100 times normal, although the degree of increase does not reflect the severity of the disease. Following these enzyme levels does provide important information about the progression of the liver failure. Sustained elevations may reflect a continued ability of the liver to synthesize these enzymes, but a sudden decrease may indicate the child's imminent death.[34]

Although the serum enzymes reflect the integrity of the hepatic cell, hepatic function is better assessed by monitoring bilirubin, prealbumin, and coagulation. Bilirubin levels will increase to more than 20 mg/dL, and prealbumin levels will decrease to 0 mg/dL and may not respond to nutritional support. Coagulation studies such as prothrombin and partial thromboplastin times will be increased and fibrinogen levels will be decreased. Serial monitoring of these values will guide therapy for the bleeding patient. Profound bleeding should be treated with packed red blood cell, platelet, and fresh frozen plasma replacement, and vitamin K at 1 to 5 mg/dose should be administered every day. Routine correction of hepatic coagulopathy is not recommended.[36]

Hypoglycemia. Profound hypoglycemia as a result of the decrease in gluconeogenesis is common, and early identification and treatment is essential, especially in the critically ill child whose glucose stores are already low. Serum glucose should be maintained between 100 and 300 mg/dL. Alterations in serum sodium and potassium levels also occur frequently. Large doses of potassium may be necessary to maintain a normal serum potassium, and sodium must be administered to maintain the serum sodium at 130 mg/dL.

Gastrointestinal bleeding. Gastrointestinal bleeding is a complication experienced by 70% of patients with hepatic failure and the cause of death in 30% of these patients.[34] Bleeding is caused by stress ulcers and portal hypertension, both of which are exacerbated by the coagulopathies associated with hepatic failure.

The occurrence of stress gastritis can be reduced by closely monitoring the gastric pH and maintaining it at 4.5 or greater. H_2 receptor antagonists, antacids, and gentle nasogastric suction can be used to maintain the gastric pH. Cimetidine at 20 to 40 mg/kg/day in divided doses every 4 hours or ranitidine at 0.1 to 0.8 mg/kg/dose every 6 to 8 hours are the H_2 receptor antagonists of choice.

If gastrointestinal bleeding does occur, standard therapy is indicated. This includes nasogastric lavage and administering blood and fresh frozen plasma.

Nutritional support is paramount for the child in hepatic failure. Parenteral nutrition should be started as soon as possible, providing 50 to 60 kcal/kg/day and protein at 0.5 to 1.0 g/kg/day. The addition of branched-chain amino acids to hypertonic glucose may help improve the nutritional status of the child. Aromatic amino acid–containing solutions should be avoided. Fat emulsions should be restricted to the provision of essential fatty acids only.

Complications. The child with hepatic failure is prone to infections. The three most common infections are bacteremias, urinary tract infections, and aspiration pneumonias. The use of prophylactic antibiotics is not recommended, but worsening of encephalopathy, sudden development of hepatorenal syndrome, and new onset of fever or leukocytosis may indicate infection.[34] Measures to prevent infection such as meticulous hand washing and aseptic care of all lines and wounds should be employed. Appropriate antibiotic therapy should be initiated immediately when signs of infection are noted.

Cardiovascular, respiratory, and renal failure can all occur in the child with hepatic failure. Cardiovascular and respiratory failure will be treated the same as for any child with these conditions. Renal failure related to hepatic failure may respond to the use of mannitol (0.25 g/kg) and furosemide (0.5 mg/kg).

ALTERATION IN NUTRITION: LESS THAN BODY REQUIREMENTS
Age-related factors

Provision of adequate substrate for energy metabolism is critical to supporting the child with MSOF. Critically ill children are at risk for developing malnutrition because of increased energy requirements and increased protein catabolism associated with MSOF. In addition, age-related factors make nutritional depletion more likely when adequate nutritional support is not provided. Children have larger obligate energy needs and lower macronutrient stores than adults.[37] The combination of these two factors makes the child less likely to withstand nutritional depletion when nutritional support is not provided.[38]

Several studies have demonstrated that malnutrition does exist in critically ill children. Malnutrition and fat and protein depletions are common, especially in children under 2 years of age.[38] Also, acute malnutrition in critically ill children is associated with increased physiologic instability and increased requirements for care as evidenced by higher Physiologic stability index (PSI) and Therapeutic intervention scoring system (TISS) scores.[39]

Assessment

Nutritional needs for the child with MSOF must be addressed before complications and potentially irreversible changes related to malnutrition take place. The nurse plays an important role as the child's advocate for nutritional support. Performing the initial nutritional assessment by obtaining the child's height, weight, and head circumference, if appropriate, and obtaining a diet history as part of the data base will help identify the patient at risk for nutrition-related complications.

By obtaining daily weights the nurse can monitor weight loss in the critically ill child. An unexplained weight loss of greater than 5% of the child's admission weight places the child nutritionally at risk. A weight loss of greater than 10% is associated with increased morbidity, and weight loss of greater than 30% is associated with increased mortality.[37]

The child's assessment should include noting signs of possible nutritional deficiencies such as muscle wasting or weakness, dermatitis, tetany, growth retardation, central nervous system depression, and bleeding tendencies. Mortality is increased from 3% to 33% in children with malnutrition severe enough to depress cell-mediated immunity.[37] Other clinical parameters to note are hair, eyes, mouth, lips, tongue, skin, and extremities. Dryness, pallor, thinness, and other abnormalities

are often signs of malnutrition. An in-depth nutritional assessment will include anthropometric measurements and laboratory studies such as serum albumin, serum transferrin, serum protein, and total lymphocyte count.

Therapeutic management

Nursing interventions start with advocating early nutritional support. In critically ill patients, a short ebb phase is followed by a long flow phase in which the stress hormone response is followed by a long course of enhanced metabolic activity.[40] Critically ill children need nutritional support to maintain lean body mass and host defense, promote growth and development, and gain time for reversal of organ failure and eradication of sepsis. Nutritional support should be provided based on the child's nutrient needs as listed in Table 15-8.

Enteral feedings are preferable because they are physiologically normal and more efficient. There are a variety of enteral formulas available, including specialized pediatric formulas for infants less than 12 months of age and for children between the ages of 1 and 5 years. Older children usually can receive enteral formulas developed for adults. Potential complications related to enteral feedings are intolerance as evidenced by vomiting, diarrhea, abdominal distention and/or gastric retention, aspiration, infection, and fluid and electrolyte imbalances.

If the child is unable to tolerate enteral feedings, then total parenteral nutrition must be initiated.

Table 15-8 Estimated Daily Nutrient Needs for Children

Age (yr)	Calories (kcal/kg)	Protein (g/kg)
0 to 0.5	115	2.2
0.5 to 1	105	2.0
1 to 3	100	1.8
4 to 6	85	1.5
7 to 10	85	1.2
Male		
11 to 14	60	1.0
15 to 18	42	0.85
Female		
11 to 14	48	1.0
15 to 18	38	0.85

Modified from Walker W, Hendricks K: Manual of pediatric nutrition. Philadelphia, WB Saunders, 1985:53.

Table 15-9 Parenteral Nutrient Doses in Critically Ill Children

Nutrient	Initial dose	Approximate maintenance dose
Protein	0.5 to 1.5 g/kg/day*	3 to 4 g/kg/day†
Dextrose	5 to 7 mg/kg/min	To obtain calorie/nitrogen ratio of 150 to 200:1 in low stress and 80 to 125:1 in high stress 70 to 90 kcal/kg/day‡
Lipid	1 g/kg/day	2 to 4 g/kg/day§

From Steinhorn DM. Nutritional strategies in organ system failure. In: Blumer JL, ed. A practical guide to pediatric intensive care. 3rd ed. St Louis, Mosby–Year Book, 1990:617.
*Decrease dose for renal or hepatic insufficiency.
†Decrease dose for renal or hepatic function; desired end point is stable or increasing transferrin.
‡Caloric intake may be increased with calorimetric evidence of increased resting energy expenditure.
§Follow plasma triglycerides 4 hours after discontinuing total parenteral nutrition for evidence of clearance.

Table 15-9 lists appropriate doses for parenteral nutrients in the critically ill child. As noted in the table, special considerations must be taken for the child in renal or hepatic failure.

Complications related to total parenteral nutrition are infection, liver dysfunction, hyperlipidemia, metabolic problems such as hyperglycemia and electrolyte imbalances, and technical problems such as air emboli, pneumothorax, and catheter occlusion or breakage. Close monitoring and meticulous nursing care are essential to prevent these complications.

As the critically ill child begins to tolerate enteral feedings again, total parenteral nutrition should be slowly discontinued. The weaning process should occur over 1 to 3 days with close monitoring of serum glucose to prevent hypoglycemia.

HIGH RISK FOR INFECTION
Age-related factors

MSOF, medical and nursing interventions, nutritional status, and stress all lead to an increased risk of infection for the critically ill child. Pediatric anatomic and physiologic differences in the immune system also place the child at increased risk for infection. The infant has fewer neutrophils and is less able than the older child to replace white blood cells in the face of an overwhelming infection. Complement levels are low in the infant and do not come within normal adult range until 3 to 6 months of age, which affects the infant's chemotactic and opsonic activity. The infant is able to synthesize small amounts of immunoglobin, but most is received through placental transfer.[41] The lowest immunoglobin concentration occurs at approximately 4 to 5 months of age, during which time the infant is most susceptible to infections caused by viruses, *Candida* organisms, and certain bacteria. The infant and young child do have all the components to mount an immune response, but since the exposure to many antigens has not occurred, a vigorous response to certain bacteria, viruses, and fungi does not occur.[41]

Immunosuppression

Many of the conditions that trigger MSOF are known to cause immunosuppression in children. Injury as the result of thermal, mechanical, or surgical trauma affects humoral immunity more in children than it does in adults.[42] Hemorrhagic shock has been demonstrated to cause profound depression in several immune functions in children. Depressed neutrophil motility exists at low temperatures, and the movement of immune cells and proteins in the heart-lung machine has been shown to cause cell destruction, complement activation, and other changes that lead to depressed immunity.[42] When a child sustains a severe insult such as surgery, hypoxia, sepsis, hemorrhage, or trauma, immune cells are mobilized and activated as a result of this stress, and they release inflammatory mediators. Secondary injury results from overactivation of these mediators, and the inflammatory immune response becomes exaggerated and uncontrolled.[42] An unregulated inflammatory/immune response may be involved in a number of complications, including MSOF.

Since environmental, anatomic, and physiologic factors place the child at risk for infection, nursing assessment for signs of infection is critical. Because of the immaturity and alterations in the infant's immune system, the child may experience an overwhelming infection without the normal systemic signs such as fever and an increased white blood cell count. The nurse should observe for other signs of infection, such as temperature instability, hyperglycemia, hemodynamic instability, and changes in the level of consciousness.

Therapeutic management

Nursing interventions must begin with good hand washing before all procedures and aseptic care of all lines and wounds. Wounds and invasive line sites should be inspected daily, and surveillance cultures should be obtained. Skin and mucous membranes should be kept as intact as possible. Frequent skin and mouth care, turning every 2 hours, and keeping the skin clean will help protect the first-line defense against infection. Antibiotics should be administered as appropriate, and the child's response should be closely observed and documented.

IMPAIRED SKIN INTEGRITY
Age-related factors

The integumentary system is not mature at birth; therefore, it is not a very effective barrier against physical elements or microorganisms. The skin is thinner at birth and more permeable because of smaller amounts of stratum corneum. The skin pH is more alkaline at birth, which increases susceptibility to infection, since a more acidic skin pH discourages microorganisms.[43] The infant possesses less subcutaneous fat than the older child, so there is increased sensitivity to environmental changes.

Assessment

Nursing assessment of the skin should be conducted with adequate lighting so all areas can be viewed thoroughly. Mucous membranes, scalp, hair, and nails should be included in skin assessment. Areas of dryness should be noted since dry, cracked skin provides a portal of entry for bacteria. Areas where invasive lines are inserted and areas of breakdown must be observed closely for signs of infection. In infants and young children, the diaper should be removed and the perineal and buttock area observed for diaper rash, which can quickly lead to a severe skin breakdown.

Therapeutic management

Skin care must be provided at least every 8 hours and more often, if appropriate, to keep the skin clean and moist. Providing air flotation or EGGCRATE mattresses and turning the child every 2 hours will help prevent skin breakdown. Mouth care should include lubricating the mouth and cleaning the teeth every shift. Eye care in the unconscious child should be provided by applying an ophthalmic ointment at least every 2 hours.

Infants and young children have larger body surface areas in proportion to their body weight and are more sensitive to environmental changes. These factors place them at risk for hypothermia, which can result in physiologic instability. Hypothermia will shift the oxyhemoglobin curve to the left, prevent the release of oxygen to the tissue, and increase oxygen consumption and glucose use in order to maintain the body's core temperature. The child's temperature must be closely monitored and measures taken to maintain a normal body temperature. Radiant warmers and hyperthermia blankets are useful for warming a child. Cooling blankets can be used for those children who are febrile and not responding to antipyretic medications. Shivering should be avoided because it increases body heat production and oxygen consumption.

ALTERATION IN COMFORT: PAIN
Age-related factors

Pain management is a very important part of every nurse's role in the pediatric intensive care unit (PICU). Pain is a complex, subjective, and elusive phenomenon.[44] The International Association for the Study of Pain describes it as "an unpleasant sensory and emotional experience with actual or potential tissue damage, as described in terms of such damage."[45] McCaffery[46] believes that pain exists if the child says it does, even if a physical reason cannot be found. Most definitions depend on the child's ability to verbalize pain, but this is frequently not the case when dealing with infants, young children, and critically ill patients.

Many beliefs that exist about children and pain have interfered with adequate pain management. One of these beliefs is that infants and children do not feel or remember pain and therefore are unable to communicate about their pain. Evidence exists to refute this statement, and numerous studies have documented the infant's physiologic and behavioral response to painful stimuli.[47-49] These studies show that infants respond to stress with increased heart rates, blood pressures, and intracranial pressures.

They also demonstrate simple motor responses, changes in facial expressions, and intense crying. The idea that complete nerve myelinization is necessary to experience pain is no longer supported by many clinicians. Current thinking is that the process of myelinization begins in utero, and the cortical and subcortical centers are well developed late in gestation.[50] This supports the idea that the newborn is capable of experiencing pain. There is much evidence to support the idea that infants and children do remember pain. Savedra et al[51] report that children remember pain from many years earlier. Several studies have documented that children are able to accurately describe the location and nature of their pain, often using graphic words.[52,53]

Perception of pain in older children appears to be related to their level of cognitive development.[44] In theory the preoperational child (age 2½ to 6 years) is unable to understand cause and effect relationships and will be more afraid and distressed by medical procedures than older children. The operational child (7 to 10 years), who is able to think more logically and realistically, should understand the need for procedures and exhibit less anxiety. As children get older (12 to 17 years), they can think more abstractly and give meaning to pain. This has been shown to increase their pain sensitivity.[54] Based on these perceptual differences, it is critical that the nurse consider the child's development level when assessing and managing pain (Fig. 15-1).

Assessment

Assessment of pain usually involves collecting physiologic and behavioral data. The process should be ongoing and must precede and follow all interventions to relieve or eliminate pain.[55] Physiologic responses indicate activation of the sympathetic nervous system, and commonly include increased heart rate, blood pressure, respi-

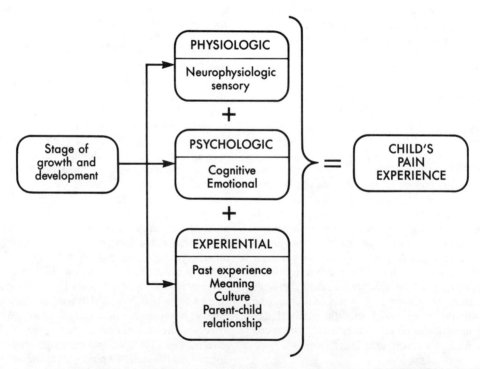

Fig. 15-1 Effect of stage of growth and development on the child's pain experience. (From Stevens B, Hunsberger M, Browne G. Pain in children: Theoretical, research, and practice dilemmas. J Pediatr Nurs 1987, 2:159.)

ratory rate, diaphoresis, hyperventilation, pupil dilatation, and nausea and vomiting. Nurses cannot infer or rule out pain strictly based on these parameters. Behavioral responses to pain must also be considered if a thorough assessment is desired. These responses might include crying, moaning, screaming, and facial and body expressions such as grimacing and rigidity. Behavioral observation tools have been developed that assist nurses in assessing pain. Instruments such as the Pediatric Pain Inventory,[52] Observational Scale of Behavioral Distress,[53] and CHEOPS[56] are designed for use with specific age groups to measure pain perceptions and behaviors. Other assessment tools such as the Body Outline,[57] Pain Ladder,[58] Heat Thermometer,[59] Stewart Color Scale,[60] and the McGill Pain Questionnaire[61] are age specific and are used to describe the location, intensity, and quality of pain. Although these tools can be very valuable, their use is often impractical in the critical care environment, and they do not replace the skilled observations of the ICU nurse.

Therapeutic management

Interventions for pain are generally classified as nonpharmacologic and pharmacologic. Pharmacologic interventions must never be withheld if that is the most appropriate means to alleviate a child's pain. When administering pain medication to children, it is essential to monitor vital functions such as airway patency, ventilatory adequacy, heart rate and rhythm, and blood pressure. Pain relief must be achieved without profound respiratory or central nervous system (CNS) depression. Opiates are the most commonly used sedation in the critical care setting, and intravenous administration is the preferred route. Morphine sulfate (0.1 to 0.2 mg/kg) has predictable analgesic and euphoric properties with an onset within 1 minute of administration.[62] It does cause histamine release and the potential for hypotension, tachycardia, and respiratory depression. Fentanyl (1 to 2 μg/kg) is a very potent, synthetically derived narcotic. Onset is very rapid, duration is short, and side effects include respiratory and CNS depression, severe nausea and vomiting, and muscle rigidity. Meperidine (1 to 2 mg/kg) is also widely used to manage pain in children. The onset and duration are similar to morphine sulfate, and the potential for respiratory and CNS depression also exists. Tremors, muscle

twitches, and seizures sometimes occur. Diazepam (0.2 to 0.5 mg/kg) is frequently used in children to achieve sedation and amnesia. Side effects include apnea, respiratory depression, and hypotension. Other drugs, such as chloral hydrate, thiopental, and diphenhydramine, can also play important roles in pediatric pain management. Combinations of drugs can be used very successfully and can reduce undesirable side effects. The response to combinations, however, may be less predictable than the response to single agents. Continuous drug infusions are also very effective and provide a more constant level of sedation instead of the uneven control provided by bolus doses.

Nurses and parents can often use nonpharmacologic techniques such as relaxation, distraction, guided imagery, and cutaneous stimulation in the critical care setting.[55] Relaxation is used to reduce the muscle tension that accompanies pain and may include simple techniques such as cuddling, holding, and rocking. Distractions are very effective with children and may include games, pop-up books, toys, songs, or stories. Guided imagery works well with children, because they can actively imagine. This technique requires that the child focus on a pleasant experience or place and then talk about the experience. Cutaneous stimulation measures are often used with children and include massage, pressure, and the use of heat and cold. Parents should be encouraged to participate in these interventions and should be taught how to perform them. Often a combination of nonpharmacologic and pharmacologic interventions will be the most effective approach to pain management in the child.

Minimizing the effects of the critical care environment by eliminating excess light, noise, and interruptions can also help alleviate pain. No matter what intervention is used, an ongoing assessment of the child's response is vital in order to accurately assess the effectiveness of pain management.

FEAR AND ANXIETY/ALTERATION IN GROWTH AND DEVELOPMENT

A critical care unit can be a horrifying experience for the child. The child with MSOF requires intensive technology and numerous, painful procedures that are completely foreign. The child's ability to understand and develop means to cope with the experience is highly dependent on the developmental level, and nursing interventions to help the child cope must address these developmental differences.

Infants

Infants (birth to 12 months) are at a stage where, according to Erikson, they are developing a sense of trust vs. mistrust. They are not able to care for themselves and are totally dependent on those around them to meet their needs. Sight and sound provide stimulation, and play is important in their development. Stressors for this age group include separation from parents or primary caregivers, pain and intrusion, and immobilization. Immobilization is stressful because the infant uses motor activity as a means of exploration as well as a coping mechanism.

Nursing interventions for the infant are focused upon providing a sense of trust. Infants are so acutely aware of their environment that calm, quiet, comforting surroundings are very important. Infants should be spoken to quietly, and stroking and cuddling can be used to soothe. Nurses should involve the parents or primary caretaker as much as possible in the child's care. Caretakers should be consistent to provide a sense of security. Sudden movements should be avoided, since these will startle the infant, and hands should always be warm before touching the infant. Exploration of the environment should be allowed, and mobiles should be at the bedside for the infant to look at as well as toys for the infant to hold. Mirrors can provide hours of enjoyment since babies like to look at themselves.

Toddlers

Toddlers (1 to 3 years) are working at their developmental task of developing autonomy vs. shame and doubt. They are assertive in expressing their will, though they are still very dependent upon their parents. They see the world from their view only. They are developing language skills quickly, though their receptive language skills are more advanced than their expressive skills. Their major stressors are separation from their parents or primary caretakers, pain and intrusion, and disruption of their rituals.[63] Ritualistic behavior provides a sense of self-control for toddlers as they develop new physical skills and abilities. Toddlers require active play as a means of furthering their social and motor development.

Toddlers need interventions that allow them to be dependent but maintain their autonomy. Parents should be permitted to stay with their child and encouraged to play with their child. Parents should also be encouraged to bring objects from home that will provide comfort. As the critically ill toddler becomes more stable, he or she should be allowed to play with and explore appropriate equipment such as stethoscopes, tongue blades, and syringe barrels and continue rituals. The child should be encouraged to talk about or draw pictures of the experience, if able, to have an outlet for frustration. When possible, the child should also be given choices. Explain to parents that the toddler often regresses as a means of coping when faced with stressful circumstances and that lost skills will be regained quickly.

Preschoolers

The preschooler (3 to 5 years) is developing a sense of initiative vs. guilt. The child is acquiring more language skills, and there is a strong sense of self. The imagination is vivid and magical thinking is frequent. Major stressors for this age group are being alone, loss of self-control, pain and intrusion, and fear of mutilation.[63]

Effective nursing interventions for the preschooler include good explanations of equipment and procedures. Procedures should be explained immediately before they take place, and the nurse can help the child cooperate by explaining what is expected of him or her. Realistic limits on behavior should be set, and the child needs to be reassured that the procedure is necessary and is not punishment. The child should be encouraged to ask questions and discuss feelings, using the ability to fantasize constructively. When possible, the child should participate in care. Like the toddler, the preschooler is comforted by favorite items from home.

School-age children

The school-age child (6 to 12 years) is developing a sense of industry vs. inferiority. The child has well-developed language skills and is capable of verbalizing concerns and responding to reason and compromise. The child has a strong need to accomplish and will feel inferior if unable to achieve. The school-age child has an incomplete understanding of death. Major stressors for the school-age child include separation from parents and peer group, loss of self-control, loss of privacy, fear of the unknown, pain and intrusion, fear of disfigurement, and fear of death.[63]

The school-age child requires concrete answers to questions and can usually understand pathophysiology and treatment. Procedures should be explained well beforehand, and, if possible, the child should be offered choices. The child should be encouraged to discuss his or her understanding of the event, which can help the child retain a sense of worth. Parents should be encouraged to visit, though the child may not want them present during procedures. Communication from siblings and schoolmates should also be suggested. At all times, the child's sense of modesty should be respected.

Adolescents

The adolescent (12 to 19 years) is seeking identity vs. role confusion. Adolescence is characterized by rapid growth and emotional lability related to hormone changes. The adolescent cognitive level is comparable to an adult, yet adolescents have not had the adult life experiences that bring their thinking to a more mature level. They are usually able to and want to make their own decisions. Their peer group is very significant, since they are attempting to establish their own sense of belonging and self-esteem. Major stressors for adolescents include separation from their peers, loss of group status and acceptance, dependency, loss of self-control, and permanent disability and death.[63]

The autonomy of the adolescent needs to be respected at all times. Choices and control should be permitted as much as possible. Adolescents should be encouraged to maintain contact with their peers and family, although parents may need assistance in understanding their child's wish to be independent of them. Adolescents should be prepared for procedures as far in advance as possible to allow for questions and corrections of any misconceptions. Nurses should help the adolescent verbalize fears. Privacy must be maintained, and flexibility with hospital routines should be provided when possible.

ALTERATION IN FAMILY PROCESSES/ PARENTAL ROLE CONFLICT

Having a child with MSOF in the critical care unit is an extremely stressful experience for the family. The child is critically ill with a dramatically changed appearance, and the family must cope with this frightening situation in a world of strangers. Nurses play a critical role in helping family members cope with this crisis. If the parents or primary caretakers are unable to cope with the hospitalization, then their ability to support and comfort their child will be disrupted.[64]

Parental needs

Miles and Carter[65] assessed parental needs and identified stressors in the pediatric critical care unit. Stressors identified were the environment, the child's appearance, procedures, communication with staff, staff behavior, and changes in the parental role. Eberly et al[66] studied parents of children in the pediatric ICU and found that the areas of highest stress were parental role, communication, and response to their child's behavior and appearance. Philichi[64] identified other parental needs in the pediatric critical care unit including the need to be with the child, to receive accurate and truthful information, to have a place to sleep and rest near the unit, to participate in the child's care, and to feel assured that the child's care and treatment are appropriate.

Therapeutic management

Based on these and many other research findings, there are many nursing interventions that can help the parents of a child in MSOF in the critical care unit. Parents must be allowed to visit and stay with their child on a continuous, 24-hour-a-day basis. Questions should be answered honestly and accurately. The child's primary nurse should be with the parents when the physician talks to them to explain any issues that they may not understand. Nurses should guide parents to where they can sleep, bathe, and eat, and they should facilitate these activities as much as possible. Nurses can assist parents in touching and talking to their critically ill child. Encouragement to bathe and massage their child, read a story, and bring familiar items from home helps the parents feel that they are still maintaining their parental role. Sibling visitation should be an option especially if the parents request it. This requires careful preparation of the sibling by both the nurse and the parents.

A study conducted by Curley[67] validates the importance of nursing interventions in reducing parental stress. Parents were assigned randomly to two groups. One was a control group that received routine nursing contact. The treatment group received nursing intervention designed to allow the parents to participate in their child's care to the extent that the parents wished and that the child's condition permitted. The parents in the intervention group reported significantly lower stress scores than the control group for four of the seven dimensions that have been reported as stressful for parents. An important finding in this study was that the nursing intervention was effective in reducing stress and that time, alone, did not account for stress reduction.

Parental grief

Mortality rates are high for children with MSOF, so nurses will often be supporting parents whose child has died. At this time, care shifts entirely to the family, and support from the nursing staff must continue. It is important to assure parents that all possible measures were taken to save their child and that their child did not suffer. Further conversation can be guided by the parent's need for information. The presence of the nurse while the parents begin to experience the tremendous loss is helpful. Parents will often not remember the exact words that were said, but they will remember that someone cared enough to be with them during their grief. Parents should be allowed to spend as much time as they need to say goodbye to their child, and expressions of grief such as crying or screaming should not be discouraged.

It is helpful to the parents if the nurse who cared for the child makes contact with them shortly after the child's death. Usually the child with MSOF was a patient in the critical care unit for a number of days or weeks, and the primary nurse has developed a relationship with the parents. Talking to the nurse gives the parents the opportunity to ask questions and express feelings that may have developed since the child's death. Many parents need continued reassurance and support as they experience the various stages of grief, and the nurse can play a key role in providing that support. Also, the nurse can recommend grief support groups for the parents if appropriate.

CONCLUSION

MSOF is the result of a variety of conditions in the critically ill child. In the child with MSOF, the normal equilibrium between organ systems and protective responses does not exist. Disruption of organ function occurs, and the body attempts to compensate and regain equilibrium. Compensation and intervention will benefit certain organs but harm others, and when compensation and regulatory mechanisms fail, organ dysfunction occurs.

The pathophysiology of MSOF in the child is not tremendously different from the pathophysiology in adults. Anatomic and physiologic differences in each child, however, will affect his or her response to organ dysfunction and to treatment. No single therapy is based on treating MSOF as a primary entity; therefore nursing and medical interventions focus on maximizing oxygen delivery, providing nutritional support, and supporting individual organ systems. The interventions must be based on reversing the primary entity, minimizing infection and inflammation, and preventing cellular damage.[4]

Although overall mortality rates are high, children have a better chance for survival than do adults. Expert nursing management is essential to maximize the potential for a positive outcome. More research in the area of MSOF in children is necessary, especially in the area of nurisng interventions and their effect on patient outcomes.

REFERENCES

1. Wilkinson JD et al. Outcomes of pediatric patients with organ system failure. Crit Care Med 1986;14:271-274.
2. Wilkinson JD et al. Mortality associated with multiple organ system failure and sepsis in pediatric intensive care. J Pediatr 1987;111:324-328.
3. Faist E et al. Multiple organ failure in polytrauma patients. J Trauma 1983;23:775-787.
4. Toro-Figuera L. Multiple organ system failure. In: Levin DL, Morriss FC, eds. Essentials of pediatric intensive care. St Louis: Quality Medical Publishing, Inc., 1990:186-193.
5. Lyrene RK, Truog WE. Adult respiratory distress syndrome in a pediatric intensive care unit: Predisposing conditions, clinical course, and outcomes. Pediatrics 1981;67:790-795.
6. Witte M. Acute respiratory failure. In: Blumer J, ed. A practical guide to pediatric intensive care. 3rd ed. St Louis: Mosby–Year Book, 1990:95-103.
7. Eigen H. Adult respiratory distress syndrome. In: Blumer J, ed. A practical guide to pediatric intensive care. 3rd ed. St Louis: Mosby–Year Book, 1990:348-352.
8. Boegner E. Modes of ventilatory support and weaning parameters in children. Clin Issues Crit Care Nurs 1990;1:378-386.
9. Wetzel R. Dysrhythmias and their management. In: Rogers M, ed. Textbook of pediatric intensive care. Baltimore: Williams & Wilkins, 1987:459-482.
10. Blumer J. Shock. In: Blumer J, ed. A practical guide to pediatric intensive care. 3rd ed. St Louis: Mosby–Year Book, 1990:71-81.

11. Crone R. Acute circulatory failure in children. Pediatr Clin North Am 1980;27:527-538.

12. Rimar J. Recognizing shock syndromes in infants and children. MCN 1988;13:32-37.

13. Zimmerman JJ, Dietrich KA. Current perspectives on septic shock. Pediatr Clin North Am 1987;34:131-163.

14. Schleien CL, Zahka KG, Rogers MC. Principles of postoperative management in the pediatric intensive care unit. In: Rogers MC, ed. Textbook of pediatric intensive care. Baltimore: Williams & Wilkins, 1987:411-458.

15. Rekate H. Increased intracranial pressure. In: Blumer J, ed. A practical guide to pediatric intensive care. 3rd ed. St Louis: Mosby–Year Book, 1990:239-246.

16. Aumick JE. Head trauma guidelines for care. RN 1991; 54(4):27-31.

17. Dean JM et al. Theories of brain resuscitation. In: Rogers MC, ed. Textbook of pediatric intensive care. Baltimore: Williams & Wilkins, 1987:557-596.

18. Hahn YS et al. Factors influencing posttraumatic seizures in children. Neurosurgery 1988;22:864.

19. Moloney-Harmon PA. Pediatric issues in multisystem trauma. Crit Care Nurs Clin North Am 1989;1:85-94.

20. Luchka S. Working with ICP monitors. RN 1991; 54(4):34-37.

21. Shapiro K, Giller CA. Increased intracranial pressure. In: Levin DL, Morriss FC, eds. Essentials of pediatric intensive care. St Louis: Quality Medical Publishing Inc., 1990:49-53.

22. Andrus C. Intracranial pressure: Dynamics and nursing management. J Neurosci Nurs 1991;23:85-91.

23. Mitchell P, Mauss N. Relationships of patient/nurse activity to intracranial pressure variations: A pilot study. Nurse Res 1978;27:4-10.

24. Muwaswes M. Increased intracranial pressure and its systematic effects. J Neurosurg Nurs 1985;17:238-243.

25. Walleck Ca. 1983 National Teaching Institute, unpublished data.

26. Gordon JB et al. Hematologic disorders in the pediatric intensive care unit. In: Rogers MC, ed. Textbook of pediatric intensive care. Baltimore: Williams & Wilkins, 1987:1181-1222.

27. Kedar A, Gross S. Disseminated intravascular coagulation. In: Blumer J, ed. A practical guide to pediatric intensive care. 3rd ed. St Louis: Mosby–Year Book, 1990:517-519.

28. Fry DE et al. Multiple system organ failure. Arch Surg 1980;115:136-140.

29. Bell RC et al. Multiple organ system failure and infection in adult respiratory distress syndrome. Ann Intern Med 1983;99:293-298.

30. Ferraris VA. Exploratory laparotomy for potential abdominal sepsis in patients with multiple organ failure. Arch Surg 1983;118:1130-1133.

31. Pine RW et al. Determinants of organ malfunction or death in patients with intraabdominal sepsis. Arch Surg 1983; 118:242-249.

32. Stork J. Acute renal failure. In: Blumer J, ed. A practical guide to pediatric intensive care. 3rd ed. St Louis: Mosby–Year Book, 1990:429-437.

33. Maxwell LG, Fivush BA, McLean RH. Renal failure. In: Rogers MC, ed. Textbook of pediatric intensive care. Baltimore: Williams & Wilkins, 1987:1001-1056.

34. Rogers EL, Perman JA. Gastrointestinal and hepatic failure. In: Rogers MC, ed. Textbook of pediatric intensive care. Baltimore: Williams & Wilkins, 1987:979-998.

35. Halpin TJ. Acute hepatic failure. In: Blumer J, ed. A practical guide to pediatric intensive care. 3rd ed. St Louis: Mosby–Year Book, 1990:135-139.

36. Belknap WM. Acute hepatic failure. In: Levin DL, Morriss FC, eds. Essentials of pediatric intensive care. St Louis: Quality Medical Publishing, Inc., 1990:137-143.

37. Pollack M. Nutritional failure and support in pediatric intensive care. In: Shoemaker WC, Ayres S, Grenvik A, Holbrook PR, Thompson WL, eds. Textbook of critical care. Philadelphia: WB Saunders, 1989:1125-1128.

38. Pollack M et al. Malnutrition in critically ill infants and children. JPEN 1982;6:20-24.

39. Pollack M, Ruttimann U, Wiley J. Nutritional depletions in critically ill children: Associations with physiologic instability and increased quantity of care. JPEN 1985;9:309-313.

40. Benotti P, Blackburn G. Protein and caloric or macronutrient metabolic management of the critically ill patient. Crit Care Med 1979;7:520-523.

41. Rosenthal CH. Immunosuppression in pediatric critical care patients. Crit Care Nurs Clin North Am 1989;1:775-784.

42. Hauser GJ, Holbrook PR. Immune dysfunction in the critically ill infant and child. Crit Care Clin 1988;4:711-729.

43. Foster RL. Nursing strategies: Altered skin integrity. In: Foster RL, Hunsberger M, Anderson J, eds. Family centered nursing care of children. Philadelphia: WB Saunders, 1989:1612-1637.

44. Stevens B, Hunsberger M, Browne G. Pain in children: Theoretical, research, and practice dilemmas. J Pediatr Nurs 1987;2:154-164.

45. Merskey H and the International Association for the Study of Pain Subcommittee on Taxonomy. Pain terms: A list with definitions and notes on usage. Pain 1979;6:249-252.

46. McCaffery M. Nursing management of the patient with pain. Philadelphia: JB Lippincott, 1979:10-21.

47. Owens ME, Todt EH. Pain in infancy: Neonatal reaction to heel lance. Pain 1984;20:77-86.

48. Johnston CC, Strada ME. Acute pain response in infants: A multidimensional description. Pain 1986;24:373-382.

49. Anand KJ, Aynsley-Green A. Measuring the severity of surgical stress in newborn infants. J Pediatr Surg 1988;23:297-305.

50. Gilles FJ, Shankle W, Dooling EC. Myelinated tracts: Growth patterns. In: Gilles FJ, Leviton A, Dooling EC, eds. The developing human brain growth and epidemiologic neuropathy. Boston: John Wright, 1983:117-183.

51. Savedra M et al. Description of the pain experience: A study of school-age children. Issues Compr Pediatr Nurs 1981;5:373-380.

52. Lollar DJ, Smits SJ, Patterson DL. Assessment of pediatric pain: An empirical perspective. J Pediatr Psychol 1982;7:267-277.

53. Jay SM et al. Behavioral management of children's distress during painful medical procedures. Behav Res Ther 1985;5:513-520.

54. Ross DM, Ross SA. Childhood pain: The school-aged child's viewpoint. Pain 1983;20:179-191.

55. Savedra M, Eland J, Tesler M. Pain management. In: Craft MJ, Denehy JA, eds. Nursing interventions for infants and children. Philadelphia: WB Saunders, 1990:304-325.

56. McGrath P et al. CHEOPS: A behavioral scale for rating postoperative pain in children. Adv Pain Res Ther 1985;9:387-402.

57. Margolis RB, Tait RC, Krause SJ. A rating system for use with patients with pain drawings. Pain 1986;24:57-65.

58. Jeans ME, Johnston CC. Pain in children: Assessment and management. In: Lipton S, Miles J, eds. Persistent pain: Modern methods of treatment. Vol 5. London: Grune & Stratton, Inc, 1985:111-127.

59. Molsberry D. Young children's subjective qualifications of pain following surgery [master's thesis]. Iowa City, Iowa: University of Iowa, 1979.

60. Stewart ML. Measurement of clinical pain. In: Jacox AV, ed. Pain: A source book for nurses and other health professionals. Boston: Little, Brown & Co, 1977:107-138.

61. Melzak R. The McGill pain questionnaire: Major properties and scoring methods. Pain 1975;1:277-299.

62. Marx C. Sedation and analgesia. In: Blumer J, ed. A practical guide to pediatric intensive care. St Louis: Mosby–Year Book, 1990:292-308.

63. Smith JB. Nursing process in pediatric critical care. In: Smith JB, ed. Pediatric critical care. New York: J. Wiley & Sons, 1983:1-25.

64. Philichi LM. Supporting the parents when the child requires intensive care. Focus Crit Care 1988, 15:34-37.

65. Miles MS, Carter MC. Assessing parental stress in the intensive care unit. MCN 1983;8:354-359.

66. Eberly TW, Miles MS, Carter MC. Parental stress after the unexpected admission of a child to the intensive care unit. Crit Care Q 1986:57-65.

67. Curley MAQ. Effects on the nursing mutual participation model of care on parental stress in the pediatric intensive care unit. Heart Lung 1988;17:683-688.

16 Conclusion: Collaborative Management and Overview of Multisystem Organ Failure

Virginia Byrn Huddleston

Although single organ failure and severe, simultaneous failure of all organ systems (as seen following profound shock or arrest) have been recognized for decades, multisystem organ failure (MSOF) as a distinct clinical syndrome has only been recognized since the mid-1970s when Baue[1] and others[2-4] described a sequential organ failure related to both the insult itself and associated therapeutic interventions. Through the years since its initial description, MSOF has become known as the final common pathway to death in the 20th-century ICU, although several paradoxes remain concerning its development and progression (see box at top). With damage occurring to organs often remote from the site of injury or inflammation, numerous hypotheses have been developed to explain the interrelationship among the failure of various organs[5-19] (see box at bottom).

Significant interest in the inflammatory/immune response (IIR) exists at both the laboratory and clinical levels of investigation. Many investigators believe the common thread among the different patient populations that progress to MSOF is the dysregulation of the IIR.[10,19,20-27] Control is lost in the systems initially designed to protect and defend the patient. Exaggerated and overwhelming inflammation ensues, leading to maldistribution of circulating volume, imbalance of oxygen supply/demand, and alterations in metabolism[28-32] (Fig. 16-1).

OVERVIEW OF PATHOPHYSIOLOGY
Primary events and pathophysiologic changes

In Chapter 1, predisposing factors and primary events triggering mediator release are presented. Sepsis, perfusion deficits, persistent inflammatory foci, and preexisting factors such as chronic dis-

---

CLINICAL PARADOXES IN MULTISYSTEM ORGAN FAILURE

Organs that fail frequently are not directly injured in the initial insult.

There is a lag period of days to weeks between the initial insult and the development of clinical organ failure.

Not all patients having clinical sepsis with MSOF have microbiologic evidence of infection (septic syndrome).

No septic focus can be identified clinically or at autopsy in more than 30% of patients with bacteremia dying of clinical sepsis and MSOF.

Identification and treatment of suppurative infections in patients with MSOF may not improve survival.

From Deitch EA. Multiple organ failure: Summary and overview. In: Deitch EA, ed. Multiple organ failure: Pathophysiology and basic concepts of therapy. New York: Thieme Medical Publishers, 1990;287.

HYPOTHESES FOR MULTISYSTEM ORGAN FAILURE

Uncontrolled bacterial invasion of lungs, peritoneum, blood, and other tissue

Overwhelming systemic host defense activation

Severe inflammation, no evidence of sepsis

Altered gastrointestinal barrier function

Injury, shock, and sepsis produce ischemia, which triggers the four preceding events

From Baue AE. Multiple organ failure. Patient care and prevention. St Louis: Mosby–Year Book, 1990;484.

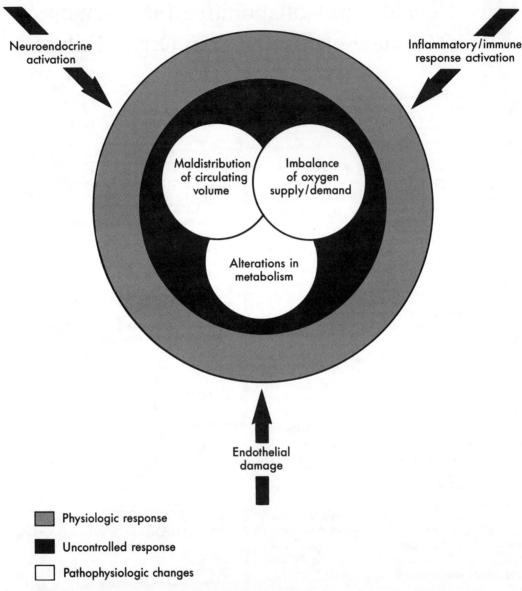

Fig. 16-1   Failure of host defense homeostasis. Once insulted, primary events such as neuroendocrine activation, IIR activation, and endothelial damage trigger the release of an elaborate system of mediators. Under proper regulation *(outer circle)*, many effects are local and specific. If control is lost *(dark circle)*, the cycle becomes self-propagating, and the mediators initially released to protect the host actually provoke the three major pathophysiologic changes *(light circle)*. (From Huddleston VB. Multisystem organ failure: A pathophysiologic approach, Boston, 1991;5.)

ease, age, and nutritional status are common physiologic insults and conditions associated with the development of MSOF.* Primary events such as neuroendocrine activation, endothelial damage, and activation of the IIR occur with the insult or following resuscitation, and these events trigger the release of numerous mediators.[35-37] Under tight control, the IIR protects the host and promotes rapid healing of involved tissue; however, if control is lost, pathophysiologic changes develop (Fig. 16-1). Chapter 2 presents an overview of the IIR, with a special emphasis on the immunosuppressant roles of trauma, stress, hemorrhage, blood transfusions, general anesthesia, and malnutrition. Key assessment findings including both the role of natural host defenses and laboratory values are also discussed.[38] An increasing amount of evidence points to ineffective macrophage/T-cell interaction as a source of this immunosuppression.[39-43] Liberation of glucocorticoids, decreased antibody production, decreased lymphokine production, and increased T-cell suppressor activity are also implicated in the immunosuppression seen in critically ill patients.†

Chapter 3 presents an in-depth explanation of both the physiologic role and pathophysiologic effects of the major mediators implicated in the pathophysiology of sepsis and/or MSOF.[47-49] Tumor necrosis factor (TNF), interleukin-1 (IL-1), oxygen-derived free radicals (ODFR), arachidonic acid metabolites (AA), and proteases are dominant mediators. Consequently, their presence implicates the neutrophil (source of ODFRs, AA, and proteases) and macrophage (source of TNF and IL-1) as principal elements in the pathogenesis of MSOF.[50]

In Chapter 4, Bell comprehensively examines the role of DIC in MSOF progression, showing endothelial damage and microvascular thrombi as key factors in the development and progression of ischemic organ damage and dysfunction.[36] Removal of the underlying pathologic conditions in DIC remains the definitive therapy.

The cyclical, self-activating nature of the IIR and endothelial damage constitutes the major danger in MSOF and contributes to the self-propagation of the major pathophysiologic changes (Table 16-1). Robins extensively describes maldistribution of volume at the systemic, organ, and local levels in Chapter 5, emphasizing that despite a hyperdynamic circulation and increased cardiac output, perfusion may be submaximal in some tissue beds. Patchy areas of low flow may exist in an organ even when the organ's overall flow is normal or increased.[19,51] The elegant balance of oxygen supply and demand and autoregulatory capacities are often lost, thus setting the stage for organ dysfunction and failure. Increased capillary permeability, vasodilatation, selective vasoconstriction, and vascular obstruction all contribute to the maldistribution of volume. Without volume delivery, no oxygen delivery occurs, which exacerbates the balance between oxygen supply and demand. In

---

*References 6, 7, 10, 12, 33, and 34.
†References 35, 39, 40, 42, and 44-46.

Table 16-1 Definition of Pathophysiologic Changes

Maldistribution of circulating volume	Imbalance of oxygen supply and demand	Alterations in metabolism
Capillary permeability	V/Q mismatching	Hypermetabolism
Vasodilatation	Intrapulmonary shunting	Inadequate substrate metabolism
Selective vasoconstriction	Maldistribution of volume	Protein catabolism
Loss of autoregulation	Microcirculatory abnormalities	Liver dysfunction
Microvascular thrombi	Oxygen extraction defects	Peripheral cell dysfunction
Vascular obstruction	Increased demand	Resistance to exogenous administration
Tissue edema	Pain	
Cellular aggregation	Fever	
Microthrombi	Tachycardia	
	Restlessness	
	Increased work of breathing	

Chapter 6, Mims discusses the postulated role of pathologic oxygen supply dependency in the pathophysiology of sepsis and MSOF, and she presents several hypotheses concerning this supply dependency, including pathology at the microcirculatory level and defects in oxygen extraction and use.[52,53] An in-depth discussion of monitoring variables focusing on oxygen transport variables is also provided, accompanied by evidence citing the use of supranormal values as goals of therapy.[54,55] Because many critically ill patients are hypermetabolic and hyperdynamic, their oxygen delivery (DO_2) and oxygen consumption (VO_2) should be above normal. Therapeutically increasing DO_2 and VO_2 to supranormal values has been shown to increase survival,[55] although this therapeutic philosophy remains controversial.

Another factor in both the pathophysiology and survival rates of MSOF is the nutritional status of the patient, both before and after admission. Kimbrell presents the hypermetabolic state as a primary pathophysiologic mechanism in MSOF.[7,32] In Chapter 7, she addresses inadequate substrate metabolism of carbohydrates, proteins, and lipids. As gluconeogenesis increases, muscle mass is severely depleted, and visceral protein stores fall prey to the metabolic machine. Immunocompetence is affected, along with diaphragmatic muscle strength, mobility, and organ system integrity. Liver dysfunction compounds the immune dysfunction and metabolic abnormalities. Lohrman presents evidence in Chapter 8 implicating liver involvement as a major determinant of MSOF development and progression.[7,15] Although controversy exists concerning the exact etiology and pathogenesis of the liver dysfunction (ischemic vs. cell-to-cell interaction), the failure does occur much earlier than previously thought.[5,56] Cerra[7] and others believe that the severity of MSOF parallels the severity of the liver dysfunction; therefore, when the liver can no longer meet the metabolic demands of the body, the patient dies.

Role of the individual organ

The systemic pathophysiologic derangements (Chapters 5, 6, and 7) set the stage for malfunction in each organ. Although each organ may have varying degrees of damage related to numerous factors, MSOF is NOT a series of isolated failures. Although each of the organs may be a victim or target of the

syndrome, each organ also has the potential to affect the process and contribute to failure of other organs, thus perpetuating the explosive nature of the syndrome (Fig. 16-2). As O'Neill points out in her discussion on gastrointestinal involvement (Chapter 9), the gut may be a predominant source of microbial contamination. Bacteria, fungi, or endotoxin may translocate across the injured gut barrier into the lymphatics and portal circulation.[57-59] If the hepatic Kupffer cells do not adequately clear this foreign debris, systemic infection results. The patient may also develop nosocomial pneumonia from bacteria colonized in the stomach and esophagus or by aspirating contaminated oropharyngeal secretions.[60,61]

The pancreas is also an initiating factor in the development of MSOF. McMillan provides an indepth overview of the etiology and pathophysiologic derangements seen in acute pancreatitis (Chapter 14). A chief problem related to pancreatitis is the massive necrosis and liberation of inflammatory mediators.[62,63] An interesting note is also presented: myocardial depressant factor (MDF) may be released from the ischemic pancreas, thus potentiating the myocardial depression that occurs early in the hyperdynamic state.[5]

Gates in her discussion on myocardial involvement (Chapter 10) eloquently lays out the role of myocardial depression in sepsis, integrated with a background of normal myocardial physiology. She dispels the commonly held assumption that most patients experience both the hyperdynamic and hypodynamic state during the evolution of septic shock by citing evidence showing only 10% of nonsurvivors of sepsis experience a true hypodynamic presentation. Most die from refractory hypotension and low vascular resistance or progress to MSOF.[51] The presence of a falling cardiac output is often related to inadequate fluid resuscitation, which is a common mistake in managing patients in septic shock and MSOF. Along with Robins, Gates discusses several hypotheses related to myocardial depression, including maldistribution of flow within the myocardium itself, direct mediator activity (MDF and TNF), and myocardial edema. It is important to note that myocardial depression is present early, even in the face of a high cardiac output; and a high cardiac output does not guarantee sufficient oxygen delivery to all tissues because the preexisting maldistribution of volume

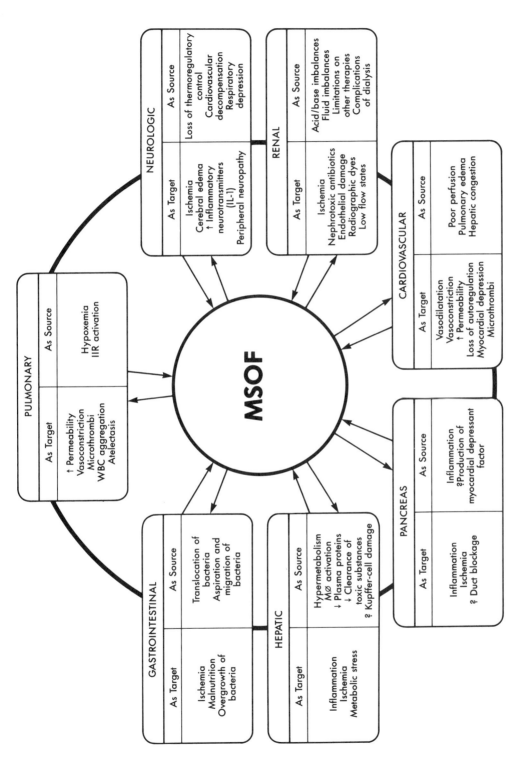

Fig. 16-2 The circle of multisystem organ failure. Each organ may be a target of damage in the process or a contributor to MSOF progression. As the number of failing organs increases, other organs are affected and mortality approaches 100%. (From Huddleston VB. Multisystem organ failure: A pathophysiologic approach, Boston, 1991;39.)

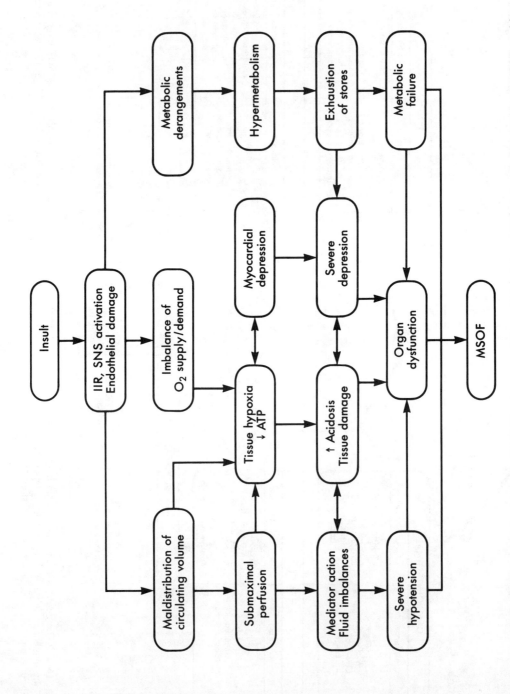

Fig. 16-3 Pathophysiologic cascade mechanism of multisystem organ failure. Abbreviations: *ATP*, Adenosine triphosphate; *MSOF*, multisystem organ failure. (From Huddleston VB. Multisystem organ failure: A pathophysiologic approach, Boston, 1991;24.)

precludes adequate flow to all regions.[19,51]

In Chapter 11, Morris discusses the adult respiratory distress syndrome (ARDS). Often the first organ to fail in MSOF, acute lung injury represents a major insult to the body. The inability of the lungs to adequately oxygenate the cardiac output coming from the right side of the heart potentiates hypoxemia that is often refractory to therapy. V/Q mismatching and intrapulmonary shunting are the mechanisms responsible for the hypoxemia. Although ARDS can occur in isolation, it is more frequently associated with sepsis and the MSOF syndrome; therefore the lung failure occurring in MSOF manifests as ARDS.

Although isolated failure was a common finding in casualties of war and trauma patients in the 1950s and 1960s, improvement in fluid resuscitation techniques and aggressive monitoring have greatly reduced the incidence of single organ failure, particularly prerenal failure. Today renal failure is more commonly associated with ischemic acute tubular necrosis and nephrotoxic factors such as antibiotic administration, vasopressor therapy, and inflammatory mediator activity. Lancaster examines the categories of renal failure, differential diagnosis, clinical progression, and common assessment findings in Chapter 12.

In relation to other organs, little is known concerning the nervous system and MSOF. Dasch (Chapter 13) points out that shock and sepsis frequently induce ischemic brain injury. Autoregulatory mechanisms fail, and the blood-brain barrier becomes more permeable to toxic substances. As in other organs, reperfusion may actually exacerbate the damage because petechial and subarachnoid hemorrhage and transudation of colloid occur secondary to increased capillary permeability and restoration of flow.[64] Recent studies also identify peripheral neuropathies in MSOF.[65]

Summary

MSOF represents failure of host defense homeostasis. Physiologic insults, early primary events, and pathophysiologic derangements are involved in a cascade of events ultimately leading to organ dysfunction, failure, and death (Fig. 16-3). Currently, therapeutic intervention remains primarily supportive. A 100% mortality has been noted by some investigators if three or more organs have failed, particularly with renal involvement.[11,16,66]

ASSESSMENT AND NURSING DIAGNOSES

The box on p. 300 outlines the criteria developed by Knaus et al[67] to define failure of each specific organ. The patient with MSOF has numerous problems and complications, and most of the accepted nursing diagnoses could be applied to the MSOF patient sometime during the clinical course. The box on p. 301 lists the more frequently cited nursing diagnoses with associated causes. To deliver effective care, the nurse must constantly interact with all levels of the health care delivery team to coordinate and deliver the therapy required by the patient to reach the therapeutic goals necessary for recovery.

THERAPEUTIC MANAGEMENT
Goals

The management of MSOF remains difficult and controversial. It requires a multidisciplinary approach including nursing, medicine, respiratory therapy, nutritional support, physical therapy, occupational therapy, social services, and rehabilitation. Collaborative management concentrates on four major goals[5,9]:

1. Prevention and early identification of infectious/inflammatory stimuli
2. Restoration of oxygen supply and demand balance
3. Provision of nutritional support and metabolic requirements
4. Individual organ support

Prevention

Once triggered, the systemic IIR continues with minimal exogenous stimuli. Even aggressive treatment of the initial insult may not halt the vicious cycle of inflammation once it becomes malignant. Therefore the ultimate and most effective weapon against MSOF is prevention. Early interventions must focus on infection control, early identification of complications, and prompt, aggressive resuscitation and ongoing therapy.[38,68] Often referred to as "front-loading" therapy, complications are prevented or minimized by early intervention rather than treated only when compromise and decompensation occur.

Upon admission, all treatable injuries should be managed. Removal of all necrotic tissue, early debridement of burn eschar, and prompt stabilization of fractures minimize further soft tissue damage, inflammation, and infection.[5,69] A secure airway

---

KNAUS' CRITERIA FOR DETERMINATION OF ORGAN FAILURE

Cardiovascular failure (presence of one or more of the following):
Heart rate $\leq 54/$min
MAP ≤ 49 mm Hg
Ventricular tachycardia or fibrillation
Serum pH ≤ 7.24 with a $PaCO_2 \leq 49$ mm Hg
Respiratory failure (presence of one or more of the following):
Respiratory rate $\leq 5/$min or $\geq 49/$min
$PaCO_2 \geq 50$ mm Hg
$AaDO_2 \geq 350$ mm Hg ($AaDO_2 = 713$ (FiO_2) $- PaCO_2 - PaO_2$) with $FiO_2 = 1.0$
Dependent on ventilator or CPAP on the second day of organ failure
Renal failure (presence of one or more of the following):
Urine output ≤ 479 mL/24 hr or ≤ 159 mL/8 hr
Serum BUN ≥ 100 mg/dL
Serum creatinine ≥ 3.5 mg/dL

Hematologic failure (presence of one or more of the following):
WBC $\leq 1000/$mm^3
Platelets $\leq 20,000/$mm^3
Hematocrit $\leq 20\%$
Neurologic failure
Glasgow Coma Score ≤ 6 (without sedation)
Other indicators not included in Knaus' criteria:
Liver failure
Total bilirubin ≥ 2 mg/dL
Clinical jaundice
Elevated liver enzymes (SGOT, SGPT, alkaline phosphatase, and LDH)
Elevated blood ammonia
Blood albumin ≤ 3.0 g/dL
Gastrointestinal failure
Upper/lower gastrointestinal bleeding
Mucosal ulceration/erosion
Diarrhea
Ileus
Bacterial overgrowth in stool culture

From Knaus WA, Wagner DP. Multiple systems organ failure: Epidemiology and prognosis. Crit Care Clin 1989;5:223. Abbreviations: *mm Hg*, millimeter of mercury; *mg*, milligram; *dL*, deciliter; *mm*, millimeter; *WBC*, white blood count; *BUN*, blood urea nitrogen; *PaCO₂*, partial pressure of carbon dioxide in arterial blood; *PaO₂*, partial pressure of oxygen in arterial blood; *AaDO₂*, alveolar-arterial oxygen difference; *FiO₂*, fraction of inspired oxygen; *CPAP*, continuous positive airway pressure; *mL*, milliliter; *SGOT*, serum glutamic oxaloacetic transaminase; *SGPT*, serum glutamic pyruvic transaminase; *LDH*, lactic acid dehydrogenase.

and frequent oral care are crucial in reducing aspiration and nosocomial pneumonia. Meticulous line, site, and catheter care and observation, along with aggressive wound and skin care, decrease iatrogenic complications. Hand washing remains a key factor in prevention of nosocomial colonization and infection.

Antibiotic therapy is based on initial Gram's stain results and the patient's clinical status, and it is altered according to patient response and culture reports. The use of empiric antibiotics and empiric laparotomy remains controversial.[70,71] Although corticosteroids are potent antiinflammatory agents, they are not routinely used in sepsis and MSOF.[72] Because their immunosuppressant effects are so great, corticosteroids actually predispose the patient to greater infectious complications.[73-75]

Restoration of oxygen supply/demand balance

A major focus of both monitoring and intervention involves restoration of the oxygen supply/demand balance by either increasing oxygen supply or decreasing oxygen demand. Although arterial blood gases (ABGs) provide crucial patient information, they only assess the amount of oxygen brought into the body, not what is actually delivered to the tissues. As Mims points out in Chapter 6, oxygen transport formulas such as oxygen delivery (DO_2) and oxygen consumption (VO_2) provide the clinician with much more valid information concerning oxygen delivery and tissue oxygenation. An arterial saturation (SaO_2) of 99% matters little if cardiac output is so low that oxygen cannot be delivered to the tissues. Likewise, assessing oxygen delivery without considering the

NURSING DIAGNOSES IN MULTISYSTEM ORGAN FAILURE

Alteration in tissue perfusion related to maldistribution of circulating volume secondary to capillary permeability, tissue edema, microvascular thrombi, hemorrhage, vascular plugging with platelets and white blood cells, loss of autoregulation, vasodilatation, vasoconstriction, myocardial depression, and low perfusion pressures.

Fluid volume deficit related to vasodilatation, increased capillary permeability, hemorrhage, decreased intake, inadequate fluid resuscitation, increased insensible losses (NGT, ETT, and diaphoresis), excessive wound drainage, fistulas, and diarrhea.

Fluid volume excess related to renal failure, congestive heart failure, liver failure (ascites), endocrine disorders (SIADH), and iatrogenic volume overload.

Impaired gas exchange related to vasoconstriction, increased capillary permeability, alterations in pulmonary endothelium, atelectasis, decreased functional residual capacity, secretion accumulation, intrapulmonary shunting secondary to ARDS, and pulmonary edema secondary to biventricular failure and pneumonia.

Ineffective airway clearance secondary to diaphragmatic muscle weakness, pain, artificial airway, decreased level of consciousness, tenacious secretions, and fatigue.

High risk for infection related to invasive techniques, immunocompromise, antibiotic administration, and immunosuppressant therapy.

Alteration in nutrition: less than body requirements, related to hypermetabolism secondary to mediator systems and inadequate nutritional support.

Alteration in skin integrity related to malnutrition, invasive devices, immobility, volume status, dehydration, edema, obesity, excessive diaphoresis, poor perfusion, frequent dressing changes, neuropathies, and preexisting chronic diseases such as peripheral vascular disease or diabetes.

Impaired mobility related to ICU environment, restraints, extent of injury, muscle atrophy, and neuromuscular blockade.

Decreased cardiac output related to hypovolemia, ischemic dysfunction, and myocardial depression secondary to mediators, acidosis, and exhaustion.

Anxiety related to prognosis, ICU environment, procedures, neuromuscular blockade, and pain.

Pain-related injuries, invasive devices, immobility, invasive procedures, hyperthermia, and hypothermia.

Hyperthermia related to mediator activity in the hypothalamus and increased metabolic rate.

Hypothermia related to hypothalamic dysfunction and decreased metabolic rate.

Impaired communication related to artificial airway and decreased level of consciousness secondary to head injury, poor cerebral perfusion, liver failure, and sedation.

Ineffective family coping related to prognosis, severity of insult, ICU environment, infrequent visiting hours, previous coping strategies, financial burdens, and fear.

Abbreviations: *NGT,* nasogastric tube; *ETT,* endotracheal tube; *SIADH,* syndrome of inappropriate secretion of antidiuretic hormone; *ARDS,* adult respiratory distress syndrome; *ICU,* intensive care unit.

amount of oxygen that tissues actually consume (VO_2) leads to misinterpretation of assessment findings and clinical condition. All parameters of oxygenation must be assessed, including the variables that define those parameters. Cardiac output, hemoglobin, and arterial saturation are principal variables in both DO_2 and VO_2 formulas; therefore, aggressive efforts are aimed at optimizing cardiac output, hemoglobin, and arterial saturation in MSOF.

Cardiac output. Pulmonary artery catheterization is often necessary to accurately monitor fluid status and cardiac function. Because of the low SVR, large volumes of fluid are usually necessary to maintain adequate preload. Adequate preload also increases the accuracy of pulmonary artery measurements taken during mechanical ventilation.[76] Removing intubated patients from the ventilator during pulmonary artery measurements often compromises ventilatory status, gas exchange, and arterial saturation; therefore the patient should remain on the ventilator during measurements. The crystalloid/colloid controversy concerning the optimal fluid for fluid resuscitation continues (see Chapter 5). Crystalloids tend to have fewer complications, but they do third-space more easily. On the other hand, if the capillaries are very permeable (as they often are), colloids not only move to the interstitium but draw more fluid with them secondary to the osmotic effect. Because each patient has different underlying pathologic conditions and complications, choice of fluid should be guided by individual patient response to fluid challenge.

Along with volume infusion, inotropic agents are used to counteract myocardial depression and increase cardiac output. Dobutamine is the first-line drug of choice and has been used to drive cardiac output up to levels of 15 to 20 L/min in some institutions in an effort to increase DO_2 and VO_2, particularly if pathologic supply dependency is suspected (Chapter 6). As patients progress through the septic state and MSOF, they exhibit a decreased responsiveness to catecholamines and adrenergic stimulation. Because dopamine, dobutamine, and other inotropic agents require adrenergic responsiveness to achieve desired effects, researchers are attempting to develop positive inotropic agents that are not dependent on adrenergic receptor sensitivity. Although digoxin meets these criteria, its use

---

COMPLICATIONS OF SODIUM BICARBONATE ADMINISTRATION

Paradoxical intracellular acidosis

Induction of hyperosmolar and alkalotic states

Fluid overload secondary to increased sodium and hyperosmolar state

Shift of oxyhemoglobin dissociation curve to the left leading to increased affinity and decreased release of oxygen by hemoglobin at the tissue level

Hypocalcemia and hypokalemia secondary to rapid changes in pH, which induce extracellular/intracellular shifts in electrolytes

Induction of respiratory acidosis secondary to increased CO_2 generation:

$$H^+ + HCO_3^- \leftrightarrow H_2CO_3 \leftrightarrow CO_2 + H_2O$$

---

is limited because of renal and hepatic failure and predisposition toward digoxin toxicity. Severe acidosis also increases myocardial depression, and bicarbonate administration may partially alleviate the decrease in cardiac output secondary to acidosis. Bicarbonate is not a benign drug, and care should be taken in choosing both dosage and speed of administration. Rapid changes in pH potentiate rapid electrolyte shifts and other complications (see box above). The "best" time to treat acidosis remains controversial. Although acidosis is associated with complications such as myocardial depression, electrolyte shifts, and enzymatic dysfunction, acidosis shifts the oxyhemoglobin dissociation curve to the right. In a shift to the right, the affinity between oxygen and hemoglobin decreases, which assists in the release of oxygen at the tissue bed. Therefore acidosis actually enhances oxygen unloading at the tissue level.[77]

If fluid and inotropic therapy do not maintain adequate cardiac output and perfusion pressures, vasopressor therapy may be instituted. The low SVR assists in maintaining a high cardiac output; therefore vasopressor agents are used judiciously to maintain mean arterial pressure above 70 mm

Hg. Extreme vasoconstriction hinders flow to select organs, especially in the splanchnic and renal circulation. Increasing the afterload also increases myocardial oxygen demands and contributes to myocardial fatigue and ischemia. Although dopamine remains the first-line drug of choice, some clinicians now favor dopamine at low doses to enhance renal and splanchnic perfusion. Other vasopressor agents such as phenylephrine (Neo-Synephrine) and levarterenol (Levophed) are then used to induce vasoconstriction and increase SVR. For the rare patient who does develop an elevated SVR, nitroprusside may be used to reduce afterload and myocardial oxygen demands.[78] Robins and Gates provide an overview of commonly used vasoactive agents in Chapters 5 and 10, respectively.

Hemoglobin. An optimal hemoglobin level contributes to adequate oxygen delivery, although concentrated hemoglobin levels increase transit time and sludging in the microcirculation, which promote the development of microthrombi. Conversely, a low hemoglobin level decreases capillary transit time and concomitantly decreases oxygen extraction. As Robins notes in Chapter 5, optimal tissue oxygenation must be balanced with promotion of flow through the microcirculation. A hemoglobin of 10 to 12 g/dL is frequently recommended.

Arterial saturation. The third major variable in the oxygen transport formulas is SaO_2. Measures to improve oxygen saturation include ventilatory support, prevention of nosocomial pneumonia, and frequent position changes.[79] Supplemental oxygen by mask or ventilator, along with CPAP or PEEP, is usually required to increase the driving pressure of oxygen across the alveolocapillary membrane, achieve adequate minute ventilation, and maintain $SaO_2 > 90\%$. If increasing FiO_2 is not adequate, PEEP is instituted to stabilize functional alveoli and recruit collapsed alveoli. An FiO_2 of greater than 50% is associated with increased oxygen toxicity to the lung parenchyma, particularly in acute lung injury and ARDS. Although increasing FiO_2 can alleviate hypoxemia related to venous admixture and dead space ventilation, true shunt is not affected by a higher FiO_2, and PEEP must be used to improve gas exchange[80] (see Chapter 11). Turning and repositioning also aid in redistribution of flow through the lungs, enhancing V/Q matching

and preventing venous stasis.[81]

If secretions are thick or the patient does not have the strength to mobilize them, suctioning is indicated. Both secretions and suctioning predispose the patient to atelectasis and pneumonia, so care must be taken to ensure absolute sterile technique in the suctioning procedure. Recent research supports the use of ventilator breaths for hyperoxygenation and hyperventilation over the use of manual resuscitation bags in maintaining SaO_2 during routine suctioning.[82] A closed ventilator circuit also minimizes contamination. The complications of hypoxemia, airway collapse, and increased risk of infection preclude the use of mandated (every 2 hours) suctioning in every patient. Careful auscultation of the lungs will clue the critical care nurse or respiratory therapist to the necessity of suctioning.

Because standard stress bleeding prophylaxis of H_2-blockers and antacids has been associated with an overgrowth of bacteria in the stomach and increased incidence of nosocomial pneumonia secondary to migration of these bacteria and gastric reflux, clinicians are examining other therapies for mucosal protection. In several studies, sucralfate and/or continuous infusions of H_2-blockers have decreased the incidence of nosocomial pneumonia in the intubated patient in comparison with standard therapy.[83,84] Sucralfate provides mucosal protection without greatly altering the gastric pH. Interventions minimizing aspiration of glucose-laden enteral feeding may also decrease the incidence of nosocomial pneumonia.

Decrease in oxygen demand. Because oxygen demand is greater than supply, any patient condition that increases demand such as fever, pain, shivering, and tachycardia places a severe strain on an already compromised balance. Interventions that decrease demand are as vital as those aimed at increasing supply. Although fever shifts the oxyhemoglobin dissociation curve to the right and also enhances immune system function, excessive body temperatures (greater than 102° F, or 39° C) need to be reduced and controlled. Antipyretics are preferred over hypothermia units because they are less likely to induce shivering. Pain medication and antianxiety medication not only increase patient comfort, but also decrease restlessness, tachycardia, and work of breathing, thus "freeing up" additional oxygen for use by the major organ beds. Analgesics also enhance toleration of invasive procedures and interventions such as turning, suctioning, dressing changes, and line insertions; therefore desaturation in minimized.

Provision of nutritional support

Nutritional support must be provided early. For every day the patient goes unfed, several days are often required to "make up the difference" as the hypermetabolism and muscle catabolism continue

unabated. Kimbrell discusses the advantages and complications of total parenteral nutrition and enteral feedings along with nutritional assessment and investigational therapies in Chapter 7. Goals of nutritional support include:

1. Supporting organ structure and function
2. Preventing substrate limited metabolism
3. Supporting metabolic pathways
4. Maintaining nitrogen equilibrium

Increasing evidence points to enteral feedings as superior in both number of complications and

---

GENERAL THERAPEUTIC GOALS AND INTERVENTIONS FOR MSOF[5,9,38,68]

Prevention and early identification of inflammatory stimuli

Obtain thorough history and physical to prevent overlooking injuries or other significant information.

Use rapid resuscitation to decrease shock and ischemic time.

Perform surgical debridement/drainage of necrotic tissue or abscesses.

Stabilize fractures early to prevent further tissue damage and promote early ambulation.

Replace lines inserted in the field within 12 to 24 hours.

Secure airway to prevent aspiration and enhance oxygen delivery.

Perform frequent oral care to minimize oropharyngeal contamination and risk of silent aspiration.

Perform meticulous line, site, and catheter care and observation and documentation.

Maintain closed systems: capped ports, fewer stopcocks, inline suctioning, manual ventilator breaths for hyperoxygenation/hyperventilation.

Perform meticulous wound care.

Recognize changes promptly: cultures, WBC, fever, and radiographic changes.

Administer intravenous antibiotics based on Gram's stain, patient condition, culture reports, and patient response.

Remove potential contaminants such as cut flowers or standing water.

Ensure proper terminal cleaning of bedside and other reusable equipment

Ensure early, aggressive supportive therapy: nutrition, intravenous fluids, mobilization, and pulmonary toilet.

Wash your hands before and after patient contact.

Restoration of oxygen supply and demand

Optimize cardiac output
  Pulmonary artery catheterization
  Fluid resuscitation
  Inotropic therapy
  Vasoactive therapy
  Control severe acidosis
Optimize hemoglobin
  Maintain level at 10 to 12 g/dL
  Monitor CBC
Optimize Sao_2
  Ventilatory support
  Prevent nosocomial pneumonia
    Sterile technique with suctioning
    Frequent oral care
    Consider sucralfate for stress bleeding prophylaxis
    Monitor for aspiration of gastric contents, tube feedings, and oral secretions
    Frequent position changes and early mobility

Nutritional support

Early tube feedings if possible
Total parenteral nutrition as necessary to meet metabolic needs

Individual organ support as indicated

Mechanical ventilation
Hemodialysis/continuous arteriovenous hemofiltration
Inotropic and vasoactive agents
Therapeutic beds

Abbreviations: *WBC*, white blood count; *mg/dL*, milligrams per deciliter; *CBC*, complete blood count.

maintenance of gut barrier function.[58,85,86] Advantages of early enteral feedings include:

1. Enhancement of enteral immune function
2. Prevention of GI atrophy and maintenance of mucosal integrity, thus aiding in prevention of bacterial translocation
3. Decrease in bile sludging, which contributes to cholestasis and cholecystitis
4. Decrease in incidence of stress ulceration
5. Support of hepatic function

Individual organ support

The fourth major goal of therapy is support of individual organs, but the treatment of the patient must focus on the entire disease process and halting the stimulus of the IIR. Supportive care treats manifestations and does not remove the underlying problem. Monitoring must include parameters such as oxygen delivery and consumption that measure the effects of therapy on more than one system. The box on p. 304 summarizes the general therapeutic goals and interventions for MSOF.

INVESTIGATIONAL THERAPIES

Investigational therapies for MSOF are extremely broad in scope. Everything from tube feedings to cutting-edge immunotherapeutics has the potential to affect the MSOF process. Numerous organ-specific therapies are discussed in Section Three.[87-90] Other investigational therapies such as immunomodulation therapy are more "syndrome-specific" rather than targeting any particular organ.[91-96] Steadily making its way from the basic science laboratory to the clinical arena, immunomodulation focuses on inhibiting or controlling the IIR and minimizing damage after inflammation and resuscitation.

Monoclonal antibodies

One of the biggest breakthroughs to move from the bench to the bedside is the clinical application of monoclonal antibody techniques. Monoclonal antibodies (mAbs) against endotoxin, endotoxin receptors, TNF, and TNF receptors are currently under investigation. In the case of actual mediators such as TNF, the mAb binds to the mediator and neutralizes the mediator's ability to impair host tissues. In the case of receptors, the mAb competes with the mediator at the target cell and blocks the receptor so that the mediator cannot bind and cause

damage. Because white blood cell/endothelial cell interaction and adhesion can cause significant endothelial damage secondary to oxygen-derived free radical and protease activity, mAbs to WBC adhesion molecules are also being examined. If the adhesion molecule on the WBC is bound with the mAb, the white blood cell cannot adhere to the endothelial wall and injure it.[97,98]

Development. Each B cell is genetically dedicated to binding only with a specific antigenic determinant.[99] The binding of antigen with a B cell stimulates that particular B cell to proliferate (clonal selection) and ultimately differentiate into antibody-producing cells and memory cells. Many foreign agents are complex and contain many antigenic determinants, each capable of stimulating a different B-cell clone; therefore a heterogeneous mixture of antibodies (polyclonal) is produced as different B cells bind with different determinants[100] (Fig. 16-4).

In 1975, Köhler and Milstein[101] developed the mAb technique that produced homogeneous, specific antibodies. Before this discovery, production of therapeutic antibodies required volunteers to be injected with an antigen. A response then occurred in which antibodies with several different specificities (idiotypes) were formed. The volunteer's blood was then drawn, and serum containing the different antibodies was collected. Because the response was variable, it was difficult to reproduce from one collection to the next. Conversely, mAbs are specific for one antigenic determinant; therefore their specificity and affinity are more potent in effect, and toxic interactions are minimized.[102,103] See the box on p. 307 for advantages of monoclonal therapy.

At present, the most developed mAb for use in sepsis and MSOF is the antiendotoxin antibody.[104-106] Known as HA-1A (Centoxin) and E5, they have recently been recommended for approval by the FDA. Initial multicenter trials of HA-1A performed by Ziegler and the HA-1A Sepsis Study Group[104] reported a 39% decrease in mortality. Greenman and the Xoma sepsis study group[105] reported a 2.3-fold improvement in survival for those patients receiving E5. Therefore it appears that mAbs represent a major breakthrough in the therapeutic management of gram-negative sepsis.

HA-1A is a human monoclonal IgM antibody directed against the lipid A domain of endotoxin.

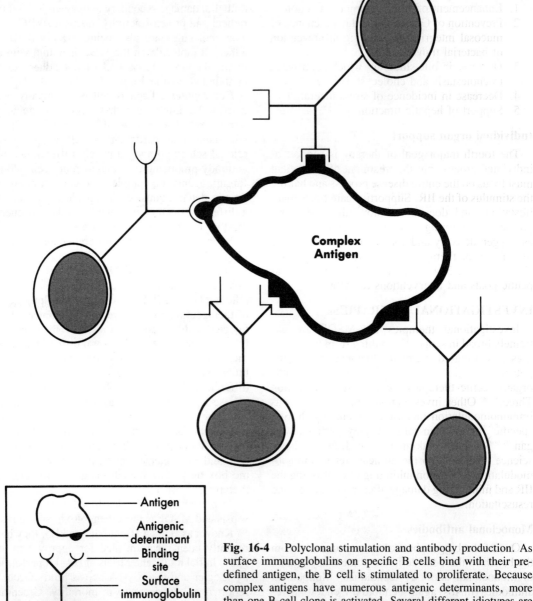

Fig. 16-4 Polyclonal stimulation and antibody production. As surface immunoglobulins on specific B cells bind with their predefined antigen, the B cell is stimulated to proliferate. Because complex antigens have numerous antigenic determinants, more than one B-cell clone is activated. Several different idiotypes are produced, yielding serum with polyclonal antibodies. (From Huddleston VB. Multisystem organ failure: A pathophysiologic approach, Boston, 1991;52.)

The lipid A region is highly conserved among different species of gram-negative bacteria, and therefore the antiendotoxin antibody is useful against a broad range of gram-negative organisms.[107]

Although antiendotoxin antibodies show significant promise, they are only effective against gram-negative septicemia. Gram-negative sepsis is a major etiologic factor in the development of MSOF, but it is not the only factor. Overwhelming inflammation without a septic source is documented in 30% to 50% of the cases.[8] Anti-TNF or anti-TNF receptor mAbs may be more helpful in these patients, when ischemia and other conditions in addition to endotoxemia trigger the systemic inflammatory response and TNF release.[108-113] The potential for mAbs in clinical therapy is promising, but future research is necessary to define their therapeutic role. Other therapies have also shown promise against the negative systemic effects of inflammation (see box below).

Receptor antagonists

Receptor antagonists also block the effects of select mediators.[114-116] IL-1 acting in isolation or in concert with TNF inflicts cellular and tissue injury.[50,117] By binding and blocking the receptor on the target site, the IL-1 receptor antagonist inhibits IL-1-induced activity. Wakabayashi et al[114] document a significant reduction in the severity of *Esch-*

ADVANTAGES OF MONOCLONAL ANTIBODIES[102-107]

Increased availability (do not require frequent immunization and phlebotomy of donors)

Minimal transmission risk of hepatitis, AIDS, CMV, and other serum-acquired viruses

Reproducible specificity and affinity; thus greater potency

Ability to standardize therapeutic reagent

Abbreviations: *AIDS*, acquired immunodeficiency syndrome; *CMV*, cytomegalovirus.

INVESTIGATIONAL THERAPIES

Monoclonal antibodies
  Endotoxin
  Endotoxin receptors
  Tumor necrosis factor
  Tumor necrosis factor receptors
  White blood cell adhesion molecules
Receptor antagonists
  Interleukin-1
Vasodilatory mediators
  PGE_1
  PGI_2
Eicosanoid inhibitors
  Ibuprofen
  Thromboxane synthetase inhibitors
  Indomethacin
Antioxidants (oxygen-derived free radical scavengers, xanthine oxidase inhibitors, and iron chelators)
  Ibuprofen
  Allopurinol
  Deferoxamine

  Superoxide dismutase
  Catalase
  Mannitol
  Vitamins C and E
  Synthetics
Calcium antagonists
Pentoxifylline
Selective decontamination of the gut
ECMO, $ECCO_2R$
Plasmapheresis
Other mediator inhibitors
  Antiproteases
  PAF antagonists
Tissue and immune stimulators
  Colony-stimulating factors
  Glucan
  Growth factors and hormones
  Glutamine
  Erythropoietin
  Thymopentin-5
  Interleukin-2

Abbreviations: *PG*, prostaglandin; *ECMO*, extracorporeal membrane oxygenation; *ECCO₂R*, extracorporeal carbon dioxide removal; *PAF*, platelet activating factor.

erichia coli–induced sepsis in laboratory animals given recombinant IL-1 receptor antagonist.[114]

Antioxidant therapy

Another large area of interest and research concentrates on oxygen-derived free radical production and damage during WBC activation and reperfusion injury. In the body, several mechanisms generate free radicals (oxidants) following insult and injury, including increased xanthine oxidase activity seen with reperfusion injury and histamine release, activated neutrophils undergoing respiratory burst activity, and increased arachidonic acid metabolism. Chapters 3 and 5 provide in-depth discussions on reperfusion injury, WBC respiratory burst, and free radical production and damage. The release of intracellular iron from injured cells also increases production of the more toxic oxidant hydroxyl radical (see Fig. 3-6).

Free radicals incite lipid peroxidation of cell membranes and cell damage, which may contribute to local and systemic tissue inflammation and organ dysfunction. Whether lipid peroxidation incites cell and tissue damage and increased capillary permeability or the tissue damage induces increased lipid peroxidation remains controversial.[118] Lipid peroxidation also generates arachidonic acid, leading to increased production of eicosanoids (prostaglandins, thromboxanes, leukotrienes). Antioxidants, including free radical scavengers, xanthine oxidase inhibitors, and iron-chelating agents, are under investigation (see box on p. 307).

Ibuprofen. Ibuprofen and allopurinol both attenuate inflammatory changes seen after an insult,[118-121] although the exact physiologic mechanism of action is not completely defined. Proposed antiinflammatory effects of ibuprofen include cyclooxygenase inhibition leading to decreased production of prostaglandins and thromboxane, stabilization of neutrophils leading to decreased production of free radicals, and decreased lipid peroxidation leading to membrane stability.[118-120,122] Other recent research by Demling and LaLonde[118] and others highlights ibuprofen's iron-chelating activity as an important antiinflammatory mechanism. Because continued hydroxyl radical generation requires iron, iron-chelating agents such as ibuprofen and deferoxamine inhibit production of free radicals and may decrease cell and tissue injury caused by free radical–induced lipid peroxidation of cell membranes.[120]

Allopurinol. Allopurinol inhibits xanthine oxidase and thus free radical production, but it has also been shown to scavenge free radicals as well.[123] Unlike other antioxidants, such as superoxide dismutase and catalase, which only act in the extracellular space when exogenously administered, allopurinol has the ability to inhibit both intracellular and extracellular xanthine oxidase activity.[124] Because ischemic cells are more sensitive to oxidant injury, pharmacologic agents that reduce free radical production have the potential to decrease inflammatory changes associated with sepsis, MSOF, and other ischemic conditions. Allopurinol has been shown to decrease the oxidant damage occurring in the patient after a coronary artery bypass graft.[125,126]

Calcium antagonists

Calcium is thought to migrate into ischemic cells and impair cellular structure and function,[42,127] particularly during resuscitation[128]; therefore, calcium antagonists may confer cellular protection in ischemic events.[42,129] Immune cells such as macrophages may be a target for excess intracellular calcium influx, thus potentiating cellular dysfunction and immunosuppression. By giving calcium antagonists during resuscitation, Ertel et al[42] have demonstrated an increased macrophage/T-cell interaction through increased antigen presentation, MHC Class II expression, and IL-1 synthesis in laboratory animals. Other therapeutic effects of calcium channel blockers include vasodilatation and increased tissue perfusion, particularly in the splanchnic bed; improved myocardial performance; antagonism of renal vasoconstriction; and maintenance of intracellular magnesium levels.[130]

Pentoxifylline

Pentoxifylline, a methylxanthine used to decrease blood viscosity in chronic vascular disease, has shown promise in the treatment of tissue perfusion and oxygenation in sepsis and MSOF.[131,132] Noel et al[133] report that pentoxifylline decreases the sequestration of neutrophils, inhibits TNF activity, and decreases severe morbidity in animals given intravenous endotoxin. Waxman et al[134] report improved tissue oxygenation and oxygen consumption after hemorrhage with pentoxifylline administration. Improved microcirculatory blood flow and possible decreased neutophil adherence to the endothelium are hypothesized mechanisms of action.[134]

Summary

As clinical investigation progresses, only a few of these investigational therapies will actually prove feasible and effective for use in the general patient population. Others will be dismissed, and new therapies will surface. Many therapies may appear inadequate only because they were implemented too late in the course of the disease. Timing may be just as crucial as the therapy itself. Investigations are difficult to conduct in the patient with MSOF because of the complexity of the syndrome and the number of confounding variables involved. Therefore initial studies involve laboratory animals under controlled conditions. Although this is necessary to control confounding variables and protect the patient from unforeseen complications, caution must be taken in extrapolating all animal findings to the human response.

One major drawback in immunomodulation therapy is the potential to actually inhibit not only the uncontrolled aspect of the IIR response but the protective aspect as well. Corticosteroid therapy is a perfect example: by blocking specific mediator functions and activities, protective host mechanisms are impaired, predisposing the patient to overwhelming microbial invasion. Knowledge of the IIR is not only vital for understanding the pathophysiology of clinical conditions but also for ensuring safe, effective delivery of pharmacologic agents and accurate assessment of the patient's response to therapy.[135,136]

ETHICAL CONSIDERATIONS

With a mortality approaching 100% in many patients with MSOF, numerous ethical dilemmas surface in the ICU. As controls over availability of resources tighten and critical care costs skyrocket, care decisions regarding limiting or withdrawing treatment are being made at an earlier time. Costs approaching $200,000 have been quoted for a 21-day stay in the ICU. Rehabilitation costs for the survivor may approach $300,000 during the year following discharge from the unit. What role does cost-benefit ratio play in our decisions? When is enough enough? Or too much? It is hoped that these decisions will continue to be made by compassionate health care professionals in conjunction with patient and family wishes and not by legis-

lative bodies. Unfortunately, many end-stage patients are comatose and cannot verbalize their desires. The weight of the decision often falls on distraught and anxious family members who have emotional and psychologic needs as well.[137] The development of a comprehensive supportive care team for hopelessly ill patients with MSOF was recently reported.[138] The multidisciplinary team consists of a clinical nurse specialist, staff physician, chaplain, social worker, respiratory therapist, and the patient's bedside nurse. The team assumes patient responsibility in accordance with patient and/or family wishes for those patients deemed hopelessly ill by Knaus' organ failure criteria.[67] Patient and family preferences regarding heroic measures, physical comfort, psychosocial comfort, and family support were incorporated into decision-making. Although mortality did not decrease (100% as expected), length of ICU stay and number of therapeutic interventions decreased significantly. The high technologic maintenance of hopelessly ill patients presents a psychologic burden to family and staff, a financial burden to the family and the health care industry, and a gross intrusion into the patient's privacy and death. Moving patients out of the ICU greatly increases patient/family interaction and enhances patient dignity and privacy.

CONCLUSION

Assessment and treatment of this complex syndrome focus primarily on minimizing infectious/inflammatory stimuli, maintaining adequate preload and circulating volume, enhancing oxygen delivery and consumption, minimizing oxygen demand, and meeting metabolic requirements. Individual organ support and other standard critical care regimens are used to maintain the patient during this state although they often do not treat the underlying problem.[139,140] Unfortunately, many therapies treat one problem only to initiate a new one. Standard stress bleeding prophylaxis with antacids and H_2-receptor antagonists protects against gastric ulceration but predisposes the patient to overgrowth of bacteria in the stomach. Total parenteral nutrition increases the risk of infection, gut atrophy, and fatty liver. Positive end-expiratory pressure (PEEP) decreases venous return and cardiac output, affecting renal function and renin secretion. Benefits and risks of routine therapies and investigational interventions must be carefully weighed for each patient. Moloney-Harmon and Czerwinski discuss specific management strategies for the pediatric population in Chapter 15. Although the pathophysiology follows a similar cascade of events to the adult population, the anatomic and physiologic differences in infants and young children require specialized assessment skills and alterations in therapy.

New attention is being diverted from the classic cardiopulmonary etiologies to more novel sources of complications, such as the role of the gut and wound in MSOF. Are they the ultimate culprit, or at the very least, a major contributor to continual inflammation?* Until newer therapies are readily available that can control the inflammatory process without increasing the risk of infection, efforts must be focused on *prevention* and *early identification*.

As Deitch states in his text on the syndrome: "Although many facets of MSOF remain shrouded in mystery, confusion, or controversy, progress is being made. Testable hypotheses on the cause and pathophysiologic features of organ failure have been generated and a consensus has been reached on multiple aspects of the care of these patients."[69] Although the morbidity and mortality of MSOF remain high, major breakthroughs in our understanding of the physiologic response to insult, resuscitative techniques, and the role of the IIR in MSOF promise a brighter future for the critically ill patient at risk for the development of MSOF. The future will not only test our ability to aggressively and appropriately intervene but also our willingness to appropriately limit or withdraw that intervention when the patient's condition and wishes warrant such action.

---

*References 5, 57, 58, 141, and 142.

REFERENCES

1. Baue AE. Multiple, progressive, or sequential systems failure: A syndrome of the 1970s. Arch Surg 1975;110:779-781.
2. Tilney NL, Bailey GL, Morgan AP. Sequential system failure after rupture of abdominal aortic aneurysms: An unsolved problem in postoperative care. Ann Surg 1973;178:117-122.
3. Eiseman B, Beart R, Norton L. Multiple organ failure. Surg Gynecol Obstet 1977;144:323-326.
4. Polk HC, Shields CL. Remote organ failure: A valid sign of occult intra-abdominal infection. Surgery 1977;81:310-313.
5. Baue AE. Multiple organ failure: Patient care and prevention. St Louis: Mosby–Year Book; 1990.
6. Carrico CJ et al. Multiple-organ-failure syndrome [Panel discussion—Surgical Infection Society]. Arch Surg 1986;121:196-208.
7. Cerra FB. Hypermetabolism, organ failure, and metabolic support. Surgery 1987;101:1-14.
8. DeCamp MM, Demling RH. Posttraumatic multisystem organ failure. JAMA 1988;260:530-534.
9. Deitch EA, ed. Multiple organ failure. New York: Thieme Medical Publishers; 1990.
10. Dorinsky PM, Gadek JE. Multiple organ failure. Clin Chest Med 1990;11:581-591.
11. Fry DE. Multiple system organ failure. Surg Clin North Am 1988;68:107-122.
12. Goodwin CW. Multiple organ failure: Clinical overview of the syndrome. J Trauma 1990;30:S163-S165.
13. Hotter AN. The pathophysiology of multi-system organ failure in the trauma patient. Clin Issues Crit Care Nurs 1990;1:465-478.
14. Huddleston VB. Multisystem organ failure. In: Mims BC, ed. Case studies in critical care nursing. Baltimore: Williams & Wilkins; 1990:494-499.
15. Lekander BJ, Cerra FB. The syndrome of multiple organ failure. Crit Care Nurs Clin North Am 1990;2:331-342.
16. Marshall JC, Meakins JL. Multiorgan failure. In: Wilmore DW, ed. American College of Surgeons: Care of the surgical patient. Vol. 1. Critical Care. New York: Sci Am; 1989.
17. Meakins JL. Etiology of multiple organ failure. J Trauma 1990;30:S165-S168.
18. Nelson K, Herndon B, Reisz G. Pulmonary effects of ischemic limb reperfusion: Evidence for a role of oxygen-derived radicals. Crit Care Med 1991;19:360-363.
19. Pinsky MR, Matuschak GM. Multiple systems organ failure: Failure of host defense homeostasis. Crit Care Clin 1989;5:199-220.
20. Anderson BO, Harken AH. Multiple organ failure: Inflammatory priming and activation sequence promote autologous tissue injury. J Trauma 1990;30:S44-S49.
21. Border JR. Hypothesis: Sepsis, multiple systems organ failure, and the macrophage [editorial]. Arch Surg 1988;123:285-286.
22. Goris RJ et al. Multiple organ failure: Generalized autodestructive inflammation. Arch Surg 1985;120:1109-1115.
23. Goris RJ et al. Multiple organ failure and sepsis without bacteria. Arch Surg 1986;121:897-901.
24. Goris RJ. Multiple organ failure: Whole body inflammation? Schweiz Med Wochenschr 1989;119:347-353.
25. Nuytinck HKS et al. Whole-body inflammation in trauma patients. Arch Surg 1988;123:1519-1524.
26. Hyers TM, Gee M, Andreadis NA. Cellular interactions in the multiple organ injury syndrome. Am Rev Respir Dis 1987;135:952-953.
27. Pinsky MR. Multiple systems organ failure: Malignant intravascular inflammation. Crit Care Clin 1989;5:195-198.
28. Bersten A, Sibbald WJ. Circulatory disturbances in multiple organ failure. Crit Care Clin 1989;5:233-254.
29. Cunnion RE, Parrillo JE. Myocardial dysfunction in sepsis. Crit Care Clin 1989;5:99-118.
30. Dantzker D. Oxygen delivery and utilization in sepsis. Crit Care Clin 1989;5:81-98.
31. Gutierrez G, Lund N, Bryan-Brown CW. Cellular oxygen utilization during multiple organ failure. Crit Care Clin 1989;5:271-288.

32. Barton R, Cerra FB. The hypermetabolism, multiple organ failure syndrome. Chest 1989;96:1153-1160.

33. Darling GE, Duff JH, Mustard RA, Finley RJ. Multiorgan failure in critically ill patients. Can J Surg 1988;31:172-176.

34. Abraham E. Physiologic stress and cellular ischemia: Relationship to immunosuppression and susceptibility to sepsis. Crit Care Med 1991;19:613-618.

35. Axelrod J, Reisine TD. Stress hormones: Their interaction and regulation. Science 1984;224:452-459.

36. Müller-Berghaus G. Pathophysiologic and biochemical events in disseminated intravascular coagulation: Dysregulation of procoagulant and anticoagulant pathways. Semin Thromb Hemost 1989;15:58-87.

37. Roitt I, Brostoff J, Male D, eds. Immunology. 2nd ed. London: Gower Medical Publishing; 1989.

38. Hoyt NJ. Host defense mechanisms and compromises in the trauma patient. Crit Care Nurs Clin North Am 1989;1:753-766.

39. Faist E et al. Mediators and the trauma induced cascade of immunologic defects. Prog Clin Biol Res: Second Vienna Shock Forum 1989;308:495-506.

40. Faist E et al. Immunoprotective effects of cyclooxygenase inhibition in patients with major surgical trauma. J Trauma 1990;30:8-18.

41. Ertel W et al. Dynamics of immunoglobin synthesis after major trauma. Arch Surg 1989;124:1437-1442.

42. Ertel W et al. Immunoprotective effect of a calcium channel blocker on macrophage antigen presentation function, major histocompatibility class II antigen expression, and interleukin-1 synthesis after hemorrhage. Surgery 1990;108:154-160.

43. Ayala A, Perrin MM, Chaudry IH. Defective antigen presentation following hemorrhage is associated with the loss of MHC class II (Ia) antigens. Immunology 1990;70:33-39.

44. Brunson ME, Alexander JW. Mechanisms of transfusion-induced immunosuppression. Transfusion 1990;30:651-658.

45. Browder W, Williams D. Immunosuppression in the surgical patient. J Nat Med Assoc 1988;80:531-536.

46. Waymack JP et al. Effect of blood transfusion and anesthesia on resistance to bacterial peritonitis. J Surg Res 1987;42:528-535.

47. Stroud M, Swindell B, Bernard GR. Cellular and humoral mediators of sepsis syndrome. Crit Care Nurs Clin North Am 1990;2:151-160.

48. Littleton MT. Complications of multiple trauma. Crit Care Nurs Clin North Am 1989;1:75-84.

49. Littleton MT. Pathophysiology of sepsis and septic shock. Crit Care Nurs Quart 1988;11:30-47.

50. Tracey KJ, Lowry SF. The role of cytokine mediators in septic shock. Adv Surg 1990;23:21-56.

51. Parillo JE et al. Septic shock in humans: Advances in the understanding of pathogenesis, cardiovascular dysfunction, and therapy. Ann Intern Med 1990;113:227-242.

52. Cain SM, Curtis SE. Experimental models of pathologic oxygen supply dependency. Crit Care Med 1991;19:603-612.

53. Gutierrez G. Cellular energy metabolism during hypoxia. Crit Care Med 1991;19:619-626.

54. Mims BC. Physiologic rationale of Svo₂ monitoring. Crit Care Nurs Clin North Am 1989;1:619-627.

55. Shoemaker WC, Appel PL, Kram HB. Oxygen transport measurements to evaluate tissue perfusion and titrate therapy: Dobutamine and dopamine effects. Crit Care Med 1991;19:672-688.

56. Wang P, Hauptman JG, Chaudry IH. Hepatocellular dysfunction occurs early after hemorrhage and persists despite fluid resuscitation. J Surg Res 1990;48:466-470.

57. Deitch EA. Bacterial translocation of the gut flora. J Trauma 1990;30(Suppl 12):S184-S189.

58. Deitch EA. Gut failure: Its role in the multiple organ failure syndrome. In: Deitch EA, ed. Multiple organ failure: Pathophysiology and basic concepts of therapy. New York: Thieme Medical Publishers; 1990:40-59.

59. Bounous G. The intestinal factor in multiple organ failure and shock. Surgery 1990;107:118-119.

60. Driks MR et al. Nosocomial pneumonia in intubated patients given sucralfate as compared with antacids or histamine type 2 blockers. N Engl J Med 1987;317:1376-1382.

61. Meijer K, van Saene HK, Hill JC. Infection control in patients undergoing mechanical ventilation: Traditional approach versus a new development—selective decontamination of the digestive tract. Heart Lung 1990;19:11-20.

62. Fan ST et al. Prediction of severity of acute pancreatitis: An alternative approach. Gut 1989;30:1591-1595.

63. Beger HG et al. Hemodynamic data pattern in patients with acute pancreatitis. Gastroenterology 1986;90:74-79.

64. Hotter AN. The pathophysiology of shock brain. Crit Care Nurs Clin North Am 1989;1:123-130.

65. Witt NJ et al. Peripheral nerve function in sepsis and multiple organ failure. Chest 1991;99:176-184.

66. Crump JM, Duncan DA, Wears R. Analysis of multiple organ system failure in trauma and nontrauma patients. Am Surg 1988;12:702-708.

67. Knaus WA, Wagner DP. Multiple systems organ failure: Epidemiology and prognosis. Crit Care Clin 1989;5:221-232.

68. Hoyt NJ. Preventing septic shock: Infection control in the intensive care unit. Crit Care Nurs Clin North Am 1990;2:287-298.

69. Deitch EA. Multiple organ failure: Summary and overview. In Deitch EA, ed. Multiple organ failure: Pathophysiology and basic concepts of therapy. New York: Thieme Medical Publishers; 1990:285-299.

70. Dunn DL. Role of infection and the use of antimicrobial agents during multiple system organ failure. In: Deitch EA, ed. Multiple organ failure: Pathophysiology and basic concepts of therapy. New York: Thieme Medical Publishers; 1990:150-171.

71. Christou NV. Pros and cons of empiric laparotomy in multiple organ failure. In: Deitch EA, ed. Multiple organ failure: Pathophysiology and basic concepts of therapy. New York: Thieme Medical Publishers; 1990:275-284.

72. Nicholson DP. Review of corticosteroid treatment in sepsis and septic shock: Pro or con. Crit Care Clin 1989;5:151-155.

73. Bernard GR et al. High-dose corticosteroids in patients with the adult respiratory distress syndrome. N Engl J Med 1987;317:1565-1570.

74. Veterans Administration Systemic Sepsis Cooperative Study Group. Effect of high-dose glucocorticoid therapy on mortality in patients with clinical signs of systemic sepsis. N Engl J Med 1987;317:659-665.

75. Bone RC et al. A controlled clinical trial of high-dose methylprednisolone in the treatment of severe sepsis and septic shock. N Engl J Med 1987;317:653-658.

76. Lookinland S. Comparison of pulmonary vascular pressures based on blood volume and ventilator status. Nurs Res 1989;38:68-72.

77. Guyton AC. Textbook of medical physiology. 8th ed. Philadelphia: WB Saunders;1991.

78. Burns KM. Vasoactive drug therapy in shock. Crit Care Nurs Clin North Am 1990;2:167-178.

79. Huddleston VB. Postoperative pulmonary problems. Crit Care Nurs Clin North Am 1990;2:527-536.

80. Reischman RR. Impaired gas exchange related to intrapulmonary shunting. Crit Care Nurse 1988;8:35-49.

81. Reischman RR. Review of ventilation and perfusion physiology. Crit Care Nurse 1988;8:24-30.

82. Stone KS. Ventilator versus manual resuscitation bag as the method for delivering hyperoxygenation before endotracheal suctioning. Clin Issues Crit Care Nurs 1990;1:289-299.

83. Siepler JK, Trudeau W, Petty DE. Use of continuous infusion of histamine 2-receptor antagonists in critically ill patients. DICP 1989;23:S40-S43.

84. Tryba M. Side effects of stress bleeding prophylaxis. Am J Med 1989;86:85-93.

85. Cerra FB. Metabolic manifestation of multiple systems organ failure. Crit Care Clin 1989;5:119-131.

86. Bessey PQ. Nutritional support in critical illness. In: Deitch EA, ed. Multiple organ failure: Pathophysiology and basic concepts of therapy. New York: Thieme Medical Publishers; 1990:126-149.

87. Burns SM. Advances in ventilator therapy. Focus Crit Care 1990;17:227-237.

88. Hartenauer U et al. Effect of selective flora suppression on colonization, infection, and mortality in critically ill patients: A one-year prospective consecutive study. Crit Care Med 1991;19:463-473.

89. Peterson KJ. Extracorporeal membrane oxygenation in adults: A nursing challenge. Focus Crit Care 1990;17:40-49.

90. Reidy JJ, Ramsay G. Clinical trials of selective decontamination of the digestive tract: Review. Crit Care Med 1990;18:1449-1456.

91. Silverman HJ et al. Effects of prostaglandin E_1 on oxygen delivery and consumption in patients with the adult respiratory distress syndrome. Results from the prostaglandin E_1 multicenter trial. Chest 1990;98:405-410.

92. Russell JA, Ronco JJ, Dodek PM. Physiologic effects and side-effects of prostaglandin E_1 in adult respiratory distress syndrome. Chest 1990;97:684-692.

93. Bihari DJ, Tinker J. The therapeutic value of vasodilator prostaglandins in multiple organ failure associated with sepsis. Intens Care Med 1988;15:2-7.

94. Barzilay E et al. Use of extracorporeal supportive techniques as additional treatment for septic-induced multiple organ failure patients. Crit Care Med 1989;17:634-637.

95. Cairo MS et al. Prophylactic or simultaneous administration of recombinant human granulocyte colony stimulating factor in the treatment of group B streptococcal sepsis in neonatal rats. Pediatr Res 1990;27:612-616.

96. Hudson-Goodman P, Girard N, Jones MB. Wound repair and the potential use of growth factors. Heart Lung 1990;19:379-386.

97. Tuomanen EI et al. Reduction of inflammation, tissue damage, and mortality in bacterial meningitis in rabbits treated with monoclonal antibodies against adhesion-promoting receptors of leukocytes. J Exper Med 1989;170:959-968.

98. Mileski WJ et al. Inhibition of CD18-dependent neutrophil adherence reduces organ injury after hemorrhagic shock in primates. Surgery 1990;108:206-212.

99. Male D, Roitt I. Adaptive and innate immunity. In: Roitt I, Brostoff J, Male D, eds. Immunology. 2nd ed. London: Gower Medical Publishing; 1989:1.1-1.10.

100. Steward M. Antigen recognition. In: Roitt I, Brostoff J, Male D, eds. Immunology. 2nd ed. London: Gower Medical Publishing; 1989:7.1-7.10.

101. Köhler G, Milstein C. Continuous cultures of fused cells secreting antibody of predefined specificity. Nature 1975;256:495-497.

102. Fisher CF et al. Initial evaluation of human monoclonal anti-lipid A antibody (HA-1A) in patients with sepsis syndrome. Crit Care Med 1990;18:1311-1315.

103. Teng NNH et al. Protection against gram-negative bacteremia and endotoxemia with human monoclonal IgM antibodies. Proc Natl Acad Sci 1985;82:1790-1794.

104. Ziegler EJ et al. Treatment of gram-negative bacteremia and septic shock with HA-1A human monoclonal antibody against endotoxin. N Engl J Med 1991;324:429-436.

105. Greenman RL et al. A controlled clinical trial of E5 murine monoclonal IgM antibody to endotoxin and the treatment of gram-negative sepsis: the XOMA sepsis study group. JAMA 1991;266:1097-1102.

106. MacIntyre NR et al. Xoma Sepsis Study Group. E5 antibody improves outcome from multi-organ failure in survivors of gram-negative sepsis [abstract]. Crit Care Med 1991;19(4 suppl):S14.

107. Priest BP et al. Treatment of experimental gram-negative bacterial sepsis with murine monoclonal antibodies directed against lipopolysaccharide. Surgery 1989;106:147-155.

108. Tracey KJ et al. Anticachectin/TNF monoclonal antibodies prevent shock during lethal bacteraemia. Nature 1987;330:662-665.

109. Hinshaw LB et al. Survival of primates in LD100 septic shock following therapy with antibody to tumor necrosis factor (TNF alpha). Circ Shock 1990;30:279-292.

110. Shalaby MR et al. Binding and regulation of cellular functions by monoclonal antibodies against human tumor necrosis factor receptors. J Exp Med 1990;172:1517-1520.

111. Espevik T et al. Characterization of binding and biological effects of monoclonal antibodies against a human tumor necrosis factor receptor. J Exp Med 1990;171:415-426.

112. Exley AR et al. Monoclonal antibody to TNF in severe septic shock. Lancet 1990;335:1275-1277.

113. Stellin G et al. Hypoxia stimulates release of tumor necrosis factor from human macrophages [abstract]. Crit Care Med 1991;19(4 suppl):S57.

114. Wakabayashi G et al. A specific receptor antagonist for interleukin-1 prevents *Escherichia coli*-induced shock in rabbits. FASEB J 1991;5:338-343.

115. Ohlsson K et al. Interleukin-1 receptor antagonist reduces mortality from endotoxin shock. Nature 1990;348:550-552.

116. Opp MR, Krueger JM. Interleukin 1-receptor antagonist blocks interleukin 1-induced sleep and fever. Am J Physiol 1991;260:R453-R457.

117. Dinarello CA. Biology of interleukin 1. FASEB J 1988;2:108-115.

118. Demling RH, LaLonde C. Identification and modification of the pulmonary and systemic inflammatory and biochemical changes caused by a skin burn. J Trauma 1990;30(Suppl 12):S57-S62.

119. Demling RH, LaLonde C. Early postburn lipid peroxidation: Effect of ibuprofen and allopurinol. Surgery 1990;107:85-93.

120. Kennedy TP et al. Ibuprofen prevents oxidant lung injury and in vitro lipid peroxidation by chelating iron. J Clin Invest 1990;86:1565-1573.

121. Evans DA et al. The effects of tumor necrosis factor and their selective inhibition by ibuprofen. Ann Surg 1989;209:312-321.

122. Bernard GR et al. Prostacyclin and thromboxane A2 formation is increased in human sepsis syndrome: Effects of cyclooxygenase inhibition. Am Rev Respir Dis 1991;144:1095-1101.

123. Moorhouse CB et al. Allopurinol and oxypurinol are hydroxyl radical scavengers. FEBS Lett 1987;213:23-28.

124. Brigham KL. Oxidant stress and adult respiratory distress syndrome. Eur Resp J 1990;3(suppl 11):482s-484s.

125. Johnson WD et al. A randomized controlled trial of allopurinol in coronary bypass surgery. Am Heart J 1991;121:20-24.

126. Tabayashi K et al. A clinical trial of allopurinol (Zyloric) for myocardial protection. J Thorac Cardiovasc Surg 1991;101:713-718.

127. Siesjoe BK. Calcium and death. Magnesium 1989;8:223-237.

128. Yano Y et al. Calcium-accented ischemic damage during reperfusion: The time course of the reperfusion injury in the isolated working rat heart model. J Surg Res 1987;42:51-55.

129. Horton JW. Calcium-channel blockade in canine hemorrhagic shock. Am J Physiol 1989;257:R1012-R1019.

130. Parratt JR. Calcium antagonists in shock: A minireview of the evidence. Prog Clin Biol Res: Second Vienna Shock Forum 1989;308:1065-1074.

131. Schade UF. Pentoxifylline increases survival in murine endotoxin shock and decreases formation of tumor necrosis factor. Circ Shock 1990;31:171-181.

132. Haas F et al. Pentoxifylline improves pulmonary gas exchange. Chest 1990;97:621-627.

133. Noel P et al. Pentoxyifylline inhibits lipopolysaccharide-induced tumor necrosis factor and mortality. Life Sci 1990;47:1023-1029.

134. Waxman K et al. Pentoxifylline in resuscitation of experimental hemorrhagic shock. Crit Care Med 1991;19:728-731.

135. Byram DA. Future expectations for critical care nurses: Competence in immunotherapy. Crit Care Nurs Clin North Am 1989;1:797-806.

136. Tribett D. Immune system function: Implications for critical care nursing practice. Crit Care Nurs Clin North Am 1989;1:725-740.

137. Jillings CR. Shock: Psychosocial needs of the patient and family. Crit Care Nurs Clin North Am 1990;2:325-330.

138. Field BE, Devich LE, Carlson RW. Impact of a comprehensive supportive care team on management of hopelessly ill patients with multiple organ failure. Chest 1989;96:353-356.

139. Sheagren JN. Mechanism-oriented therapy for multiple systems organ failure. Crit Care Clin 1989;5:393-409.

140. Macho JR, Luce JM. Rational approach to the management of multiple systems organ failure. Crit Care Clin 1989;5:379-392.

141. Baxter CR. Future prospectives in trauma and burn care. J Trauma 1990;30(Suppl 12):S208-S209.

142. Baker JW et al. Hemorrhagic shock induces bacterial translocation from the gut. J Trauma 1988;28:896-906.

APPENDICES

A Inflammatory Mediators

Plasma Enzyme Cascades

Component	Function	Source	Stimulated by	Action

Complement	Activation and enhancement of IIR
	
	Induction of inflammation through anaphylatoxin formation (C3a, C5a)
	
	Mediator between tissue injury and cellular activation
		Circulating pool — complex series of proteins and proteases produced by macrophages and endothelial cells of the liver and gut	Classic pathway: Ag/Ab complex (IgG and IgM only)
			
			Alternate pathway:
			tissue trauma
			cell debris
			kinins
			endotoxin
			plasmin
				Opsonization
				Cellular activation:
				  PMN chemotaxis, phagocytosis, and aggregation
				  Stimulate PMN oxidative metabolism and release of mediators
				  Stimulate degranulation of mast cells and basophils → histamine and serotonin release
				Direct target cell lysis
				Vasodilatation
				↑ Capillary permeability
				Activation of kinin cascade
				↑ Arachidonic acid metabolism
				? Induction of TF expression by PMN and MØ

Continued.

Plasma Enzyme Cascades — cont'd

Component	Function	Source	Stimulated by	Action
Coagulation	Prevent hemorrhage and isolate injury site	Circulating pool — complex series of proteins produced by liver, endothelium, MØ, and megakaryocytes	Intrinsic pathway: endothelial damage and collagen exposure → activation of Hageman factor (XII) activation Extrinsic pathway: tissue trauma and long bone fracture → release of tissue factor	Fibrin formation and deposition
Fibrinolysis	Promotes clot breakdown Works in concert with other natural anticoagulants to prevent intravascular thrombosis	Circulating pool — proteins produced by liver	Plasminogen → plasmin activated by: tPA thrombin activated Hageman kallikrein lysosomal enzymes	Clot degradation
Kallikrein/kinin (bradykinin)	Enhance IIR activity Enhance fibrinolytic cascade Possible role in renal blood flow and blood pressure regulation	Circulating pool — protein precursors produced in liver	Hageman factor Tissue trauma Complement WBCs and their mediators	Potent vasodilatation ↑ Capillary permeability PMN chemotaxis, respiratory burst, and mediator release Smooth muscle contraction

Cellular Components

Component	Function	Origin and/or Location	Stimulated by/ Attracted by	Action
Lymphocytes	Inflammatory/immune response Regulation of IIR	Bone marrow/thymus Lymphatic tissue Circulating pool	APCs with antigen + MHC Interleukin-1 and 2 Cancerous cells Foreign donor tissue Intracellular infections Virally infected cells	T cell: Helper (T4) activity via mediator release: enhance B-cell proliferation and antibody production enhance MØ activity enhance further T-cell activity Suppressor activity (T8)-regulator Cytotoxic activity (T8) against cancer cells, virally infected cells, and intracellular infections B cell: Antibody production Memory response Antigen presentation
Mast cells and basophils	Inflammatory/immune response	Bone marrow Mast cell: body tissues, primarily those near external environment Basophil: circulating pool	Direct injury Endotoxin Complement Bradykinin	Induction of inflammation via mediator release: Histamine Proteases Eicosanoids Heparin Chemotactic factors

Continued.

Cellular Components—cont'd

Component	Function	Origin and/or Location	Stimulated by/ Attracted by	Action
Monocyte/ Macrophage family	Inflammatory/immune response Link between nonspecific and specific responses Wound microdebridement	Bone marrow Circulating pool Lymphatic tissue Marginal pool Peripheral tissue	Endotoxin Complement Lymphokines Monocyte chemotactants; complement fragments PMN fragments Bacterial fragments Lymphokines	Phagocytosis Antigen processing and presentation Mediator release: IL-1 TNF Proteases Eicosanoids Colony stimulating factors ODFR Interferon PAF Plasminogen activator Complement proteins Coagulation factors
Neutrophil (PMN)	Inflammatory/immune response	Bone marrow Marginal pool Circulating pool	Complement Kinins TNF IL-1 PAF Endotoxin Cell debris Clotting factors Eicosanoids Proteases	Phagocytosis Mediator release: ODFR Proteases PAF Eicosanoids Interleukins Tissue factor
Platelets	Coagulation Inflammatory/immune response	Bone marrow Spleen Circulating pool	Vessel wall components Exposed collagen Thrombin Fibrin PAF Immune complexes Epinephrine	Aggregation and plug Release of mediators: Eicosanoids, particularly thromboxane Serotonin Chemotactants PAF Histamine Enhance PMN aggregation Fibrinogen binding site

Biochemical Mediators

Mediator	Function	Source	Release stimulated by	Action
Arachidonic acid metabolites (eicosanoids), including prostaglandins, thromboxane, and leukotrienes	Inflammatory/immune response Physiologic homeostasis	Cell membrane phospholipids (made by all cells except RBCs)	Catecholamines, tissue injury, hypoxia, ischemia, endotoxin, neurogenic and hormonal stimulation, collagen, thrombi, bradykinin, Ag/Ab complexes, and ODFRs Cell membrane disruption → Phospholipid available → arachidonic acid → lipoxygenase pathway → leukotrienes cyclooxygenase pathway → prostaglandins and thromboxane	Biologic targets: Vasomotor tone Microvascular permeability Platelet aggregation Macrophage/T-cell interaction Temperature regulation Cellular activation and mediator release Bronchial smooth muscle tone
PGI₂ (prostacyclin)	Major vascular AA metabolite	Endothelium most active producer		Vasodilatation ↓ Platelet aggregation
Thromboxane	IIR and coagulation	Platelets Macrophages		Vasoconstriction ↑ Platelet aggregation
PGE₂	Feedback inhibition of macrophage response	Macrophages		Inhibition of MØ/T-cell interaction Induction of T-cell suppressor activity

Continued.

Abbreviations: *IIR*, inflammatory/immune response; *PMN*, polymorphonuclear granulocyte (neutrophil); *Ag*, antigen; *Ab*, antibody; *TF*, tissue factor; *MØ*, macrophage; *t-PA*, tissue plasminogen activator; *WBC*, white blood cell; *TNF*, tumor necrosis factor; *IL*, interleukin; *PAF*, platelet activating factor; *ODFR*, oxygen-derived free radicals; *APC*, antigen presenting cell; *MHC*, major histocompatibility complex; *RBC*, red blood cell; *AA*, arachidonic acid; *PG*, prostaglandin; *SRS-A*, slow releasing substance of anaphylaxis; *NK*, natural killer.

Biochemical Mediators—cont'd

Mediator	Function	Source	Release stimulated by	Action
Leukotrienes (SRS-A)	Inflammatory/immune response			↑ Vascular permeability Pulmonary vasoconstriction Smooth muscle contraction Activation of IIR cells

Hageman factor	Activation of coagulation and kinin systems
	Link between coagulation and IIR
		Circulating pool
		Produced by the liver
			Endotoxin
			Contact with damaged tissue:
			  collagen
			  cartilage
			  basement membrane
			Contact with Ag/Ab
			Kallikrein
			Contact with negatively charged particles
				Conversion of prekallikrein to kallikrein
				Initiate intrinsic coagulation cascade

Histamine	Induction of inflammation	Mast cells Basophils Platelets Gastric mucosa Skin	Binding of complement, antigen, and endotoxin to cells Direct cell trauma Neurogenic stimulation	Vasodilatation ↑ Capillary permeability Smooth muscle contraction Gastric acid secretion
Interferon-gamma	Inflammatory/immune response	T cells Virally infected cells NK cells Fibroblasts Macrophages	Interleukin-2 Viral infections	Weak antiviral properties Induces MHC II expression on APC Stimulates T-cell, B-cell, MØ, and NK activity
Interleukin-1 (IL-1)	Inflammatory/immune response Synergistic activity with TNF	Macrophages Blood monocytes Natural killer cells ?PMN Fibroblasts Perturbed endothelium	Phagocytosis of foreign debris T-cell lymphokines or TNF acting on MØ Hemorrhage Thrombin	↑ PMN/endothelium adhesion Links IIR with neuroendocrine system, such as fever induction Leukocytosis Enhance T cell, B cell, NK, MØ, PMN activity and proliferation Enhance antibody production Stimulates production of acute-phase reactants

Mediator	Function	Source cells	Stimulus	Physiologic effects
Interleukin-2 (IL-2)	Inflammatory/immune response	T4-helper T cells NK cells	Interleukin-1 MO/T-cell interaction	Stimulates hematopoiesis ↑ PMN/endothelium adhesion Stimulates release of IL-2 from T cell ↑ Amino acid flux and muscle proteolysis Stimulates endothelium to express mediators and procoagulant activity ↑ Fibroblast activity and wound healing ↑ T-cell proliferation and mediator release, such as interferon gamma ↑ T-cell receptors for IL-2 Enhance B-cell proliferation Further activation of MØ and NK
Oxygen-derived free radicals	Killing of microorganisms	PMN and MØ oxidative metabolism (respiratory burst) By-product of reperfusion Arachidonic acid metabolism Xanthine oxidase systems	Perfusion deficit Inflammatory cellular activity Reperfusion ↑ FiO$_2$	Endothelial damage Lipid peroxidation of cell membranes → loss of membrane fluidity, secretory function, and ionic gradients ↑ Capillary permeability Altered cell receptor function Denaturation of proteins, including antiproteases
Platelet activating factor (PAF)	Inflammatory/immune response Coagulation	Platelets Mast cells Basophils Monocytes Macrophages PMNs Endothelium	Anything stimulating source cells Decreased coronary artery flow Hypotension Renal dysfunction	Platelet shape change → platelet aggregation Serotonin release PMN activation → respiratory burst and degranulation ↑ Capillary permeability Smooth muscle contraction Vasodilatation and vasoconstriction Bronchoconstriction Myocardial depression

Continued.

Biochemical Mediators—cont'd

Mediator	Function	Source	Release stimulated by	Action
Proteases (elastase and collagenase)	Inflammatory/immune response Tissue remodeling	PMNs Macrophages Mast cells	PMN, macrophage, and mast cell activation secondary to tissue trauma, ischemia, necrosis, microorganisms, and other foreign matter	Degradation of tissue for wound healing and remodeling Degradation of vasculature and parenchyma → damage and fibrosis
Serotonin	Vasoactive amine Neurotransmitter	Intestinal tissue Central nervous system Platelets	Activated platelets Neurogenic stimulation	Vasodilatation and vasoconstriction Inhibition of pain pathways
Tumor necrosis factor (TNF)/cachectin	Inflammatory/immune response, particularly against parasitic infections	Macrophages	Endotoxin Microorganisms Ischemic tissue Tissue debris	Induces fever Enhance MØ, PMN, eosinophil, and lymphocyte function and mediator release ↑ Hepatocyte resistance to infection, particularly parasitic infection ↑ WBC/endothelium adhesion Suppression of lipoprotein lipase→ ↓ fat uptake Anorexia/wasting Stimulates ↑ collagenase production Endothelial damage ↑ Procoagulant activity of endothelium ↓ Vascular responsiveness to catecholamines

B Abbreviations

AA .... arachidonic acid
Ab .... antibody
ABG .... arterial blood gas
ADH .... antidiuretic hormone
Ag .... antigen
APC .... antigen presenting cell
ARDS .... adult respiratory distress syndrome
ARF .... acute renal failure
AT III .... antithrombin III
ATN .... acute tubular necrosis
ATP .... adenosine triphosphate
BUN .... blood urea nitrogen
C3a, C5a .... complement split products
CaO₂ .... arterial oxygen content
CAVH ...... continuous arteriovenous hemofiltration
CBC .... complete blood count
CI .... cardiac index
CO .... cardiac output
CO₂ .... carbon dioxide
CPP .... cerebral perfusion pressure
CRRT .... continuous renal replacement therapy
CSF .... cerebral spinal fluid
CSF .... colony stimulating factor
CvO₂ .... mixed venous oxygen content
CVP .... central venous pressure
DIC .... disseminated intravascular coagulation
DO₂ .... oxygen delivery
EDRF .... endothelial-derived relaxation factor
EDV .... end-diastolic volume
EF .... ejection fraction
ESV .... end-systolic volume
FDP .... fibrin/fibrinogen degradation product
FiO₂ .... fraction of inspired oxygen
GALT .... gut-associated lymphoid tissue
GFR .... glomerular filtration rate
GI .... gastrointestinal
HLA .... human leukocyte antigen
HMWK .... high molecular weight kininogen
HR .... heart rate
ICP .... intracranial pressure
IIR .... inflammatory/immune response
IL-1, IL-2 .... interleukin-1(-2)
ITP .... idiopathic thrombocytopenic purpura
LDH .... lactate dehydrogenase
LT .... leukotriene

LV .... left ventricle
LVAD .... left ventricle assist device
LVEF .... left ventricular ejection fraction
LVSWI .... left ventricular stroke work index
MØ .... macrophage
MAb .... monoclonal antibody
MAP .... mean arterial pressure
MDF .... myocardial depressant factor
MDO₂ .... myocardial oxygen delivery
μg .... microgram
MHC .... major histocompatibility complex
MSOF .... multisystem organ failure
MVO₂ .... myocardial oxygen consumption
NK .... natural killer
ODFR .... oxygen-derived free radical
PA .... pulmonary artery
PAD .... pulmonary artery diastolic
PAF .... platelet activating factor
PAP .... pulmonary artery pressure
PCWP .... pulmonary capillary wedge pressure
PEEP .... positive end-expiratory pressure
PF-3 .... platelet factor-3
PG .... prostaglandin
PMN .... polymorphonuclear granulocyte
PVR .... pulmonary vascular resistance
RES .... reticuloendothelial system
RV .... right ventricle
RVAD .... right ventricular assist device
RVEF .... right ventricular ejection fraction
RVSWI .... right ventricular stroke work index
SaO₂ .... arterial oxygen saturation
SDD ... selective decontamination of digestive tract
SNS .... sympathetic nervous system
SOD .... superoxide dismutase
SV .... stroke volume
SvO₂ .... mixed venous oxygen saturation
SVR .... systemic vascular resistance
SWI .... stroke work index
TF .... tissue factor
TNF .... tumor necrosis factor
t-PA .... tissue plasminogen activator
TX .... thromboxane
VO₂ .... oxygen consumption
V/Q .... ventilation/perfusion ratio
WBC .... white blood cell

C Glossary*

agonist A substance that promotes a given system's normal biologic activity.

anaphylatoxin Active complement peptides (C3a, C5a) that cause mast cell degranulation (release of mediators such as histamine) and smooth muscle contraction.

antagonist A substance that opposes a given system's activity.

arachidonic acid A fatty acid derived from the phospholipid of most cell membranes. Its metabolism produces three distinct groups of mediators, collectively known as eicosanoids.

autocatalytic A reaction or series of reactions whose by-products continue to stimulate (catalyze) the reaction so that a continuous cycle is established.

cascade A reaction in which the product of one step serves as the catalyst for the next step.

catabolism Phase of metabolism involved in the degradation of nutrient molecules.

chemotaxis Cells sensing and moving toward a specific biochemical agent.

cofactor A small molecular weight substance required for the action of an enzyme. Magnesium and calcium ions are important cofactors in ATP production and coagulation.

cytokines A generic term for mediators (usually peptides) involved in signalling between cells. Factors formed by one cell that induce activity in other cells.

down regulation Decrease in cell surface receptor density (number), usually resulting from an increase in the circulating concentration of the endogenous agonist for that receptor. If a cell is down regulated, it is not as responsive to the mediator that usually stimulates the receptor on the cell.

Down regulation serves to limit and control the response.

effector cell Cells involved in the activity of certain biologic responses, which produce the end-effect. For example, immune effector cells carry out the functions of the immune system.

eicosanoids Group of substances derived from arachidonic acid, including the prostaglandins, thromboxane, and leukotrienes.

endogenous Originating within the organism. Endorphin is an endogenous opioid.

enzyme A protein specialized to catalyze a specific metabolic reaction.

exogenous Originating outside the organism. Morphine sulfate is an exogenous opioid.

gluconeogenesis The biosynthesis of new carbohydrate from noncarbohydrate precursors. Occurs primarily in the liver. For example: amino acids →glucose.

glycolysis The reactions involved in breaking glucose down into molecules of pyruvate.

humoral Pertaining to the extracellular fluids, including the serum and lymph.

hydrolysis Cleavage of a molecule into two or more smaller molecules by reaction with water.

immune complexes The product of an antigen-antibody (Ag/Ab) reaction that may also contain components of the complement system.

interleukins A specific class of cytokines that signals between cells of the immune system.

leukotrienes Pharmacologically active metabolites of arachidonic acid metabolism.

lymphokine A cytokine produced by a lymphocyte (for example, interleukin-2). Involved in signalling between cells of the immune response.

major histocompatibility complex Surface antigens on body cells that play an important role in recognition of self vs. nonself and in regulating cell-to-cell interaction in the immune response.

mediator Generic term for bioactive substances that exert physiologic changes in body cell and tissues. For example: proteases, TNF, and interleukins.

*List of terms and definitions modified from Lehninger AL. Principles of biochemistry. New York: Worth Publishers, 1982 *and* Roitt I, Brostoff J, Male D. Immunology. 2nd ed. London: Gower Medical Publishing, 1989.

metabolism The entire set of enzyme-catalyzed reactions of metabolism.

metabolite Intermediates or end-products of enzyme-catalyzed reactions. For example, the prostaglandins are metabolites of arachidonic acid metabolism.

monokine A cytokine produced by a monocyte or macrophage (for example, TNF). Involved in signalling between cells of the immune response.

opsonization A process that facilitates phagocytosis through the deposition of specific substances (antibody, complement split products) on the pathogen.

oxidation A process involving the breakdown of substances, often for the production of energy. In aerobic metabolism, the oxidation of glucose yields ATP.

peptides Two or more amino acids covalently joined by peptide bonds.

prostaglandins Pharmacologically active metabolites of arachidonic acid.

protease An enzyme that catalyzes the hydrolysis of proteins.

substrate The specific compound acted upon by an enzyme. Glucose is the substrate in glycolysis.

ureagenesis Metabolic pathway occurring in the liver that involves the formation of urea from amino (nitrogen-containing) groups.

zymogen An inactive precursor of an enzyme. For example, pepsinogen is the zymogen; pepsin is the active enzyme.

Index*

---

*An index entry with a page number italicized indicates a ref-
erence to an illustration on that page; if a page number is
followed by a "*t*", the reference is in a table on that page.